T0356020

EXPLORING THE YOGA SŪTRAS

THE OXFORD CENTRE FOR HINDU STUDIES MANDALA PUBLISHING SERIES

General Editor
Lucian Wong

Editorial Board
John Brockington
Avni Chag
James Madaio
Valters Negribs

The Oxford Centre for Hindu Studies Mandala Publishing Series offers authoritative yet accessible introductions to a wide range of subjects in Hindu Studies. Each book in the series aims to present its subject matter in a form that is engaging and readily comprehensible to persons of all backgrounds – academic or otherwise – without compromising scholarly rigor. The series thus bridges the divide between academic and popular writing by preserving and utilising the best elements of both.

EXPLORING THE YOGA SŪTRAS

Nicholas Sutton

MANDALA
San Rafael Los Angeles London

CONTENTS

PREFACE

The *Yoga Sūtras* is widely acknowledged as a seminal text for students and practitioners of Yoga alike, and is typically viewed as the foundational work of the Yoga systems, although we can be certain that its author, Patañjali, did not invent Yoga, the practice of which can be traced back to Upaniṣadic and other early sources. Despite its popularity, the *Yoga Sūtras* is far from being an easy work to comprehend, particularly on a first reading, and so the main aim of this study is to explore the layers of meaning it offers to its readers. Although Yoga is primarily about practice, the *Yoga Sūtras* itself is based on a solid foundation of Sāṁkhya philosophical doctrines and in exploring these ideas a central aim must be to show how the philosophy and the practice of Yoga are woven together in a subtle blend that typifies Patañjali's mode of exposition. In order to fulfil that goal, we take each of the *sūtras*, both individually and in the context of different passages, with the attempt being to make complex ideas more readily accessible to the modern reader who may not have any prior grounding in Indian philosophy. To assist in this attempt, I have made extensive use of the writing of some of the main traditional commentators who have offered their own insights into the meaning of the text and provide valuable explanations of the precise meaning of each *sūtra*. Study of the *Yoga Sūtras* must, I think, be undertaken in stages of progression so that one first gains a preliminary understanding and then uses that understanding as a basis for deeper exploration. I hope that the present work will fulfil that aim, although I would never suggest that this in any way represents the final word. There is always some deeper meaning to be pursued and grasped.

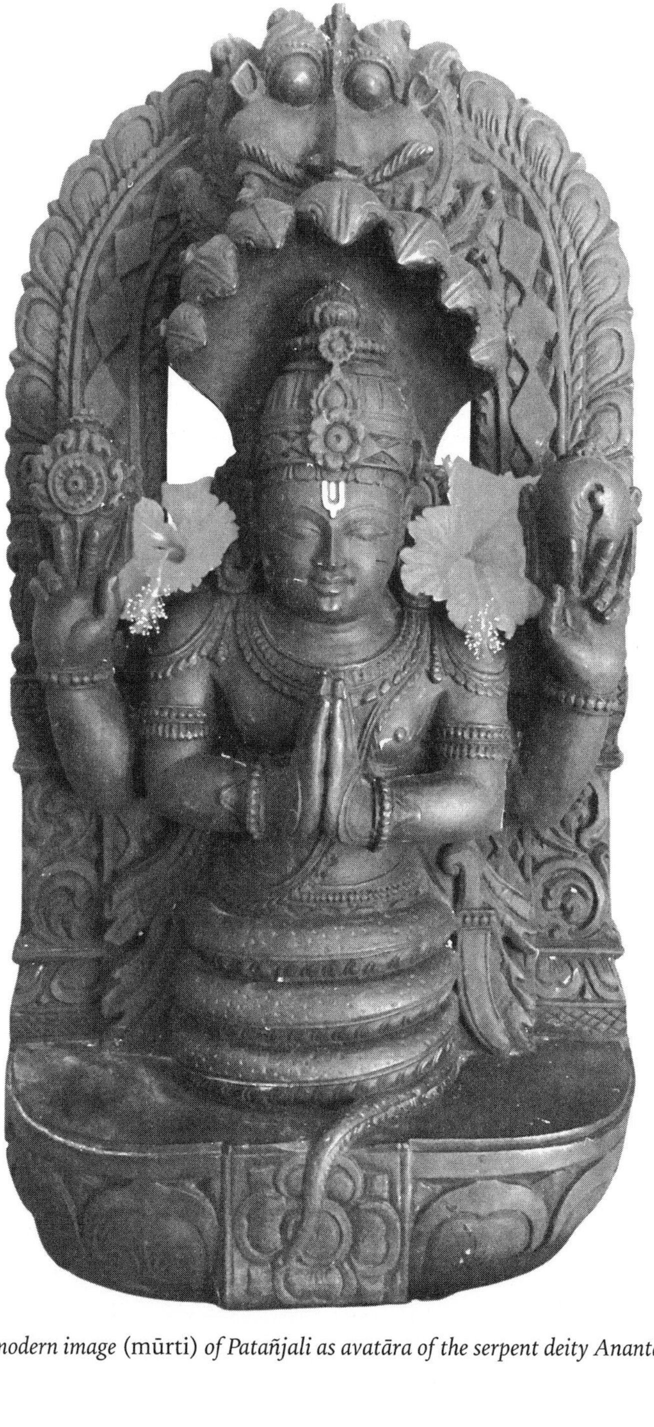

A modern image (mūrti) *of Patañjali as avatāra of the serpent deity Ananta.*

INTRODUCTION

In recent decades there has been a surge of interest in the *Yoga Sūtras* of Patañjali, which for centuries has been recognised within the Hindu tradition as the authoritative text that establishes the fundamental principles of Yoga doctrine and practice. It is widely acknowledged, though somewhat inaccurately, that there are six philosophical systems which accept the authoritative status of the Vedic revelation, and each one of these looks primarily to a single text that establishes its essential precepts. Yoga is generally included in this list of six systems, and it is Patañjali's *Yoga Sūtras* that is almost universally accepted as the foundational text for Yoga. It is also the case that the six systems are usually considered in three groups of two each, Vedānta and Mīmāṁsā, Nyāya and Vaiśeṣika, and Sāṁkhya and Yoga.

With the exception of the *Sāṁkhya-kārikā*, the foundational texts of each system are composed in the *sūtra* style, meaning that they take the form of a series of pithy aphorisms that allow for easier memorisation but can at times display less than absolute clarity. In the *sūtra* form, verbs are only very rarely included and the number of words is kept to a minimum, so that readers are at times obliged to fill in the gaps for themselves. This does mean that individual *sūtras* may be rather obscure, and the precise meaning harder to establish with absolute certainty. It seems likely that the original intention was that the *sūtras* be consigned to memory by those learning the practice of Yoga and then studied under the guidance of an experienced teacher, although we cannot be certain of Patañjali's original aims in creating his text.

The structure of this study guide exactly reflects the structure designed by Patañjali as the best means of conveying his ideas. The *Yoga Sūtras* is divided into four discrete units, although on some occasions the subject matter under consideration progresses across the lines established by these four chapters. As far as I could see, a more thematic approach, topic by topic rather than chapter by chapter, might have introduced a degree of confusion and impinged upon the integrity of the work as a whole. Therefore, after an initial review of Sāṁkhya doctrine, we start off from *sūtra* 1.1 of Chapter 1 and work our way progressively through to the conclusion of the fourth chapter. My feeling is that by adopting this approach we get the clearest possible insight into the way in which Patañjali builds on each theme of his discussion, as he works systematically towards its final conclusion. There are some variations between different manuscripts of the *Yoga Sūtras*, but these tend to be of a minor nature and to have little effect on the meaning of the *sūtra*. The text adopted and followed here is that used by most contemporary translators, although there is no established standard version. There are a good many excellent English translations of the *Yoga Sūtras* now available and different readers will no doubt have their own preferences amongst these. Personally, I very much appreciate those of T. S. Rukmani, Edwin Bryant, and P. V. Deshpande, although I have no doubt that other versions have much to recommend them.

Much of the teaching on Yoga included in the *Yoga Sūtras* and other early texts relates to practice rather than philosophical doctrine, and in many ways the Yoga system is best understood as the series of practices that have the central aim of transforming the theoretical doctrines of Sāṁkhya into experiential knowledge gained through the heightened awareness that comes to the successful practitioner. Patañjali, however, does not focus exclusively on practice, as he recognises the necessity of providing a doctrinal basis for his advocacy of specific yogic techniques. This doctrinal basis coincides almost exactly with the teachings of the Sāṁkhya system as set forth in Īśvara Kṛṣṇa's *Sāṁkhya-kārikā*. Philip Maas observes that the earliest known title of the *Yoga Sūtras* together with the earliest commentary attributed to Vyāsa is *Pātañjala-yoga-śāstra Sāṁkhya-pravacana*, the latter word meaning 'the exposition on Sāṁkhya'.[1]

In more recent centuries, and certainly in the modern era, there has been a tendency to associate Yoga with the alternative philosophical view of Advaita Vedānta. There is no reason to regard this as any sort of deviation from the purity of the primary teachings, for Yoga is constantly evolving and developing new lines of understanding, but at the same time we should be aware that the spiritual ideology of the *Yoga Sūtras* is heavily weighted towards the Sāṁkhya system, so that any suggestion that this particular text is based on an understanding of the absolute unity of all existence will probably be a good way wide of the mark. We might note that two of our commentators, Śaṅkarācārya and Vācaspati Miśra, were themselves adherents and advocates of the advaitic strand of Indian thought, but their commentaries do not reflect that orientation, as they generally follow Vyāsa's adherence to Sāṁkhya without attempting to impose any alternative reading of the *sūtras*.

It is for this reason that I have opted to start off with a relatively brief outline of the main precepts of the Sāṁkhya system, which will, I hope, enable one to undertake this study of the *Yoga Sūtras* with a firm grounding in the philosophical

1 Philipp Maas, 'A Concise Historiography of Classical Yoga Philosophy', in *Historiography and Periodization of Indian Philosophy*, ed. Eli Franco (Vienna: De Nobili Series, 2013).

basis of Patañjali's work. I would add that this is not an easy text to study or fully comprehend, simply because the ideas presented within the *Yoga Sūtras* are frequently quite complex and at times rather obscure. One might well ask if there is any need for another book on the *Yoga Sūtras* when so much has already been said and written by way of discussion and explanation. In response, I would say that my aim throughout has been to present an understanding of the *sūtras* in a manner that does full justice to that complexity and yet renders the exploration of Patañjali's teachings accessible to individuals of all backgrounds. This is by no means an easy task, and at times the attempt to find the appropriate balance between these two aims has been a trying one, but it is my hope and expectation that all those who carefully follow this study guide will embrace the unavoidable challenges presented by the core text and emerge at the end with a much deeper understanding of the principles and ideas underlying its exposition. I would not like to pretend that the progression of this study will always be a smooth one, and at times frustrations may arise due to the sheer complexity of the ideas encountered, but at the same time, I am absolutely certain that the endeavour to comprehend Patañjali's great work will be enormously beneficial to all who undertake it.

A significant element of this study guide is the use made of the insights offered by four of the principal commentaries on the *Yoga Sūtras*, those of Vyāsa, Śaṅkarācārya, Vācaspati Miśra, and Vijñāna Bhikṣu. The earliest of these is undoubtedly the commentary of Vyāsa, which subsequent commentators have all deferred to. Some (though by no means all) of the later commentators believed him to have been Veda Vyāsa, the compiler of the Vedas and the author of the *Mahābhārata*. Hence the other three commentaries take the form of a consideration of the ideas not just of Patañjali's *sūtras*, but of Vyāsa's explanations of those *sūtras* as well. For the most part, we will also defer to Vyāsa's interpretations in our consideration of the most likely reading of the text, but at times alternative meanings for the *sūtras* are suggested so that readers can review for themselves the different possibilities. It is in light of this extensive use made of Vyāsa's commentary in the present work that I have changed some of the translations from those that appeared in my earlier, shorter work on the same subject. As noted above, a number of different meanings are viable for many of the *sūtras,* so it is not that the earlier translations were wrong, but because of the more extensive and thoroughgoing use made of Vyāsa's and subsequent commentaries, it would have been confusing to include translations of the *sūtras* that differed from the understanding of the primary commentary.

As we go through the four chapters, we also make frequent reference to the teachings of the *Bhagavad-gītā* and other treatises on Yoga located within the *Mahābhārata*. My feeling is that our understanding of the *Yoga Sūtras* will undoubtedly be enhanced by gaining some insight into the wider context out of which the text emerged. Although he makes no reference to external sources, one feels that there can be little doubt that Patañjali drew on earlier teachings in constructing his work, and the passages on Yoga in the *Gītā* and *Mahābhārata* are some of the most important earlier expositions of Yoga that we have access to today. A careful reading of these texts reveals that the *Bhagavad-gītā* in particular is often pursuing the same lines of thought as the *Yoga Sūtras*, and considering very similar patterns of ideas including the *aṣṭāṅga,* or eight limbs, which are implicit in the *Gītā* although not overtly delineated as such. Hence it would certainly seem to be the case that a study of *Yoga Sūtras* would benefit from reference to parallel passages of the *Gītā*, which shed further light on the particular vision of the early Yoga traditions.

Another feature of this study guide, which some may feel adds extra difficulties to the unavoidable complexity of the text itself, is the constant emphasis placed on the original Sanskrit terminology employed by the *sūtras*. I can fully appreciate the fact that this aspect of the present work may prove to be frustrating and at times confusing, but my feeling is that an effective study of the *Yoga Sūtras* must aim to provide a broad knowledge and understanding of the specific terminology employed in early Yoga teachings. It is also the case that many of the technical terms used by Patañjali have no precise English equivalent, and hence it is my hope that repetition of these Sanskrit words within the discussions of the *sūtras* will provide a valuable level of familiarity with key terms in Yoga discourse. I hope this will not prove to be problematic as we move through the four chapters, and that there will be a recognition of the value of the insights provided by this approach.

Finally, if we were to ask the general question of what the *Yoga Sūtras* is about, or why it was written, we would have to say that Patañjali's primary aim is to offer a means by which the committed practitioner can achieve a high degree of spiritual progression, leading ultimately to enlightenment and liberation from the miseries of rebirth. From the perspective of the *Yoga Sūtras*, life in this world is beset by an existential flow of misery and frustration that can only be stemmed by enlightenment in the form of experiential knowledge of our true spiritual identity, which is always transcendent to the misery and dissatisfaction inherent in its physical and mental embodiments. The goal that is aimed at by these Yoga teachings is *kaivalya*, separation from material existence and the experience of the sense of absolute joy that is the true nature of each living being. Whatever we may seek to gain and achieve through our knowledge and practice of Yoga, it is important to keep in mind that the primary teacher of Yoga presents his system with this ultimate goal of liberation constantly in mind.

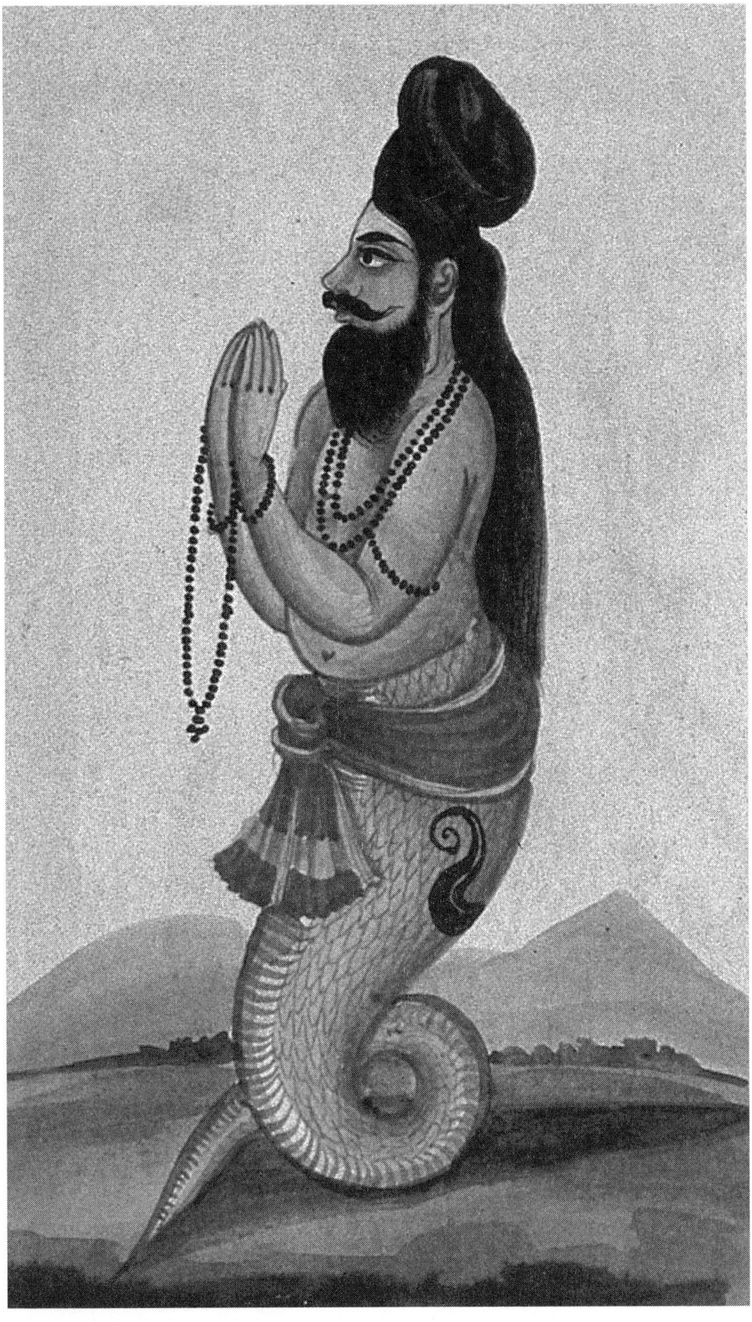

A nineteenth-century gouache of Patañjali. [Source: Wellcome Collection]

Background and Context: The Philosophy of Sāṁkhya

Background to the Yoga Sūtras

As is well known, the *Yoga Sūtras* is a relatively short treatise on Yoga practice and philosophy compiled by an author named Patañjali. As with most of the early foundational texts of the various Indian philosophical systems, the *Yoga Sūtras* presents its ideas in the form of *sūtras,* which are pithy abbreviated statements, generally made without the use of verbs. It seems likely that authors adopted this abbreviated form of presentation to allow for memorisation by students of the systems they were outlining. This does, however, present difficulties for any translator or interpreter of the text, as the meaning is not always precisely clear, and it does allow for later commentators to offer varying interpretations of the principal ideas, as we see from the commentaries on the *Vedānta Sūtras,* which are notable for the extent to which the commentaries contradict one another.

The *Yoga Sūtras* is divided into four chapters of roughly equal length apart from the final chapter, the *Kaivalya-pāda,* which is somewhat shorter. Each of these four chapters is named according to the main area of discourse it primarily focuses upon. Thus the first chapter is named the *Samādhi-pāda* as it discusses the final conclusion of the Yoga system, the second chapter is named the *Sādhana-pāda* as it focuses on the forms of practice (*sādhana*) to be undertaken, the third chapter is named the *Vibhūti-pāda* as it describes the various wondrous rewards gained by the successful adept in Yoga, and the fourth and final chapter is named the *Kaivalya-pāda* as it discusses the highest spiritual goal to be sought through Yoga practice, which is referred to as *kaivalya* rather than *mokṣa*, both of which mean liberation from rebirth.

Although there are a number of *sūtras* that consider different elements of Yoga practice, the *Yoga Sūtras* is not a Yoga manual, but rather a presentation of the understanding of the ideas that form the basis of Yoga practice. Essentially, this entails an analysis of our position in this world, which is based on the Sāṁkhya philosophical system, and then shows how Yoga techniques are effective in alleviating the existential problems of human life. Those who are familiar with contemporary Yoga practice may be surprised to notice how little attention is paid by Patañjali to *āsanas* and other postures, which today form the main features of Yoga. Here we must be aware that the *Yoga Sūtras* is the primary text of what is today referred to as 'classical Yoga', which is essentially a Yoga of the mind rather than of the body, although the body is not altogether ignored. Complex *āsanas* and other physical yoga practices start to gain prominence with the advent of Haṭha yoga from around the beginning of the second millenium CE.

We cannot be certain as to the date of the composition of the *Yoga Sūtras*, although the most common suggestion seems to be that this was some time in the fourth century CE. There can be little doubt that Patañjali drew on earlier textual sources in the construction of the *Yoga Sūtras* although we cannot be certain as to the identity of these works. We do, however, have a number of texts available to us today that are almost certainly earlier than Patañjali's exposition and these give us quite a clear

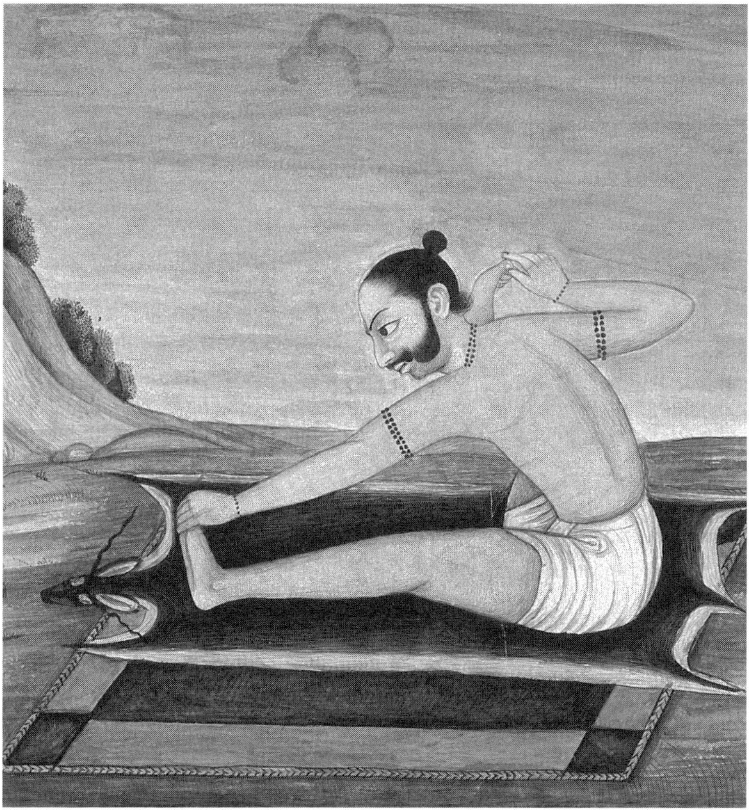

A yogin *engaged in Haṭha yogic practice.* [Source: Wellcome Collection]

insight into the wider ambience within which he was working in this early period. These potential sources would include certain passages from the Upaniṣads, certain chapters of the *Bhagavad-gītā,* and treatises on Yoga that appear in Book 12, the *Śānti-parvan,* of the *Mahābhārata.* A review of these passages reveals quite clearly that they are primarily concerned with the process of meditation that was believed to bring experiential knowledge of the true spiritual nature of our identity. Nowhere in these early works do we find instruction on postural yoga or on the subtle anatomy of *cakras* and *nāḍīs* that are an essential element of later Yoga teachings.

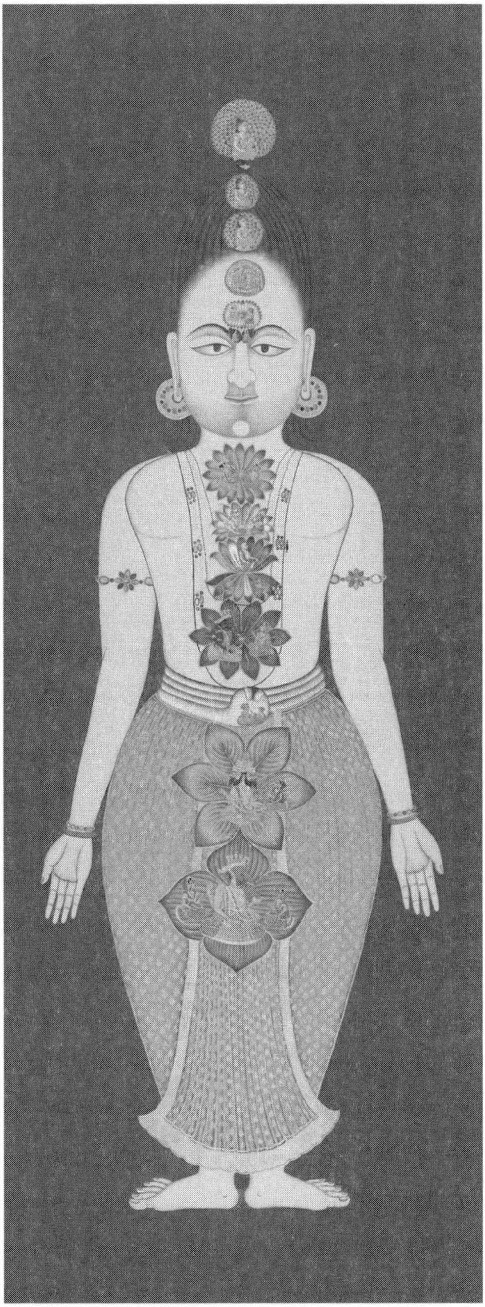

A depiction of the cakras *of the subtle body.*

Much of recent scholarship on Patañjali's yoga deal with its Buddhist background.[1] The most comprehensive of these publications is Pradeep Gokhale's book on the 'Buddhist Roots of the Yoga System'. Gokhale says that the book tries 'to show the relevance of the Abhidharma literature of Sarvāstivāda, Vaibhāṣika and Sautrāntika Buddhism, as well as Asaṅga's Yogācāra writings, for understanding the *Yogasūtra's* many aphorisms in addition to terms and passages in the *Yogabhāṣya*'.[2] The apparent references to the ideas developed by specific Buddhist thinkers, such as Vasubandu and Asaṅga, accounts for the generally accepted dating of the *Yoga Sūtras* to the fourth century CE. Gokhale further argues that 'many obscure and enigmatic terms, concepts and doctrines mentioned and used by Patañjali can be understood with greater clarity if their Buddhist background is taken into account'.[3] The *Yoga Sūtras* thus exist in a complicated historical relationship with the Buddhist tradition, which was most likely that of dialogue and mutual influence. While employing some terms that are first attested in the Buddhist literature, the *Yoga Sūtras* include polemics against Buddhist idealism and place their yogic practices in a Sāṁkhya framework.

---

1 See: Pradeep Gokhale, *The Yogasūtra of Patañjali: A New Introduction to the Buddhist Roots of the Yoga System* (London: Routledge, 2020); Philipp Maas, 'Sarvāstivāda Buddhist Theories of Temporality and the Pātañjala Yoga Theory of Transformation (pariṇāma)', Journal of Indian Philosophy, 48 (2020): 963–1003; Karen O'Brien-Kop, *Rethinking 'Classical Yoga' and Buddhism: Meditation, Metaphors and Materiality* (London: Bloomsbury, 2021); Dominik Wujastyk, 'Some Problematic Yoga Sūtra-s and their Buddhist Background', in *Yoga in Transformation: Historical and Contemporary Perspectives*, ed. Karl Baier, Karin Preisendanz, and Philipp Andre Maas (Göttingen: V&R unipress, 2018).

2 Gokhale, *The Yogasūtra of Patañjali*, 12.

3 Gokhale, *The Yogasūtra of Patañjali*, 4.

The *Yoga Sūtras* prescribes a means by which the mind can be transformed into a tool of enlightenment through which the spiritual core of the practitioner's being can be experienced. By following the ordained *yoga-sādhana*, the adept comes to the realisation of the truth of the Sāṁkhya teaching on the absolute distinction between the spiritual entity, the *ātman* or *puruṣa*, that is our true identity, and the physical and mental embodiment with which one typically identifies oneself. The perception of this spiritual truth that the expert *yogin* attains brings not only higher knowledge but also the separation of *puruṣa* from *prakṛti*, its material embodiment; this separation is the essence of *kaivalya*, 'aloneness' or 'separation', and it brings liberation from the sufferings of rebirth. Hence in technical terms, it is correct to identify the *Yoga Sūtras* as a text that has as its principal aim the liberation of the *puruṣa* from the otherwise endless cycle of death and rebirth along with all the sufferings that these repeated embodiments entail.

In terms of its more spiritual aspects, Yoga is now frequently associated with the ancient philosophy of *advaita*, non-dualism, which is the dominant system of thought based on the major Upaniṣads, such as the *Chāndogya* and *Bṛhad-āraṇyaka*. The essence of this philosophy is the idea of the identity of the individual *ātman* with the absolute reality that is Brahman. This realisation is encapsulated in the aphorism *ahaṁ brahmāsmi*, 'I am Brahman', found in the *Bṛhad-āraṇyaka Upaniṣad* (1.4.10). It is sometimes suggested that the word 'yoga' is related to this Vedāntic doctrine of absolute unity and has the meaning of union in the sense of the non-difference, the *advaita*, of *ātman* and Brahman. This, however, seems most unlikely, as the earliest teachings on Yoga that we have access to today are closely associated with the Sāṁkhya system rather than the Advaita Vedānta. As we will discuss below, the Sāṁkhya system overtly contradicts the idea of absolute unity, insisting that each *puruṣa* is an eternally individual spiritual entity and as such will remain as an individual entity even after liberation is gained. There is no doubt that the *Yoga Sūtras* bases its philosophical understanding on Sāṁkhya teachings rather than Advaita Vedānta, and hence we will shortly turn our attention to a brief exposition of the main precepts of Sāṁkhya as set out in certain treatises contained within the *Mahābhārata* and in a text known as the *Sāṁkhya Kārikā*, which provides the classical interpretation of Sāṁkhya doctrine.

As far as the author of the *Yoga Sūtras* is concerned, we have little or no real information other than the fact that his name was Patañjali. In earlier years, it was believed that this Patañjali was the same person as an author who wrote a work on grammar, probably sometime around the second or third century BCE. This view is no longer widely held, however, and many modern commentators suggest that the most likely date for the author of the *Yoga Sūtras* is some time in the late fourth century CE, although there is no absolute consensus on this point, and we cannot rule out the possibility that Patañjali lived a century or more before this. As to his life or character, we have no idea at all apart from what can be surmised from the text of the *Yoga Sūtras*, which is the only composition of his that has come down to us. Traditional sources have suggested that Patañjali was an *avatāra* of Ananta, the serpent manifestation of Viṣṇu who acts as that Deity's bed during the cosmic slumber before the creation of the world. Acceptance or otherwise of this view is of course a matter for personal faith.

Patañjali himself makes no reference to earlier works that he might have made use of, but it does not seem unreasonable to suggest that he may have had access to some of the early Yoga treatises that are still extant today, and I have a strong suspicion that he was aware of the chapters of the *Bhagavad-gītā* and at times drew on these for certain areas of his teaching. This cannot be demonstrated with any degree of certainty and is really just a subtle hunch on my part. The *Kaṭha* and *Śvetāśvatara*

Upaniṣads contain relatively brief allusions to the practice of the types of meditational Yoga that are advocated in the *Yoga Sūtras,* but these are so lacking in detail that they cannot have provided Patañjali with any meaningful guidance for the compilation of his work. The *Maitrī Upaniṣad* does contain significant teachings on Yoga, but this work is not usually considered to be one of the principal Upaniṣads and the passages and chapters that provide instruction on Yoga are almost certainly a later interpolation. Hence I think we can say that it is unlikely that the *Maitrī Upaniṣad* provided source material for the *Yoga Sūtras*.

The main Brahmanical textual sources that we should look towards in exploring the precursors of the *Yoga Sūtras* are contained within the *Śānti-parvan* (Book 12) of the *Mahābhārata*. Here the dying Bhīṣma gives extensive passages of instruction to Yudhiṣṭhira, several of which take the form of treatises on Sāṁkhya philosophy and Yoga practice. It is impossible to say with any degree of certainty whether or not Patañjali had access to these treatises or used them as source material, but what we can say is that the understanding of Yoga that they expound is of a similar nature to that encountered within the *Yoga Sūtras*. The emphasis throughout is on achieving mastery over the fluctuations of the mind so that one can gain volitional control over the thought processes and thereby fix the mind on a single point. This power of control then enables the adept to undertake the process of inward mental exploration and to thereby gain experiential knowledge of the philosophical truths contained within the Sāṁkhya treatises, specifically the distinction between the spiritual self and its mental and physical embodiment. And again we find little or nothing on the forms of Tantric, Haṭha, or postural Yoga that attain such a level of prominence in the later Yoga traditions. These treatises on Yoga contained within the *Mahābhārata* are the earliest substantial passages dealing with the subject, and hence again it is reasonable to surmise that these passages along with the

Bhagavad-gītā provided Patañjali with source material for his construction of the *Yoga Sūtras*.

The point has been made several times that the philosophical conjectures on which the *Yoga Sūtras* bases a considerable section of its teachings derive from the Sāṁkhya system, and again if we look back to the *Mahābhārata*, *Bhagavad-gītā*, and *Śvetāśvatara Upaniṣad* we will see that connection between Yoga and Sāṁkhya. The principal distinction drawn between Sāṁkhya and Yoga is that Yoga is theistic in the sense of accepting the existence of a Supreme Deity, whilst Sāṁkhya is non-theistic and presents an understanding of the world and its creation that assigns no role whatsoever to the Deity. This distinction is also apparent from a comparison of the *Yoga Sūtras*, which does refer to the existence of *īśvara*, and the *Sāṁkhya Kārikā* which makes no mention of any such Supreme Being. We could also notice that one of the passages contained in the *Mahābhārata*, the *Yoga Kathana* (*Śānti-parvan* Ch. 289), purports to show a form of debate between followers of Yoga and those who adhere to the Sāṁkhya system, with the adherents of Yoga challenging the Sāṁkhyas over their rejection of the existence of God.

This distinction is, however, relatively slight and for the most part the doctrines of Sāṁkhya and Yoga are regarded as virtually identical, as is asserted by the *Bhagavad-gītā* (5.5), *ekaṁ sāṁkhyaṁ ca yogaṁ ca*. Hence for a clearer understanding of the ideas presented by the *Yoga Sūtras*, we must start out with a brief introduction to Sāṁkhya thought, which will be of great assistance as we proceed through the *sūtras* themselves, as it will provide solid points of reference for the teachings under consideration. Of course, it is also worth bearing in mind as we proceed that Sāṁkhya is not the sole reference point for understanding the text, and that, in particular, a compelling case has recently been made by some scholars for reading the *sūtras* as also informed by Buddhist treatises on meditation such as the *Yogācāra-bhūmi* attributed to Asaṅga (fourth century CE).[4]

Sāṁkhya: A Very Brief Introduction

The Sāṁkhya system has a good number of subtleties and complexities, but for our purposes here, I have tried to isolate the main points of the doctrines it espouses with the aim of allowing a clearer insight into the more philosophical passages of the *Yoga Sūtras*, which tend to reflect the Sāṁkhya precepts outlined below.

Sources of knowledge

Sāṁkhya accepts only three of the main *pramāṇas* (sources of knowledge) considered in Indian philosophy: *pratyakṣa*, direct perception through the senses; *anumāna*, logical inference based on perception; and *śabda*, revelation or verbal testimony from a reliable source, which would include the Vedic scriptures. Although the schools of Vedānta philosophy, such as the Advaita Vedānta taught by Śaṅkarācārya, accept other secondary *pramāṇas*, the main difference from Sāṁkhya with regard to sources of knowledge relates to the reliance placed on the Vedic revelation. Whereas, theoretically at least, Vedānta bases all of its ideas on scriptural sources, Sāṁkhya prioritises reasoned inference and asserts that recourse to *śabda-pramāṇa* is only necessary for matters beyond the possible scope of perception or inference. Hence neither the *Sāṁkhya Kārikā* nor the *Yoga Sūtras* ever cite scripture in support of their arguments, whereas other early philosophical works such as the *Mīmāṁsā Sūtras* and the *Vedānta Sūtras* base their contentions primarily on the revelations of the Vedas and Upaniṣads.

---

4 Gokhale, *The Yogasūtra of Patañjali.*

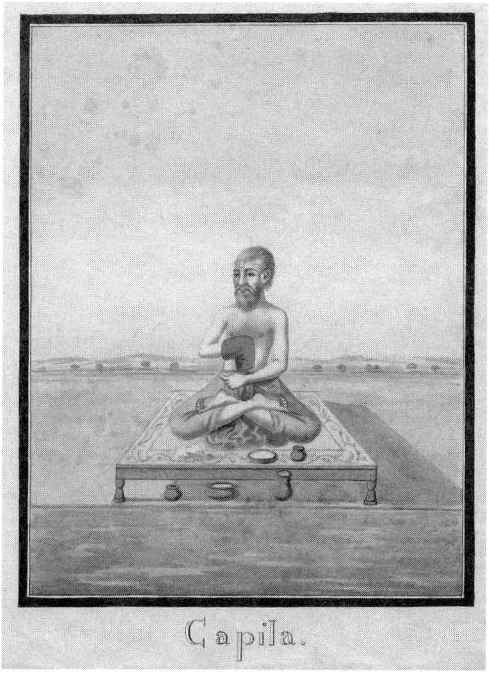

A watercolour portraying Kapila, legendary founder of Sāṁkhya.

Creation of the World

As a system that is largely non-theistic, Sāṁkhya does not present the notion of a Deity who creates the world. Rather, Sāṁkhya insists on a continual process of creation and dissolution that has neither beginning nor end. Prior to the manifestation of the world, *prakṛti* (matter) exists in an undifferentiated and non-manifest (*avyakta*) form. The three *guṇas*, or essential qualities, that pervade *prakṛti* are in a state of complete equilibrium and hence do not exert their influence. The manifestation of the world occurs when this balance is disturbed and the *guṇas* depart from their state of equilibrium. This transformation sets in motion the evolution of the elements of matter from out of the primeval, undifferentiated *prakṛti*. One might naturally ask what it is that sets this process in motion, and sources that are theistically inclined suggest that it is the work of the Deity, but most Sāṁkhya treatises insist that it is a naturally occurring process or that it takes place due to the disturbing influence of the multitude of individual spiritual entities.

The three guṇas

The idea that there are three essential qualities pervading every aspect of matter is one that originated in Sāṁkhya teachings, but was adopted by other schools of thought, notably Vedānta. This adoption was virtually inevitable given the authoritative status ascribed by Vedānta to the *Bhagavad-gītā*, which makes extensive use of this Sāṁkhya concept. These three *guṇas* are everywhere named as *sattva* (goodness, purity, truth), *rajas* (energy, passion, action), and *tamas* (darkness, ignorance, dullness), but their precise nature is not defined in the early texts, and it is only in the writings of a later interpreter of Sāṁkhya named Vijñāna Bhikṣu that we find the assertion that the *guṇas* are real objects of a super-subtle nature. We will hear more of Vijñāna Bhikṣu later on as he is one of the major commentators on the *Yoga Sūtras*. The only other possible interpretation would be that they are tendencies or qualities found in all aspects of matter, and as such, are pervasive throughout the existence of *prakṛti*, whether it be non-manifest or evolved into the world. Chapters 17 and 18 of the *Bhagavad-gītā* make extensive use of the idea of the *guṇas* in discussing the nature of this world and of human activity, but in the main Sāṁkhya texts the principal significance of the *guṇas* is in relation to their falling out of the state of equilibrium, which in turn sets the process of evolution and hence creation in motion. Once the world is manifest, each of the *guṇas* never exists alone in any object or state of mind, but in a constantly changing state of combination. Thus, for example, a person may be heavily influenced by *tamas* at one time and then become transformed by developing the attributes of *sattva*. When a person is active or agitated, it is *rajas* that comes to the fore, but this process may be impeded by a subsequent predominance of *tamas* or *sattva*, the former producing sloth and the latter a state of contentment that militates against the more passionate forms of action.

Satkārya-vāda

Sāṁkhya adheres to a philosophical concept, named the *satkārya-vāda*, which asserts that any effect is already existent within its cause. The *satkārya-vāda* indicates that all the varieties we observe in this world are already present within the primal, non-manifest state of *prakṛti*.

Elements of matter

The word *sāṁkhya* literally means a counting or an enumeration, and this is applied both to the elements of which matter is comprised and the *ātman* (*puruṣa*), the innermost self that transcends all of them. As mentioned above, Sāṁkhya theory asserts that prior to the manifestation of this world, *prakṛti* exists in a non-manifest, unevolved state in which the *guṇas* are in a condition of absolute equilibrium. When that equilibrium is disturbed, *prakṛti* begins to evolve into the twenty-four elements of which this world is comprised. The listing of these twenty-four elements differs slightly between the various Sāṁkhya treatises, and in the *Mahābhārata* we find passages that list only eight or sixteen. When primal *prakṛti* becomes agitated by the disequilibrium of the *guṇas*, a process of evolution is set in motion by which the elements of matter emerge gradually one from another. The first evolute is generally designated as *mahat*, the great element, which is equated with *buddhi,* the intellect present within all living beings. The *mahat* then evolves into *ahaṁkāra,* which is the sense of ego or I-ness that is a universal characteristic of living beings.

Here the *satkārya-vāda* is particularly significant as it reveals that *buddhi* or *mahat* is already existing within primal *prakṛti* and that *ahaṁkāra* is present within the *buddhi.* The influence of *sattva-guṇa* on *ahaṁkāra* causes it to evolve into the mind, *manas,* the five senses of perception (touch, taste, smell, sight, and hearing), and into the organs through which bodily functions are performed (feet, hands, anus, genitals, and voice). When *ahaṁkāra* is influenced by the *guṇa* known as *tamas,* it evolves into the subtle objects perceived by the senses. These five are the sensation of touch, flavour, aroma, form or colour, and sound; they are generally referred to as the five *tan-mātras.* Although they are produced by evolution, these five *tan-mātras* evolve further into what are known as the five *mahā-bhūtas,* or great elements. These are analysed as follows: sound evolves into space; sound and touch evolve into air; sound, touch, and form evolve into fire; sound, touch, form, and flavour evolve into water; sound, touch, form, flavour, and aroma evolve into earth. These five elements of space, air, fire, water, and earth are regarded as fundamental to all existence and with them the process of evolution comes to an end.

Thus we can now get a clear idea of the Sāṁkhya enumeration of the elements present within the evolved *prakṛti* that forms this world:

1. *Avyakta, prakṛti* in its unevolved form
2. *Mahat* or *buddhi,* the intellect that discriminates and makes decisions
3. *Ahaṁkāra,* ego or sense of personal identity
4. *Manas,* the mind that identifies and classifies sensory perceptions

5. The sense of taste
6. The sense of smell
7. The sense of touch
8. The sense of sight
9. The sense of hearing
10. The feet
11. The hands
12. The voice
13. The anus
14. The genitals
15. Flavour
16. Aroma
17. Touch sensations
18. Colour and form
19. Sound
20. Space
21. Water
22. Air
23. Fire
24. Earth.

The puruṣa

In addition to these twenty-four elements of which the world is comprised, Sāṁkhya also postulates the existence of a twenty-fifth element, which is eternal and untouched by *prakṛti*. This is the individual spiritual self, the *ātman* or *puruṣa*, which gives life and consciousness to the otherwise inert elements. In Sāṁkhya teachings, this innermost, eternal self is usually referred to as *puruṣa*, the person, though the terms *ātman*, the self, and *kṣetra-jña*, the knower of the field, are also used. Unlike the other twenty-four elements, *puruṣa*, the twenty-fifth, is not an evolute of *prakṛti*. It is entirely spiritual, and hence changeless and eternal. Although *buddhi* is understood as the intellect or personality of living beings, whilst *manas* is the mind that processes the information gleaned through the senses, both of these are manifestations of *prakṛti* and hence are inherently non-conscious. It is only when the *buddhi* is connected to *puruṣa* that it manifests the characteristics of consciousness.

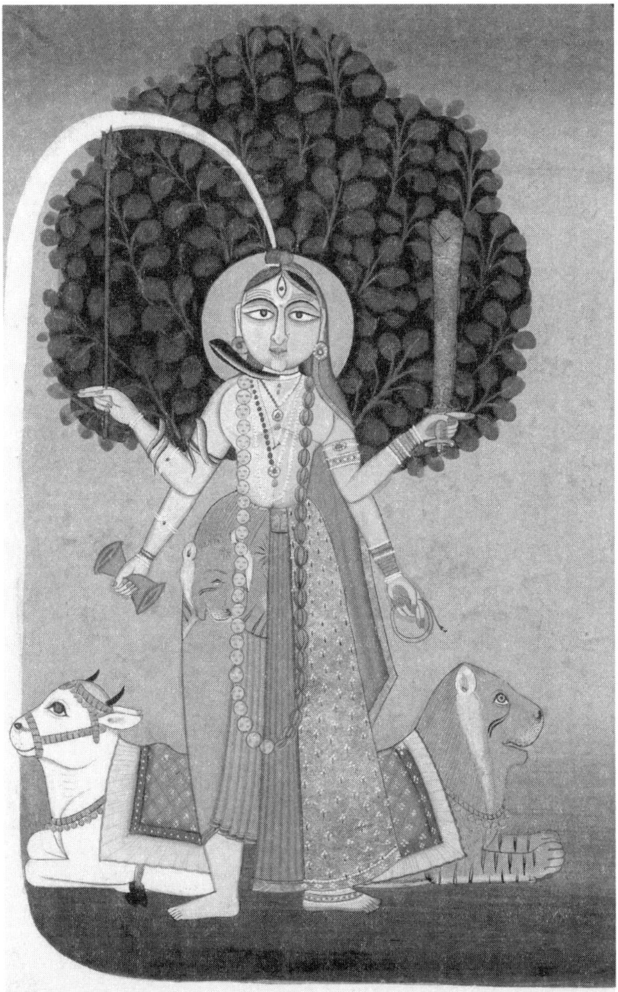

Ardhanārīśvara, the androgynous aspect of Śiva, prefigured by the foundational prakṛti-puruṣa *Sāṃkhya concept.*

There are differing opinions as to the nature of the contact between *buddhi* and *puruṣa*, notably between Vijñāna Bhikṣu and Vācaspati Miśra, another commentator on the *Yoga Sūtras* whose work we will refer to. In the view of Vācaspati Miśra, it is merely the proximity of *buddhi* to *puruṣa* that brings consciousness to the *buddhi* and hence to the living being. Vijñāna Bhikṣu, however, rejects this view and asserts that there must be direct interaction between them, although *puruṣa* is never subject to the transformations experienced moment by moment by the *buddhi*. A significant point to note here is that Sāṁkhya is insistent that each *puruṣa* is an eternally individual entity; in contrast to Śaṅkarācārya's teaching, the Advaita Vedānta, there is no absolute oneness. The world that becomes manifest due to the evolution of *prakṛti* is entirely real and the individuality of the *puruṣa* is an eternal reality even after liberation from rebirth is attained. It is primarily for this reason that both the *Vedānta Sūtras* and Śaṅkarācārya condemn the Yoga system that is based on Sāṁkhya metaphysics. During the course of our review of the *sūtras*, we will also pay attention to a commentary attributed to Śaṅkarācārya, which, by contrast, does not involve any polemic against this aspect of Sāṁkhya and Yoga doctrine.

The mental faculties

The mental faculties as defined above are *buddhi*, *manas*, and *indriya*, approximately though not precisely the intellect, the mind, and the senses. As a manifestation of *prakṛti*, these are by nature non-conscious but become conscious due either to the proximity of *puruṣa*, or even direct interaction with *puruṣa*. In that state, the senses then become active, surveying the world and bringing perceptions into the *manas* – aromas, tastes, sights, sounds, and sensations of touch.

Avidyā

The primary cause of the association between *puruṣa* and *prakṛti* is stated to be *avidyā,* ignorance of the true spiritual nature of *puruṣa*. Essentially, *puruṣa* makes the error of regarding the transformations of *buddhi* as happening to itself and it is this false identification of *puruṣa* with *buddhi* that maintains the unwanted association of *puruṣa* with *prakṛti*. According to Surendranath Dasgupta in his *A History of Indian Philosophy*:

> Buddhi resembles puruṣa in transparency, and the puruṣa fails to differentiate itself from the modifications of the buddhi, and as a result of this non-distinction the puruṣa becomes bound down to the buddhi, always failing to recognize the truth that the buddhi and its transformations are wholly alien to it. This non-distinction of puruṣa from buddhi which is itself a mode of buddhi is what is meant by *avidyā* (non-knowledge) in Sāṁkhya, and is the root of all experience and misery.[5]

We will detect the presence of this idea in the opening *sūtras* of Chapter 1 of the *Yoga Sūtras,* which refer to the true state of *puruṣa* and its false identification with the movements of the mind, which represent the constant fluctuations of *buddhi*.

Rebirth

Like most branches of Indian religious philosophy, Sāṁkhya accepts the notion of reincarnation as determined by previous actions. Good or righteous acts will produce a positive effect in the form of an elevated rebirth and good fortune in the life to

---

5 Surendranath Dasgupta, *A History of Indian Philosophy,* vol. 5 (Cambridge: Cambridge University Press, 1922–1955), 260.

come, whilst iniquitous deeds will produce the opposite result, though extremely good or extremely bad acts may produce a result in the present life. But as *puruṣa* remains completely transcendent, the question arises as to how it can be affected by acts that are performed purely within the domain of *prakṛti*. To this Sāṁkhya responds by stating that karma relates to the *buddhi* with which *puruṣa* has come into association, and it is only the false sense of identity of *puruṣa* with *buddhi* that causes it to transmigrate through bodily forms and experience the fruits of good and bad karma.

The *buddhi* is affected and transformed by the experiences it undergoes and the actions it performs, and in its state of *avidyā*, *puruṣa* identifies these transformations as relating to itself. Each experience leaves an impression on the *buddhi*, referred to as *vāsanā* or *saṁskāra*, and these resurface in the future as the process of karma unfolds. Sāṁkhya shares with Vedānta, Buddhism, and numerous other systems of Indian thought the view that life in this sphere of existence is predominated by suffering and that the ultimate aim of life is to gain release from the cycle of rebirth. This, however, can only be achieved when an individual casts off the false identity of *puruṣa* with *buddhi* and realises its true identity as transcendent to matter.

Kaivalya

In Sāṁkhya writings, this achievement of release from the suffering of rebirth is usually referred to as *kaivalya*, a term which is broadly equivalent to *mokṣa* or *mukti*, more commonly used in other systems. *Kaivalya* literally means 'aloneness', and refers to the separation of *puruṣa* from its connection with the twenty-four elements into which *prakṛti* evolves. Liberation from rebirth is achieved through the development of knowledge of the true identity of *puruṣa* as an eternal spiritual entity. At present, we understand ourselves in terms of the *buddhi*, senses, and physical body, but by gaining higher realisation, *puruṣa* recognises its true identity as distinct from *prakṛti*. In the *Mahābhārata*, we find the phrase *anyo 'ham* (12.295.20 and 12.296.10), 'I am different', denoting the realisation that awakens a living being from its state of ignorance. When this knowledge is attained, the connection between *puruṣa* and *prakṛti* is broken, and *puruṣa* comes to exist in its true state of absolute separation in which suffering and rebirth come to an end. The precise nature of this state of *kaivalya* is not fully explained, although there is an interesting statement given in Chapter 212 of the *Śānti-parvan* of the *Mahābhārata* in which Pañcaśikha, one of the original teachers of Sāṁkhya, states that it is neither existence nor non-existence. That is probably about as far as Sāṁkhya is willing to go. In this regard, Surendranath Dasgupta writes:

> Thus proceeds the course of saṁsāra. When the avidyā of a person is rooted out by the rise of true knowledge, the buddhi fails to attach itself to the purusha and is forever dissociated from it, and this is the state of mukti [liberation].[6]

Despite the aim of Sāṁkhya being to achieve the dissociation of *puruṣa* from *buddhi* (intellect), it is the *buddhi* that must be employed to achieve that goal, for the true conception of *puruṣa* as a distinct entity arises initially within the *buddhi*. Here we can readily detect the connection between Sāṁkhya and Yoga, for the Yoga system outlined by Patañjali and by the *Bhagavad-gītā* has the specific aim of gaining realised knowledge of the existence of the *puruṣa*, which is achieved by

6 Surendranath Dasgupta, *A History of Indian Philosophy*, vol. 5 (Cambridge: Cambridge University Press, 1922–1955), 261.

the *buddhi's* gaining control over the movements of the mind and then focusing constantly on the *puruṣa*. Sāṁkhya accepts the idea that liberation can be achieved even whilst a person lives in this world. This is the state of being generally referred to as *jīvan-mukti* in which one lives within the domain of *prakṛti* but remains entirely aloof from its fluctuations.

Theistic Sāṁkhya

Sāṁkhya is widely accepted as an atheistic philosophical system in the sense that it regards the manifestation of the world as a natural process brought about by the inherent nature of *prakṛti*. It does not accept the existence of a transcendent Deity presiding over the world and it understands liberation from the world as being the result of the attainment of realised knowledge rather than the grace of God. We should note, however, that in some of the early Sāṁkhya treatises found in the *Mahābhārata* a twenty-sixth element is referred to that is distinct from *puruṣa*, the twenty-fifth. This twenty-sixth element is never in contact with *prakṛti* and can perhaps be equated with the idea of *īśvara*, as revealed in the *Yoga Sūtras*. Moreover, in the *Bhagavad-gītā*, we have a text that is quite clearly substantially based on Sāṁkhya and Yoga doctrine, and yet is assertively theistic and devotional, stating overtly that the manifestation of the world from primeval *prakṛti* takes place under the direction of the Supreme Deity (9.10). We must also be aware that the later interpretations of Sāṁkhya found in the *Bhāgavata Purāṇa* and the writings of Vijñāna Bhikṣu are also theistic and even devotional. Hence, although classical Sāṁkhya as presented in the *Sāṁkhya Kārikā* is atheistic, or at least non-theistic, Sāṁkhya itself is a broad system that includes a variety of different strands, some of which accept the notion of a Supreme Deity.

Renunciation

The teachings of the Sāṁkhya and Yoga system lead naturally to an emphasis on the renunciation of worldly pleasures. Hence in many Sāṁkhya texts we find instructions to that end in terms of renouncing all attachment to family, friends, prosperity, and possessions. Similarly, in the *Bhagavad-gītā* (6.2), it is stated that the practice of Yoga must be accompanied by the renunciation of materialistic inclinations, *na hy asaṁnyasta-saṁkalpo yogī bhavati kaścana.*

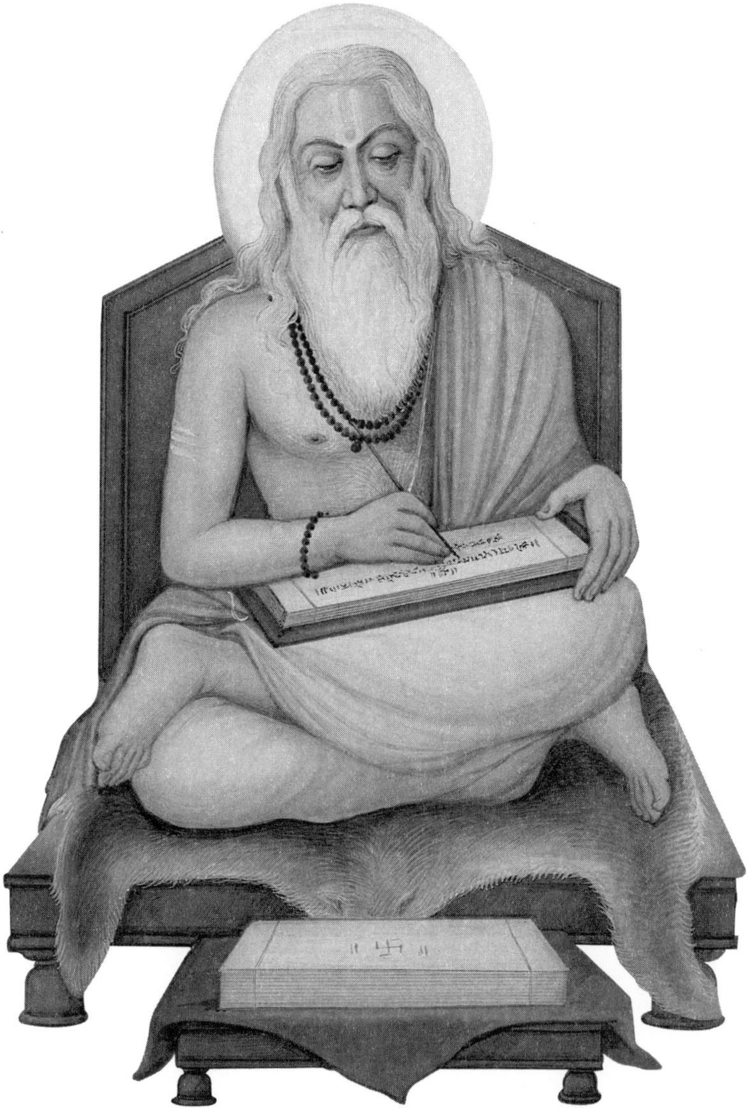

Vyāsa, legendary compiler of the Vedas.

COMMENTARIES ON THE *YOGA SŪTRAS*

Over the centuries, a number of commentaries on the *Yoga Sūtras* have been written and we will refer to some of the main ones of these as we move through the four chapters and attempt to determine the precise meaning of the *sūtras*. A lot of valuable work on the text has also been done in the modern era and we shall also consider these more recent conclusions as we move through the text. Amongst the traditional commentators, there are four in particular that we will be referring and at times deferring to. These are as follows:

1. The *Vyāsa-bhāṣya*, attributed to Vyāsa, the compiler of the Vedas, but almost certainly the work of an author who lived not long after Patañjali. Some modern writers have suggested that this commentary may have been produced by Patañjali himself as an explanation of his *Yoga Sūtras*.
2. The commentary attributed to Śaṅkarācārya, who lived in the seventh or eighth century CE. This was only discovered in the twentieth century; it is by no means certain that it is the work of Śaṅkarācārya, though some modern writers have stated their belief that it is an authentic work of his.
3. The commentary of Vācaspati Miśra who lived in the ninth century CE and was himself an adherent of Śaṅkarācārya's system of Advaita Vedānta, although he commented on other systems as well, seeking mainly to explain their main tenets without engaging in any polemical form of contradiction.

4. The commentary of Vijñāna Bhikṣu who lived in North India in the sixteenth century CE and, like Vācaspati Miśra, is to be noted as one of the greatest traditional authorities on Indian religious philosophy.

With the exception of the *Vyāsa-bhāṣya*, these commentaries frequently move some distance away from the text of the *Yoga Sūtras* itself and use that text as a starting point for an exposition of their own views on a range of different topics. As a general rule, we will not allow ourselves to be drawn too far into these tangential discussions, and for this reason, the primary focus will generally be on the *Vyāsa-bhāṣya*, which for the most part confines its discussion to explanations of the meaning of the *sūtras* and may even be Patañjali's own explanation of his primary work. Let us now say a few words about these commentaries before we move on to embark on our consideration of the first chapter, the *Samādhi-pāda*, of the *Yoga Sūtras*.

Vyāsa-bhāṣya

All traditional commentators on the *Yoga Sūtras* regard the commentary attributed to Vyāsa as being as authoritative as the primary text itself. Hence the later commentaries attempt to explain the precise meaning of both the *sūtras* themselves and of the *Vyāsa-bhāṣya* without drawing any clear distinction between them or attempting to refute this primary commentary. One reason for this is that, as mentioned above, some see this original commentary as the work of Veda Vyāsa, the compiler of the Vedas and the author of the *Mahābhārata*, who is regarded as an *avatāra* of Viṣṇu.

The acceptance of Veda Vyāsa as the author of the commentary is very much an item of faith and most modern writers would not accept that the author of the *Mahābhārata* could also have written a commentary on the *Yoga Sūtras*, as the former work is a much earlier composition. The traditional Hindu view is based on the belief that Vyāsa had incredible longevity, but again acceptance of this view is very much an article of religious faith. Nonetheless, it is certainly the case that most writers, ancient and modern, tend to regard the *Yoga Sūtras* and the *Vyāsa-bhāṣya* as a single contiguous work and present their understandings of the text from this perspective.

What is clear is that the *Vyāsa-bhāṣya* is a very early commentary on the *Yoga Sūtras* and some modern writers, notably Philipp Maas,[1] have suggested that the commentary was actually composed by Patañjali himself so as to provide a fuller elucidation of his *sūtras*. Maas indeed points out that a number of premodern scholars, such as Abhinavagupta, apparently believed that the *bhāṣya* was composed by Patañjali.[2] This is certainly a possibility, but it is a theory that is impossible to prove with any degree of certainty; hence one is drawn towards the more generic position that the *Vyāsa-bhāṣya* is an authoritative interpretation of the *Yoga Sūtras* by a highly qualified author. Nonetheless, the modern student of the *Yoga Sūtras* is still faced with the dilemma of whether or not to accept Vyāsa's commentary as the sole acceptable reading of the *sūtras* or whether to accept the viability of alternative lines of interpretation. As a general rule, I have tended to follow the *Vyāsa-bhāṣya* though without feeling obliged to do so for each and every one of the *sūtras*. There is no doubt that some of the *sūtras* can be understood in different ways and from differing perspectives, and hence I think it is right and proper that these potential alternative readings of the text should be noted and considered.

---

1 Maas, *A Concise Historiography of Classical Yoga Philosophy*.

2 Maas, *A Concise Historiography of Classical Yoga Philosophy*, 57.

An argument sometimes presented for the acceptance of Patañjali as the author of the *Vyāsa-bhāṣya* is the close proximity of the two texts in terms of the ideas they convey and the specific language they use. Moreover, the fact that the *Vyāsa-bhāṣya* rarely moves too far away from its elucidation of the *sūtras* into polemical debate or the setting forth of a tangential line of discussion reveals the very close association between the *Yoga Sūtras* and its primary commentary. From the other side of the debate, however, it might well be the case that a particular commentator opted to follow this line of approach as he had no concern other than an explanation of the *sūtras*. None of the arguments either in favour or against Patañjali's composition of the *Vyāsa-bhāṣya* are, in my view, conclusive.

The most detailed exploration of the hypothesis that Patañjali himself composed the *Vyāsa-bhāṣya* has been made by Maas.[3] Maas argues that there is no independent manuscript tradition of transmitting just the *sūtras* without the commentary attributed to Vyāsa, with manuscripts of just the *sūtras* being extracted from the commented version. The *sūtras* and the commentary now attributed to Vyāsa are presented as a single treatise on yoga called *Pātañjala-yoga-śāstra Sāṁkhya-pravacana*. According to Maas, the references to Vyāsa or to his commentary as a separate text called *Yoga-bhāṣya* are not found in the earliest version of the text that can be reconstructed from the manuscript sources. Maas also observes that among the main later commentators only Vācaspatimiśra refers to the author of the commentary as Vyāsa, and that some important Indian thinkers, such as Abhinavagupta, refer to the *sūtras* and the *Vyāsa-bhāṣya* as having been composed by a single author.

3 Maas, *A Concise Historiography of Classical Yoga Philosophy*.

This influential hypothesis is not accepted by all. Notably, Gokhale writes: 'I do not accept the advocacy of complete hermeneutic unity between *Yogasūtra* and *Yogabhāṣya*. I feel there must have been a considerable gap – an ideological and hermeneutical gap at least, and perhaps a chronological gap as well – between them'.[4] Gokhale explains his assessment by pointing out that 'many discrepancies can be found if the aphorisms are read independently of any commentary or in light of the Buddhist background'.[5]

Regardless of the identity of the author, the commentary of Vyāsa is particularly useful in gaining an understanding of the meaning of the *sūtras*, as he concentrates consistently on explaining the meaning of the words employed. Later commentators frequently use the *sūtras* and Vyāsa's commentary as a starting point from which to expound their own particular ideas, and in doing so, at times lose contact with the original wording of the *sūtra* in question. Although Vyāsa does on occasion enter into a critique of Buddhist ideas, as in *sūtra* 1.32 (and in this he is followed by later commentators, notably Śaṅkarācārya), for the most part his commentary focuses exclusively on providing an explanation of the specific *sūtra* and the precise meaning of the terms that *sūtra* employs.

The other commentators generally provide expansions on Vyāsa's interpretation, which are useful at some points but also have a tendency to distract one from the main line of discussion in the *Yoga Sūtras* itself. Hence we will refer most frequently to the *Vyāsa-bhāṣya* and less often to the other commentators, outlining their contributions only when further explanation is required or when an additional point of particular interest is raised.

---

4 Gokhale, *The Yogasūtra of Patañjali*, 9.

5 Gokhale, *The Yogasūtra of Patañjali*, 9.

Commentary on the Yoga Sūtras Attributed to Śaṅkarācārya

Ādi Śaṅkarācārya is well known as the principal teacher of the school of Indian religious philosophy known as Advaita Vedānta, which uses Upaniṣadic aphorisms such as *sarvaṁ khalv idaṁ brahma,* 'all this is Brahman alone', *ahaṁ brahmāsmi,* 'I am Brahman', and *tat tvam asi,* 'you are that', to establish a doctrine of absolute non-dualism. According to this significant strand of Hindu doctrine, the varieties we perceive in the world around us and between individual living beings

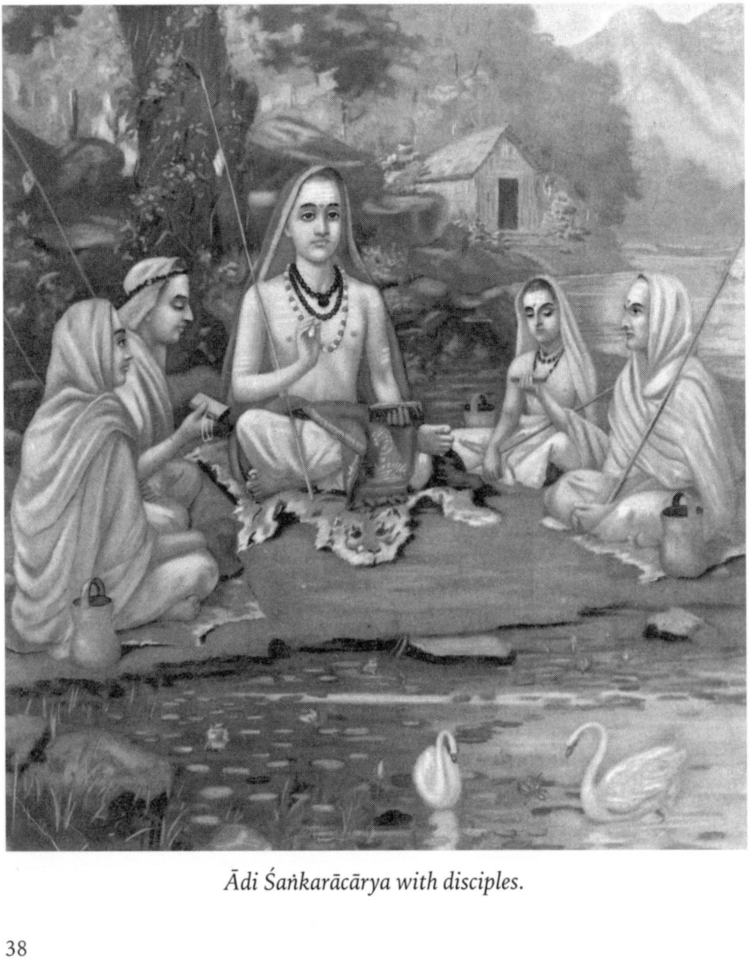

Ādi Śaṅkarācārya with disciples.

are not the absolute reality. They are a lesser reality in the way that the dream reality is a lesser reality than the waking reality. When one comes to the realisation of absolute reality, then the ultimate oneness of all existence is understood and directly perceived, for there is no variegatedness; everything is Brahman and Brahman alone.

The dates for Śaṅkara's life are uncertain but he probably lived in the seventh or eighth century CE and certainly after the composition of the *Yoga Sūtras* and the *Vyāsa-bhāṣya*. A number of works are attributed to Śaṅkarācārya, although it is uncertain how many of these were actually his own compositions. One problem is that the heads of the *maṭhas* (monasteries or religious centres) that he is said to have established are given the title of Śaṅkarācārya and it is almost certainly the case that some of the works attributed to the original Śaṅkarācārya were in fact written by his later successors. It is almost certain that the commentaries on the Upaniṣads, *Bhagavad-gītā*, and *Vedānta Sūtras* are authentic works of Ādi (first) Śaṅkarācārya, and it is highly likely that the non-commentarial works named *Viveka Cūḍāmani* and *Upadeśa Sāhasrī* are authentic as well. It is less likely, however, that the other works attributed to Śaṅkarācārya are his own compositions.

A commentary on the *Yoga Sūtras* attributed to Ādi Śaṅkarācārya was brought to light in the mid-twentieth century, although it has to be pointed out that none of the later commentators shows any awareness of this work, even though Vācaspati Miśra was a devoted follower of the Advaita Vedānta system. While some respected modern writers, including Sengaku Mayeda, have expressed the view that this commentary is indeed an authentic work of Śaṅkarācārya, I think we must be cautious in accepting this view, as the text of the commentary is in several ways quite dissimilar from Śaṅkara's other compositions.

The commentary itself is entitled the *Pātañjala-yoga-śāstra-vivaraṇa* or the *Yoga-sūtra-bhāṣya-vivaraṇa*, indicating that it is a sub-commentary on the *Vyāsa-bhāṣya*. Hence it is far more extensive than would be the case for a commentary on the *sūtras* alone. One might expect that a commentary by Ādi Śaṅkarācārya or by a later Śaṅkarācārya of one of the *maṭhas*, or indeed by an author posing as Śaṅkarācārya, would provide an advaitic interpretation of the *sūtras* and the *Vyāsa-bhāṣya*, but this is not the case and there is very little in it that would reveal the advaitic tendencies of the author.

This is not entirely surprising as we know that Vācaspati Miśra was himself a prominent teacher of the Advaita Vedānta, and yet his commentaries on the *Sāṁkhya Kārikā* and the *Yoga Sūtras* avoid any polemic against the teaching of the original text, preferring instead to focus on an explanation of the precise meaning intended by the authors. So we find that even where statements appear in the *Vyāsa-bhāṣya* that are from a Sāṁkhya perspective and in opposition to some principles of Advaita Vedānta, these are not challenged by the *Vivaraṇa*.

This is in contrast to Śaṅkara's commentary on *Vedānta Sūtras* 2.1.1–3. On 2.1.3, (which is *etena yogaḥ pratyuktaḥ*, 'hereby yoga is repudiated'), he states: 'By the repudiation of the Sāṁkhya Smṛti, it is to be understood that the Yoga Smṛti is also repudiated', though this Yoga Smṛti may be a text other than that of Patañjali, and again: 'But the followers of Sāṁkhya and Yoga are dualists, and they do not perceive the unity of the Self'. On *sūtras* 1.1.3–11, he then presents a complete denial of the Sāṁkhya view of the world as emerging by a transformation of *pradhāna*, primeval *prakṛti*, as this view is contradictory to his advaitic perspective. The point is that in his *Vedānta Sūtras* commentary, Śaṅkara assertively repudiates the Sāṁkhya system. The *Vivaraṇa*, on the other hand, lets the ideas of Sāṁkhya and Yoga pass without comment. Why?

Perhaps because he regards the *Yoga Sūtras* as a valuable text and does not want to highlight perceived flaws arising from its association with Sāṁkhya, or perhaps because this commentary is not the work of Śaṅkarācārya himself.

What we find instead is the author using the *sūtras* and the *Vyāsa-bhāṣya* as a starting point for detailed philosophical discussions on a range of different topics, often posing as an imaginary opponent who presents contrary views, and then showing how these views cannot be sustained. Thus we find Śaṅkara moving on from the text of the *Yoga Sūtras* itself into an exposition on topics such as the nature of time and on the relationship between letters and words and the objects they signify. The *Vivaraṇa* also follows the *Vyāsa-bhāṣya* by expanding on the *Bhāṣya's* polemic against Buddhist thought and, in particular, the Buddhist doctrine of momentariness, which is refuted several times over. Similarly, the reality of phenomena (*dharma*) is consistently asserted in opposition to the Buddhist view that phenomena exist only as perceptions within the mind.

Hence no firm conclusion can be reached as to whether or not the *Yoga-sūtra-bhāṣya-vivaraṇa* is in fact a written work of Ādi Śaṅkarācārya, as the evidence either way is insufficient to allow for any such conclusion to be drawn. Nevertheless we should be aware that the *Vivaraṇa* does not give us an advaitic reading of the *Yoga Sūtras* that would contradict its adherence to the precepts of Sāṁkhya thought. For the purposes of our ensuing analysis of the text, the author of this commentary on the *Yoga Sūtras* will be referred to as Śaṅkara without implying that he is necessarily the same person as Ādi Śaṅkarācārya.

The Commentary of Vācaspati Miśra

One of the commentaries most often referred to in discussions of the *Yoga Sūtras* is that of Vācaspati Miśra, known as the *Tattva-vaiśāradī*. It was probably composed sometime around 850 CE, though the dates are disputed and some suggest that he lived a century later. Surendranath Dasgupta, who was not aware of Śaṅkara's *Vivaraṇa*, refers to Vācaspati Miśra and Vijñāna Bhikṣu as 'the two great commentators on the *Vyāsabhāṣya*'.[6]

Vācaspati was himself an adherent of the school of Advaita Vedānta, following Śaṅkarācārya's non-dualism, and his commentaries on Śaṅkara's work gave rise to one of the principal later schools of Advaita, known as the Bhāmatī school, said to be named after his devoted wife whose encouragement was a frequent source of inspiration. The Bhāmatī school of Advaita Vedānta stands in opposition to several of the key precepts of Sāṁkhya and Yoga philosophy, but Vācaspati's commentaries on both the *Sāṁkhya Kārikā* and *Yoga Sūtras* do not take the form of polemical attacks on the rival schools of thought represented by these works, but seek merely to explain the meaning of the texts verse by verse or *sūtra* by *sūtra*. His commentary on the *Sāṁkhya Kārikā* is thus considered to be the most authoritative explanation of that text, despite the fact that he was not himself an adherent of that system.

Little is known about the life of Vācaspati Miśra, although it is often said that he came from Bihar in Northeast India. Over the centuries, his work has been held in high regard to the extent where he is considered to be one of the principal exponents of Indian religious philosophy. This is demonstrated by the large number of hand-written manuscripts of his work that have been collected from different areas of India, although it is likely that some of his works are no longer extant.

In his *Tattva-vaiśāradī* commentary, Vācaspati Miśra provides a careful examination of the key words used in the *Vyāsa-bhāṣya*. The commentary on each *sūtra* tends to be quite

---

6 Dasgupta, *A History of Indian Philosophy*, vol. 1, 229.

extensive because he takes the *Yoga Sūtras* and *Vyāsa-bhāṣya* almost as a single text and comments fully on both. Thus he generally starts out from the *sūtra* but moves quickly on to the *Vyāsa-bhāṣya,* directing the bulk of his commentary towards explanation and expansion of Vyāsa's statements. He does not generally attempt to introduce tangential ideas of his own, and, for the most part, his efforts seem to be directed towards giving the reader a fuller understanding of the explanation of the *sūtras* provided by Vyāsa.

The Commentary of Vijñāna Bhikṣu

The usual view is that Vijñāna Bhikṣu lived several centuries after Vācaspati Miśra, probably in the sixteenth century CE; he composed a commentary on the *Yoga Sūtras* and *Vyāsa-bhāṣya* entitled the *Yoga-vārttika*. Again we know very little about his life and it seems quite deliberate that in his written works he makes no reference to his birth, family, or origins. This was probably because, at the time of his writings, he was a renunciant, a *bhikṣu,* who had given up all connection with the world and his previous life in order to focus solely on his own spiritual progression and providing written guidance to help others towards a true understanding of the world, our place within it, and the path to liberation from rebirth. It is quite apparent from these written works that he was a vastly learned scholar in the field of Sanskrit religious literature. He was also a prolific writer and interpreter of sacred texts, although it is clear from his writing that he had a specific doctrinal view that he sought to propagate. For the accomplishment of this aim, he followed in the footsteps of earlier Vedāntists by composing commentaries on the *Vedānta Sūtras* (the *Vijñānāmṛta-bhāṣya*) and several of the major Upaniṣads, though not on the *Bhagavad-gītā*.

By the time of his writing, in the late medieval era, Hindu philosophy was dominated by Vedānta whilst, at the same time, the tendency towards devotional religious thought was also prevalent. In his commentaries on the *Vedānta Sūtras* and Upaniṣads, Vijñāna Bhikṣu rejects Śaṅkara's advaitic interpretations, often in a highly polemical manner. His own views are based primarily on the Sāṁkhya and Yoga systems, which he interprets from a theistic perspective, and it might be said that he attempts to draw together the main strands of Sāṁkhya and Vedānta in order to create a single unified system; in this sense, he could be regarded as one of the founding voices of contemporary Hindu thought, which seeks to find or create a united form of religious doctrine from out of the diverse strands of traditional thought. Moreover, Vijñāna Bhikṣu was himself a practitioner of the Yoga system taught by Patañjali in the *Yoga Sūtras*, and as such he regarded the Yoga system as the epitome of all Indian religious and spiritual teachings. According to T. S. Rukmani,

> It can be said that Vijñāna Bhikṣu represented a synthetic force in the philosophical history of India. What was achieved in the way of levelling all difference of caste, creed, and different religious sectarian ideas through bhakti was perhaps an indication and inspiration for Vijñānabhikṣu to try the same experiment in the philosophical field as well. (Vol. 1, p. 16)

Vijñāna Bhikṣu's own views differ from those of classical Sāṁkhya, as he asserts that *prakṛti* is a transformation of Brahman and likewise the *jīva* is a particular form of Brahman. The world consisting of the combination of *prakṛti* and *jīva* is therefore to be understood as wholly real and not as an illusion, as it is for Śaṅkara. Thus it can be said that his system of thought conforms most closely to *bhedābheda*, difference and non-difference, and that he forms something of a bridge between Sāṁkhya and Vedānta, whilst insisting that *asaṁprajñāta samādhi*, as taught by the *Yoga Sūtras*, is the true path to liberation, transcending even the path of *jñāna*, realised knowledge, which he regards as a step on the way towards *asaṁprajñāta samādhi*. He further differs from classical Sāṁkhya by insisting that the evolution of *prakṛti* from the single substance of *pradhāna* into the manifest world is not a natural process brought about simply by the agitation caused by the presence of *puruṣa* or the disequilibrium of the *guṇas*, but is in fact a creative process set in motion by *īśvara*, the Supreme Deity. In this view, he is in line with the teachings of the *Bhagavad-gītā* (9.10).

As a theist, Vijñāna Bhikṣu accepts the existence of *īśvara* as the Supreme Deity, but this theism does not extend to a fully developed doctrine of grace such as can be observed in Tamil Vaiṣṇavism or Tamil Śaivism, or indeed within the *Bhagavad-gītā*. *Mokṣa* can be gained only through the practice of Yoga as taught by the *Yoga Sūtras*; *īśvara* bestows his divine grace only to the extent of removing obstacles and thereby making the yogic path to liberation a little easier to traverse. According to T. S. Rukmani (Vol. 1, p. 13), 'Vijñāna Bhikṣu is first and foremost a yogī', who 'considers Yoga superior to both Sāṅkhya and Vedānta' (ibid. p. 14), and again 'Vijñāna Bhikṣu maintains that Yoga is the philosophy par excellence which contains all other philosophies within itself'.

The *Yoga Sūtras* in Translation

A very useful modern work on the *Yoga Sūtras* is that presented by Edwin Bryant, which not only includes a detailed discussion of the original *sūtras* and *Vyāsa-bhāṣya*, but also makes detailed reference to the main commentaries used in the present work. For those who wish to pursue their studies further, this work is highly recommended:

Bryant, Edwin, ed. and trans. *The Yoga-sūtras of Patañjali.* New York: North Point Press, 2009.

Other accessible English renderings of the *Yoga Sūtras* include:

Feuerstein, Georg, trans. *The Yoga-Sūtra of Patañjali: A New Translation and Commentary.* Rochester, VT: Inner Traditions International, 1989.

Miller, Barbara Stoler, trans. *Yoga: Discipline of Freedom; The Yoga Sutra Attributed to Patanjali.* Berkeley: University of California Press, 1996.

Ranganathan, Shyam, ed. and trans. *Patañjali's Yoga Sūtra.* New Delhi: Penguin, 2008.

All of the commentaries referred to in the present work are available in English translation:

The full version of the *Vyāsa-bhāṣya* is included as a part of the translations of the other three commentaries noted below. T. S. Rukmani's presentation of Vijñāna Bhikṣu's and Śaṅkara's commentaries is particularly useful as both of these also contain the Sanskrit text of the *Vyāsa-bhāṣya.*

The *Yoga-sūtra-bhāṣya-vivaraṇa* attributed to Śaṅkarācārya, available in two translations:

Leggett, Trevor, trans. *Complete Commentary by Sankara on the Yoga Sutras: A Full Translation of the Newly Discovered Text*. London: Kegan Paul International, 1990.

Rukmani, T. S., trans. *Yogasūtrabhāṣyavivaraṇa of Śaṅkara, Vivaraṇa Text with English Translation and Critical Notes along with Text and English Translation of Patañjali's Yogasūtras and Vyāsabhāṣya*. 2 vols. New Delhi: Munshiram Manoharlal, 2001.

The *Tattva-vaiśāradī* commentary by Vācaspati Miśra:

Woods, James Haughton, trans. *The Yoga-System of Patañjali, or the Ancient Hindu Doctrine of Concentration of Mind, Embracing the Mnemonic Rules, Called Yoga-Sūtras, of Patañjali and the Comment, Called Yoga-Bhāshya, Attributed to Veda-Vyāsa*. Cambridge, MA: Harvard University Press, 1914; reprinted, London: Forgotten Books, 2012.

The *Yoga-vārttika* commentary of Vijñāna Bhikṣu:

Rukmani, T. S., trans. *The Yogavarttika of Vijñanabhiksu*. 4 vols. Delhi: Munshiram Manoharlal, 1981–1989.

A Note on Translation and Sanskrit Terminology

Translation. The translations of the commentaries of Vyāsa, Śaṅkara, Vācaspati Miśra, and Vijñāna Bhikṣu produced by the scholars listed in the preceding section – Leggett, Rukmani, and Woods – are often cited in a modified form in the ensuing translation to conform with the style of this book. Such modifications are not indicated.

Sanskrit terminology. Sanskrit is an inflected language, which means that when a Sanskrit word is used in a Sanskrit sentence it takes a specific ending that indicates the role of the word in the sentence. In this book, when a Sanskrit word is mentioned in an English sentence it is usually cited without the ending, in the so-called 'stem form'. For this reason, there is a difference between the spelling of some words in the *sūtras* and in their explanations. For example, in *sūtra* 1.3, *draṣṭṛ* is the stem form of the inflected form *draṣṭuḥ*.

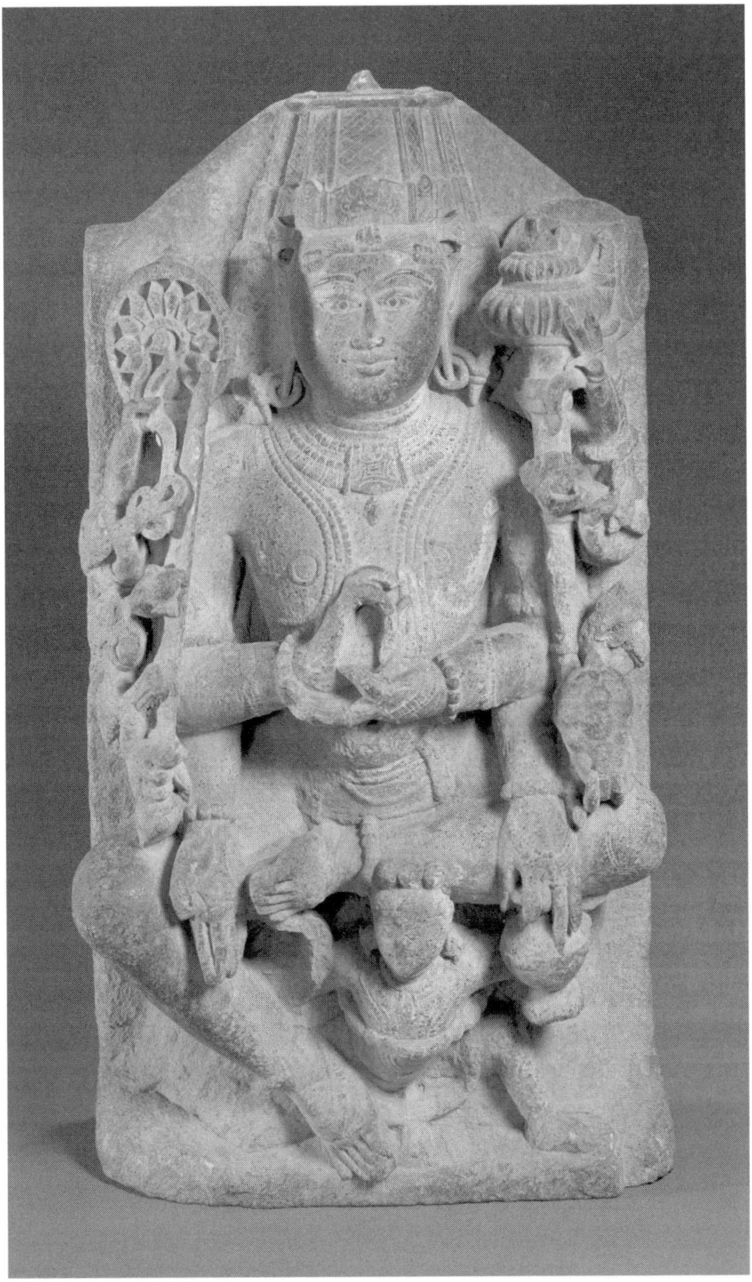

Īśvara *is a special* puruṣa, *free from the influence of affliction, action, the ripening of accumulated karma, and latent impressions.—1.24*

I
THE *SAMĀDHI-PĀDA*

We will start off our consideration of the principal ideas of the *Yoga Sūtras* by looking at the *Samādhi-pāda*, which forms the first chapter of the text as a whole. What I propose to do is take each *sūtra* in turn, consider its significance and meaning, and try to locate the ideas within the wider context of Indian religious thought. This search for meaning will be assisted by the interpretations of the main commentators previously referred to, and the primary commentary of Vyāsa in particular. So with all our introductions now complete, let us start off at the most obvious point by reviewing the opening group of *sūtras*.

SŪTRAS 1.1 TO 1.4: DEFINITION AND GOALS OF YOGA

Patañjali opens his discourse by explaining what is meant by the term Yoga and why Yoga is a worthy enterprise to embark upon. Indeed, the value of Yoga is stated to be nothing less than the spiritual liberation of the practitioner from a false position of embodiment in this world.

1.1 *atha yogānuśāsanam*

Here is the teaching on Yoga.

This opening *sūtra* is a straightforward introduction that simply announces that this treatise will provide instruction on the subject of Yoga. The *sūtra* is comprised of three words, *atha*, meaning now or here, *yoga*, which is Yoga, and *anuśāsana,* meaning teaching or instruction, thereby giving us a clear introduction.

Despite its apparently obvious meaning, all of our commentators take the opportunity to present lengthy discussions on a range of different points that are not directly related to the *sūtra* itself. Vyāsa starts his relatively short commentary by stating that the word *atha* is used to introduce a new topic of instruction (*adhikāra*). He then states that Yoga is to be understood as *samādhi,* and that this condition of *samādhi* is present in all states of consciousness. Where the mind is in a restless or agitated state, however, *samādhi* is not yogic, but when one is able to fix the mind on a single point, that is to be understood as *saṁprajñāta-samādhi,* and when even that single-pointed *samādhi* is restrained, then that is *asaṁprajñāta-samādhi.* Thus Yoga is defined by Vyāsa in relation to the two manifest forms of *samādhi.* In this state, the bonds of karma are loosened, a statement implying that Yoga is the means by which one may become liberated from the state of bondage in which we currently exist in this world.

Śaṅkarācārya builds on this point about liberation, asserting that such release from bondage can only be achieved through the acquisition of higher knowledge. If it be asked, why in that case Patañjali has not written a text on knowledge, that is because Yoga is the means by which knowledge is obtained. The ailment that afflicts us is suffering; the cure is knowledge; and Yoga is the means by which that cure can be administered. Vācaspati Miśra also discusses the word *atha,* and denies any view that this should be understood as meaning 'now the previous stage is completed'. *Atha* simply indicates the beginning of a discussion. He also makes an interesting point about the etymology of the word *yoga,* insisting that in this context, it is not related to the verbal root, *yuj,* meaning 'to join', but should rather be derived from another root, also *yuj,* which refers to the practice of concentration (*samādhi*).

Vijñāna Bhikṣu focuses on the idea of Yoga loosening the bonds of karma, pointing out that this shows that Yoga is properly understood as the means by which liberation from rebirth is achieved. Yoga has the quality of *mokṣa-hetutva*, being the cause by which liberation, *mokṣa*, is achieved.

This is all easily understood, but now in the next *sūtra* we are presented with a succinct definition of what Patañjali himself means by Yoga, and in particular the essential method through which the practice of Yoga is to be undertaken.

1.2 *yogaś citta-vṛtti-nirodhaḥ*

Yoga is the restriction of the movements of the mind.

Of the two words in this *sūtra*, namely *yoga* and the compound *citta-vṛtti-nirodha*, the first, *yoga*, is the subject of the definition offered herein. So what is it that is being referred to in Patañjali's text as Yoga? And what does *citta-vṛtti-nirodha* mean? We may recall that the Sāṁkhya analysis of the mental faculties discussed in the summary of Sāṁkhya doctrine above designates these as *buddhi*, *manas*, and *ahaṁkāra*, which collectively comprise the *antaḥ-karaṇa*, the inner organ. The word *citta* does not appear in the typical Sāṁkhya listings, though the use of the term in other texts such as the *Bhagavad-gītā* makes it clear that it refers to our mental activities. Hence when Kṛṣṇa speaks of fixing one's concentration on himself, he uses the phrase *mac-citta*. So it does not seem unreasonable to understand *citta* as used here as referring to the mind or the thought processes. The word *vṛtti* indicates activity or movement, and, in relation to *citta*, it is easy to recognise the way in which the mind constantly moves from one thought to another, never remaining still even for a moment as our sense perceptions constantly give rise to new and ever-changing patterns of thought. Then the word *nirodha* means suppression or restriction, and so we can see that the technique of Yoga being defined here is that by which our conventional mental activities are brought to a halt.

In Vyāsa's commentary on the previous *sūtra*, he referred to *saṁprajñāta-samādhi* and *asaṁprajñāta-samādhi*, and now we can see how these are related to the *citta-vṛtti-nirodha* presented here as a definition of Yoga. *Saṁprajñāta-samādhi* is where the mind is fixed unwaveringly on a single point, perhaps a *mantra* or sacred image, so that the usual wandering thought processes are reined in and all movements away from that single point are restrained. This is a practice generally referred to as *dhyāna*, meditation, and anyone can attempt it as a form of regular practice – though in most cases it will quickly become apparent that this is an extremely difficult technique to master. As Arjuna says in the *Bhagavad-gītā*: *tasyāhaṁ nigrahaṁ manye vāyur iva su-duṣkaram*, 'I think controlling the mind is as hard to achieve as controlling the wind' (6.34). And *asaṁprajñāta-samādhi* is a stage beyond even the constant focusing of the mind on a single point, as in this highest stage of Yoga perfection there is nothing at all that the mind is fixed upon. According to the sixth chapter of the *Gītā*, it is at this point that external perception is entirely nullified and internal knowledge of the true spiritual identity, knowledge of the *ātman*, comes to the fore. Clearly, this is in line with Śaṅkarācārya's view that Yoga is the means by which higher knowledge is acquired, which in turn brings liberation from suffering and rebirth.

Here Vyāsa places a particular focus on the fact that the *sūtra* does not state that all movements of the mind are to be restrained. Such movements are influenced by the three *guṇas*, but where there is a predominance of the *sattva-guṇa*, which is reflected as purity, serenity, and wisdom, then the related movements can be beneficial in the progression towards *samādhi*. The goal sought through meditation is *viveka-khyāti*, knowledge of the distinction between *sattva* and *puruṣa*. Since *sattva* is one of the three *guṇas* of *prakṛti*, this amounts to the typical Sāṁkhya goal of realising the difference between *puruṣa* and *prakṛti*. Since Vyāsa links *sattva* with clarity (*prakhyā*), it is instrumental in attaining this *viveka-khyāti*. Hence when the *vṛtti* is related to *sattva*, this should not be restrained, at least in the initial phase. Śaṅkarācārya builds upon this point and further emphasises the role of *sattva-guṇa* in bringing the aspiring practitioner to a state of *viveka-khyāti*. Vācaspati Miśra also focuses on Vyāsa's statements about the way in which the *guṇas* shape the movements of the mind, showing how it is that when these movements are influenced by *rajas* or *tamas*, there is a concomitant tendency towards the performance of unrighteous acts. It is these *vṛttis* in particular that are to be restrained by the practitioner. Vijñāna Bhikṣu comments at some length here, and he is also primarily concerned to confirm Vyāsa's emphasis on the value of *sattva-guṇa*, and to argue that where *sattva* predominates in the movements of the mind, this can have a positive influence.

1.3 *tadā draṣṭuḥ sva-rūpe 'vasthānam*

When this is achieved, the witness comes to exist in terms of its true identity.

This third *sūtra* contains four words, one of which, *sva-rūpe*, is a compound. The word *tadā* means 'then' or 'in that case' and obviously refers to the restriction of the movements of the mind from the previous *sūtra*. Then *draṣṭuḥ* means 'of the one who sees' and, in this case, almost certainly means *puruṣa*, our spiritual identity that observes the world through the senses. The compound *sva-rūpe* means 'in its own form' or 'in its own identity', and I think we must take this as referring to the separation of *puruṣa* from *prakṛti* so that it can come to exist as a purely spiritual entity free from the false sense of identity with the elements of *prakṛti* that we currently experience. *Puruṣa* is entirely spiritual by nature, but because it wrongly identifies itself with its physical and mental embodiment, it undergoes suffering and rebirth within the domain of *prakṛti*. This existential problem of the living being can only be resolved if *puruṣa* gains realisation of its true spiritual nature, untouched by *prakṛti*. It then regains its true identity, here referred to as *sva-rūpa*, so that the *sūtra* as a whole is stating that when Yoga is successfully practised, and the movements of the mind are fully restrained, *puruṣa* gains release from its association with *prakṛti* and comes to exist in a purely spiritual state of being. *Avasthāna* simply means a 'situation', 'position', or 'state of existence'. I think we can thus understand that in this *sūtra*, Patañjali is indicating that his composition is a work dealing with the subject of the means by which liberation from rebirth can be attained. This is what Yoga is.

Vyāsa gives only a short commentary in which he states that the mental state referred to here is that in which *kaivalya*, liberation, is attained. Śaṅkarācārya confirms the fact that the *draṣṭṛ*, the seer, is *puruṣa*, and that this *sūtra* is about liberation, whilst Vācaspati Miśra summarises its meaning as follows: 'The word *sva-rūpe* means that the peaceful and the cruel and the infatuated nature falsely attributed to the Self has ceased' (Trans. Woods). Vijñāna Bhikṣu adds to the discussion by stating that the word *tadā*, meaning then, in this *sūtra* refers in fact to the state of *asaṁprajñāta-samādhi*, which is the final, perfected stage of the yogic endeavour.

1.4 *vṛtti-sārūpyam itaratra*

> Otherwise, the witness assumes the identity
> dictated by the movement of the mind.

This next *sūtra* refers to the alternative state of existence where the movements of the mind are not restrained by Yoga practice, as is indicated by the word *itaratra,* which means 'otherwise' or 'alternatively'. In the previous *sūtra,* we were told that *puruṣa* exists in its own pure, spiritual form, its *sva-rūpa,* when the state of *citta-vṛtti-nirodha* is achieved and the movements of the mind are restrained. Here the phrase *vṛtti-sārūpya* means that where this restraint is not achieved, then *puruṣa* comes to adopt the form of the particular state of mind that exists at that time. In other words, when one is angry, *puruṣa* is forced into an angry state of being and when one is happy, *puruṣa* is carried into that happy identity, even though in its true nature, its *sva-rūpa,* it is untouched by these mental fluctuations.

On this *sūtra,* Vyāsa emphasises the close relationship that exists between *puruṣa* and *citta,* even though *citta,* our mental embodiment, is an element of *prakṛti.* It is because of this close interaction that *puruṣa* comes to exist in relation to the *citta-vṛtti,* the mental transformations we experience moment by moment. He writes: 'Therefore, the reason for *puruṣa*'s knowledge of the modification of the mind is the beginningless relationship with the mind' (Trans. Rukmani). Śaṅkarācārya provides us with a further explanation of how and why this takes place. It is not the case that *puruṣa* actually undergoes transformations, as its true identity is as a changeless being, but when objects are displayed to it due to its close association with the mind, then 'the apparent change is not intrinsic but projected (*adhyāropita*), like a crystal's taking on the colour of something put near it' (Trans. Leggett 1981). In other words, although *puruṣa* is not truly affected by mental fluctuations, these fluctuations are projected upon it. Vācaspati Miśra expands on this idea by using the comparison of a red rose and a crystal. The crystal is changeless and without colour, but when the red rose is adjacent to it, it appears to have a rosy hue even though it has not itself undergone any transformation. Vijñāna Bhikṣu enters into a lengthy debate on the question of how it is that the changeless *puruṣa* can be transformed by the movements of the mind, although, as we can see, a viable answer is readily supplied by the other commentators.

Sūtras 1.5 to 1.11: The Different Movements of the Mind Explained

Having started out by defining Yoga as *citta-vṛtti-nirodha,* Patañjali now seeks to explain further what is meant by that phrase. He begins that explanation in this next group of *sūtras,* which analyse the nature of the *vṛttis,* the movements of the mind, which the yogic endeavour seeks to restrain.

1.5 *vṛttayaḥ pañcatayyaḥ kliṣṭākliṣṭāḥ*

> The movements of the mind can be divided into five categories; these can either bring affliction or be free of affliction.

With the introductory passages now complete, we move into a new phase of discussion relating to the nature of the *vṛttis* referred to in the second *sūtra. Sūtra* 1.5 introduces that consideration by stating firstly that there are five types of *vṛtti,* and then that these can be either *kliṣṭa* or *akliṣṭa,* depending on whether or not they cause affliction. These statements will be explained in the *sūtras* that follow. Vyāsa here explains that the *kliṣṭa vṛttis* are those that give rise to future results, as the law of karma unfolds, whilst the *akliṣṭa vṛttis* are those that lead a person towards *viveka-khyāti,* the power of discrimination that leads to realisation of the Sāṁkhya truth of the difference between *puruṣa* and *prakṛti.* It is in this sense that the terms bringing affliction or being free of affliction should be understood, although perhaps afflictional and non-afflictional would more accurately convey the intended meaning.

Following a line of discussion started by Vyāsa, Śaṅkara reminds us that the *kliṣṭa* and *akliṣṭa* categories of mental transformation are not entirely distinct and will frequently be closely intermingled. Vācaspati Miśra goes a little further by arguing that the *akliṣṭa vṛttis* are to be regarded, at least initially, as a positive force, as these have the effect of nullifying the *kliṣṭa vṛttis*. This relates back to the statement of Vyāsa that *sūtra* 1.2 does not use the word 'all' in relation to the restraint of the movements of the mind, for those movements that take us in the direction of discriminative knowledge are to be fostered rather than restrained. Vijñāna Bhikṣu takes a more directly practical approach by explaining how the *kliṣṭa* movements of the mind are to be witnessed in the world around us. He writes: 'Overcome by greed &c. created by identification with objects, and striving to overcome that through hurting and helping others in the process *dharma* and *adharma* results are collected and from that, there is a flow of pain, that is the idea' (Trans. Rukmani). Here he is essentially confirming Vyāsa's explanation that the *kliṣṭa vṛttis* are those that perpetuate the cycle of karma and hence the pain of rebirth.

1.6 *pramāṇa-viparyaya-vikalpa-nidrā-smṛtayaḥ*

These five are right knowledge, false assessment, mental construction, sleep, and the remembrance of things past.

The sixth *sūtra* takes the form of a lengthy compound consisting of five words that are, in effect, a list of the five types of *vṛtti* experienced by the mind, as mentioned in the previous *sūtra*. As all five of these are defined and briefly explained in the next five *sūtras*, Vyāsa offers no commentary here and our other three commentators are similarly restrained.

1.7 *pratyakṣānumānāgamāḥ pramāṇāni*

> Right knowledge comes from direct perception,
> logical inference, and tradition.

Here Patañjali begins his explanation of the five types of *vṛtti* by presenting a threefold definition of what is meant by *pramāṇa*, the first of the five given in the list in the previous *sūtra*. Indian philosophy typically begins from the point of establishing a set of *pramāṇas*, which usually refers to the means by which reliable knowledge can be attained, and the threefold list given here is the usual one arrived at by most systems of thought. The question is asked as to how we know what we know, how we acquire the knowledge we possess, and the answer given here is that we gain knowledge through sensory perception (*pratyakṣa*), through the application of logical reasoning and inference (*anumāna*), and by receiving instruction from a reliable source (*āgama*). Vyāsa defines *āgama* as verbal testimony obtained from qualified individuals who themselves have obtained their knowledge by means of either perception or inference. Vācaspati Miśra argues that *āgama* also includes knowledge obtained from the scripture because even if such texts as *Manu-smṛti* are attributed to a human author, they are ultimately derived from words spoken by *īśvara* whose knowledge is still based on perception or inference and therefore reliable according to the present *sūtra*. It is interesting to note, however, that the main thrust of Patañjali's teachings herein rests on the view that true knowledge can be obtained through Yoga practice, through *citta-vṛtti-nirodha*, by means of which the external movements of the mind are stilled and knowledge of *puruṣa* can then emerge from within, without reference to any scriptural teachings. Hence one has a sense that the acceptance here of *āgama* as a valid *pramāṇa* is more formal than actual, and it is notable that at no point does the *Yoga Sūtras* cite any sacred text in order to give support to its own teachings. A certain Jaigīṣavya is nevertheless mentioned as an authority in Vyāsa's commentary on 2.55 and 3.18.

Śaṅkara takes this opportunity to present a lengthy discussion of the role of *pramāṇas* in arriving at valid conclusions, and, in so doing, moves well beyond the exposition of the *sūtra* itself or Vyāsa's commentary. Vācaspati Miśra notes that *pratyakṣa,* sensory perception, is given first in the list, and he argues that this precedence given to perception indicates the reality of the world as it is perceived. He notes alternative views on this point and then provides a detailed explanation of how knowledge of objects is gained by *puruṣa* by means of the mind and senses. Vijñāna Bhikṣu follows this same line of discussion, and one can observe that the preoccupation of the commentators with this particular point is due to the fact that *puruṣa* is regarded as entirely distinct from the senses and the mind. They are *prakṛti* whilst *puruṣa* is non-*prakṛti,* so how is it that *puruṣa* appears connected to them when gaining knowledge by means of sensory perception? Complicated arguments are considered on this point, but unfortunately the intricacies of this analysis lie beyond our present scope.

1.8 *viparyayo mithyā-jñānam atad-rūpa-pratiṣṭham*

False assessment means misunderstanding based on mistaken apprehension of the object.

Here the second of the five types of *vṛtti* is considered. This is *viparyaya,* meaning false assessment or misapprehension, which is identified as the opposite of *pramāṇa,* the first of the *vṛttis* considered in the previous *sūtra.* Hence Vyāsa explains that when the mind adopts a position contrary to the three sources of true knowledge mentioned there, that is what is meant by *viparyaya,* which can be counteracted by the proper application of one of the three *pramāṇas.* Thereby, one would obtain right knowledge about the same object. Śaṅkara then adds to the discussion by stating that *viparyaya* is to be understood as mistaking an object one sees for something else, and here one is reminded of the oft-repeated example of perceiving a rope as a snake that appears frequently in the writings of Śaṅkarācārya. Vācaspati Miśra here presents his readers with a detailed discussion of different perceptions which may overlay each other, whilst Vijñāna Bhikṣu discusses at some length the distinction or non-distinction to be drawn between different types of ignorance in relation to the world.

1.9 *śabda-jñānānupātī vastu-śūnyo vikalpaḥ*

A mental construct arises following cognition of words alone, and is devoid of a really existing object.

Here *vikalpa*, the third of the five *vṛttis*, is considered. There are a few different meanings that could be applied to the word *vikalpa*, but if we rely on Vyāsa's commentary, then the meaning intended here becomes more apparent as his commentary is quite specific. The previous two *vṛttis* related to *pramāṇa*, which is the absorption of knowledge by appropriate means, and then *viparyaya*, which is false knowledge absorbed by the mind when a *pramāṇa* is improperly applied. *Vikalpa* is the movement of the mind that occurs when it hears or reads words on a particular subject which does not really exist. As a result of that hearing, the mind forms an internal construction that is supposed to give mental substance to the words that have been heard. Since *vikalpa* depends on an object that does not really exist, it is not possible to attain either true knowledge or false impression about it, and therefore Vyāsa states, 'It is not included under true knowledge, and it is not included under false assessment', referring to the two *vṛttis* already discussed. Essentially, according to Vyāsa, *vikalpa* is a formulation created within the mind when words on any subject are heard without there being any real object or idea being described by those words. The examples given by Vyāsa are technical and pertain to philosophy of language. For example, Vyāsa considers the statement that '*puruṣa* has the quality of not having a beginning (*anutpattidharmā puruṣa iti*)'. In this case, we should understand that merely the absence of the quality of having a beginning is expressed. In other words, it is not the case that some really existing quality of *puruṣa* is being formulated here. Therefore, says Vyāsa, this quality (*dharma*) is 'formulated' or 'mentally constructed' (*vikalpita*).

1.10 *abhāva-pratyayālambanā vṛttir nidrā*

Sleep is where the movement of the mind has no object on which to focus.

Here it is the state of deep sleep rather than the dreaming state that is being referred to as *nidrā*, the fourth of the five *vṛttis* under discussion. One might naturally enough feel that this state of dreamless sleep is one in which the movements of the mind are restrained, but, according to Patañjali, one should not make the mistake of thereby equating sleep with *samādhi*. Vyāsa explains why such a distinction should be made. When one awakens from sleep, one can recall either, 'I slept very deeply', or else, 'I have slept very poorly'. He thus concludes that, 'This kind of memory in one who has awakened from sleep is not possible if there were no experience of the *vṛtti*' (Trans. Rukmani).

Śaṅkara responds to an imagined opponent by denying that the dreaming state must also be included as *nidrā*, asserting that dreams are a form of memory whereas *nidrā* is deep dreamless sleep and hence a distinctive *vṛtti*. Vācaspati Miśra discusses why it is that *nidrā* cannot be considered a cessation of all movements of the mind, whilst Vijñāna Bhikṣu makes the point that the word *vṛtti* is repeated in this *sūtra* to emphasise the understanding that deep sleep is indeed to be regarded as one of the movements of the mind.

1.11 *anubhūta-viṣayāsaṁpramoṣaḥ smṛtiḥ*

Remembrance is where the experience of an object is retained.

This *sūtra* gives a readily comprehensible definition of memory, which is simply the recollection of a previous sensory experience. Vyāsa gives a more complex analysis of what we mean by memory, stating that it is the recollection both of the object itself as perceived in the past and of the knowledge gained through that perception. In other words, memory enables us to experience both an object from the past and our own understanding of that object when it was perceived. He further goes on to state that whenever we have a mental experience of an object through perception, that leaves a *saṁskāra*, a latent impression, on the mind; memory is hence to be understood as the process by which that *saṁskāra* is brought to the fore once more.

Śaṅkara takes this opportunity to criticise the Buddhist understanding of memory by rejecting the view that all recollections are simply mental processes without reference to any specific object. This relates to the Buddhist notion of momentariness, which denies the reality of actual objects. Vācaspati Miśra emphasises the fact that memory cannot go beyond perception or a previous mental formulation, and, as such, it is limited in its range of activity. Vijñāna Bhikṣu points out that memory relates only to the *saṁskāras*, the latent impressions existing in the mind as a result of past perceptions, and hence it must be understood as a type of *vṛtti* that is distinct from that formed by direct perception of the object as it is.

Sūtras 1.12 to 1.16: The Process of Restraint

Having concluded his analysis of the *vṛttis*, the movements of the mind, Patañjali now moves his focus towards another of the terms included in his initial definition of Yoga: *nirodha,* the means by which such movements are restrained in order that the highest spiritual goals can be achieved. The discussion focuses primarily on two words, *abhyāsa* and *vairāgya,* dedicated practice and renunciation of other more worldly pursuits. If the process of *nirodha* is to be successful, then these two factors must be kept constantly to the fore.

1.12 *abhyāsa-vairāgyābhyāṁ tan-nirodhaḥ*

> The restriction of the movements of the mind is achieved through regular practice and through renunciation.

In this *sūtra,* Patañjali gives an insight into how the difficult yogic task of restricting the movements of the mind can be achieved. The means is defined by the opening compound which consists of two words, *abhyāsa* and *vairāgya,* which are given the ending *ābhyām* to provide the meaning of 'by means of'. Here one might note that in the sixth chapter of the *Bhagavad-gītā,* Kṛṣṇa gives Arjuna a similar instruction about practising Yoga by restraining the mind, a process which allows direct perception of the *ātman.* In response to this instruction, Arjuna states that he thinks restraining the mind is as difficult to achieve as restraining the wind, *vāyor iva su-duṣkaram* (v.34). Kṛṣṇa agrees that it is indeed a difficult process to follow, but insists that it is possible if one adopts the proper means, which are similarly named as *abhyāsa* and *vairāgya,* and it might be suggested that in constructing this *sūtra,* Patañjali had in mind the discussion located in the *Gītā.*

The main point of the *sūtra* is of course to affirm that the successful practice of Yoga is not an easy task or one that can be taken up lightly. It requires that regular practice be undertaken on a daily basis over a period of years, and, moreover, that one makes a commitment to abandon some of one's more worldly endeavours and aspirations. Nonetheless, lest one think that this is a process to be avoided on the grounds of its impracticability, we should again recall the progression of the conversation in Chapter 6 of the *Bhagavad-gītā*. Following on from Kṛṣṇa's advocacy of *abhyāsa* and *vairāgya*, Arjuna asks about the fate of one who starts out on the path of Yoga but falls short of final success. Does not such a person lose out in all spheres of life? On this point, Kṛṣṇa reassures him that whatever progress is made is never lost and will remain with one throughout all future forms of existence.

Vyāsa here refers to two directions in which we might project our existence; one he defines as *kalyāna*, meaning 'pure' or 'auspicious', and the other as *pāpa*, meaning 'wicked'. His point is that for the practice of Yoga one must adopt the way of *kalyāna* and avoid any tendency towards greed, malice, or anger, all of which fall under the heading of *pāpa*. Vyāsa explains that *vairāgya* prevents one from moving towards *pāpa*, whereas *abhyāsa* helps one to move towards *kalyāna*. Śaṅkara and Vācaspati Miśra add very little here by way of further explanation, and Vijñāna Bhikṣu confines himself to definitions of terms used in the *Vyāsa-bhāṣya*.

1.13 *tatra sthitau yatno 'bhyāsaḥ*

Abhyāsa means the exertion required to achieve steadiness of mind.

In his next *sūtra*, Patañjali gives an explanation of what he means by *abhyāsa*, which we have defined as 'regular practice'. The translation is not absolutely clear, but the intended meaning seems to be that *abhyāsa* is the exertion, the *yatna*, required to bring the mind to a state of steadiness, *sthiti*, which one must presume relates to the restraint of mental activities, as referred to in *sūtra* 1.2. *Sthita* means 'fixed' or 'situated', and the related state of *sthiti*, meaning 'steadiness', clearly stands in contrast to our normal state in which the mind moves constantly from one state to another. Hence we can see that *abhyāsa* means the determined effort to achieve the state of *citta-vṛtti-nirodha*, which is a primary goal of the yogic endeavour. In his short commentary, Vyāsa confirms this view, whilst Śaṅkara merely states that the grammatical form of *sthitau* indicates that steadiness is the goal to be reached through *yatna*, one's concerted efforts; Vācaspati Miśra makes exactly the same point as Śaṅkara, whilst Vijñāna Bhikṣu again seeks to define the exact meaning of Vyāsa's terminology.

1.14 *sa tu dīrgha-kāla-nairantarya-satkārāsevito dṛḍha-bhūmiḥ*

Now when the exertion is properly performed for a long time, without interruption, it becomes firmly established.

Here the final compound, *dṛḍha-bhūmi*, means 'it becomes firmly grounded' or, 'firmly established', indicating the conditions by which the endeavour towards stability of the mind becomes successful. So this *sūtra* is telling us more about what is meant by *abhyāsa*. Three components of *abhyāsa* are established herein. It must continue for a considerable period of time, *dīrgha-kāla*, it must be performed without interruption, *nairantarya*, and it must be practised with due respect in an appropriate manner, *satkārāsevita*. Vyāsa then adds to this by stating that Yoga should be undertaken with due respect for the means and the goal so that the practitioner adheres to the precepts of austerity, celibacy, knowledge, and faith in its efficacy. Otherwise, the full commitment that *abhyāsa* demands will not be apparent. Our other three commentators make only brief additions to the discussion, reiterating the points made by Patañjali and Vyāsa.

1.15 *dṛṣṭānuśravika-viṣaya-vitṛṣṇasya vaśīkāra-saṁjñā vairāgyam*

Vairāgya is known to be the self-mastery of a person who has removed the hankering arising from perceiving or learning about an object.

If we trace the course of the discussion, we can see that this and the previous three *sūtras* are offering the reader a clearer understanding of what is meant by *nirodha*. Firstly, it was explained that *nirodha* depends on *abhyāsa* and *vairāgya*, regular practice and renunciation, and now each of these two terms has been explained. The precise meaning of this *sūtra* is not absolutely clear, but it seems that *vairāgya* is being defined with reference to *vaśīkāra*, gaining control or mastery, and that control is experienced by the person, or, according to Vyāsa, by the mind (*citta*) that is free from the hankerings that typically arise from encounters with objects that might give us pleasure in a worldly sense. When we see or hear about a particular thing or object, a longing for it will often arise in the mind, but *vairāgya* means gaining sufficient self-control so that this unwanted sense of longing is restrained and suppressed. The particular word used for the suppression of hankering is *vitṛṣṇa*, which has some resonance with Buddhist thought, though, of course, it was probably a term that was in wide circulation across traditions.

Vyāsa defines this *vaśīkāra*, the power of control, as the ability to apply the discriminative knowledge that enables us to assess the true worth of any object. In this way, we can recognise that these worldly pleasures are of little value in comparison to the spiritual goals pursued by the *yogin*. Śaṅkara offers a fourfold analysis of how *vaśīkāra* is gained. First, there is a consciousness of the efforts we need to make, then a recognition of when and how we fail in these endeavours at restraint, then a consciousness of the workings of the mind, and, finally, the full attainment of self-control. Vācaspati Miśra understands *vaśīkāra-saṁjñā* as meaning an awareness of one's power of mastery rather than *vairāgya* being understood as the power of self-mastery. Both readings are equally valid, but in this latter case the meaning is that we become aware of the power that we possess over the inclinations of the mind and are thereby able to exert that power in attaining the desired state of *vairāgya*. Vijñāna Bhikṣu offers an alternative, and rather complex, fourfold analysis of the means by which one attains the control referred to as *vaśīkāra*, and also states that the attainment of superior knowledge enables us to see the objects of pleasure for what they truly are, trivial things of little importance.

1.16 *tat-paraṁ puruṣa-khyāter guṇa-vaitṛṣṇyam*

A superior form of renunciation is the lack of hankering for material attributes that arises from realisation of *puruṣa*.

In this *sūtra*, a higher form (*tat-para*) of renunciation is presented. The means to this is defined as *puruṣa-khyāti*, realisation of *puruṣa*, the spiritual part of our identity that is the true self beyond body and mind. The point here would be that in the initial stages of Yoga practice, one undertakes renunciation because it is part of the process by which a successful outcome is achieved, but when the result of Yoga practice becomes apparent in the form of *puruṣa-khyāti*, then renunciation becomes instinctive and is inherent in one's new state of consciousness. A similar point is made in the *Bhagavad-gītā* (2.59), where it is stated that when one gains the higher experience of spiritual joy, then the desire for the pleasures of this world naturally diminishes. And hence Vyāsa states,

'The uppermost limit of just this knowledge is the (highest) detachment. For liberation (*kaivalya*) is inseparably connected with this detachment' (Trans. Rukmani).

Śaṅkara makes the point that the previous *sūtra* referred to preliminary renunciation, which is in relation to individual objects, but here we find the compound word *guṇa-vaitṛṣṇyam*, which means complete detachment from the world as a whole, consisting as it does of the three *guṇas*. Vācaspati Miśra provides a slightly different perspective by arguing that one should initially promote the *guṇa* of *sattva*, as it is the purity of *sattva* that is the means by which discriminative knowledge is gained. And then that very same discriminative knowledge enables one to see oneself as one truly is, *puruṣa*, which is entirely distinct from all the *guṇas*.

Sūtras 1.17 to 1.20: The Goal of Yoga Practice

Up to this point, the discussion has focused primarily on the means by which success in Yoga can be achieved, explaining firstly the movements of the mind that are to be restrained, and then the process by which that restraint is accomplished. Now the attention moves towards the outcome that is sought, which is defined in terms of two forms of *samādhi*, or fixed concentration, which are termed *saṁprajñāta* and *asaṁprajñāta*.

1.17 *vitarka-vicārānandāsmitā-rūpānugamāt saṁprajñātaḥ*

> The concentration is known as 'conscious of an object' (*saṁprajñāta*), when it is accompanied by deliberation, reflection, joy, and the experience of selfhood.

Building on the statement of *sūtra* 1.16 regarding *puruṣa-khyāti*, realisation of our spiritual identity, *sūtra* 1.17 now takes us in a new direction by referring to one of the forms of *samādhi* which brings that realisation. This is the *saṁprajñāta-samādhi* in which the mind becomes focused exclusively on a single object, thereby restraining all other movements of the mind. As is made clear in Chapter 6 of the *Bhagavad-gītā,* once the ability to focus the mind on a single object has been acquired, it should be utilised to concentrate on the *ātman, puruṣa* in the language of the *Yoga Sūtras*. Hence Kṛṣṇa says, *viniyataṁ cittam ātmany evāvatiṣṭhate,* 'the *yogin* fixes the controlled mind on the *ātman* alone' (v. 18). It is in this way that the *puruṣa-khyāti* mentioned in *sūtra* 1.16 is achieved, along with a concomitant mood of renunciation. The *saṁprajñāta-samādhi* is accompanied by *vitarka, vicāra, ānanda,* and *asmitā*. The terms *vitarka* and *vicāra* seem to have been commonly used in early Yoga treatises as we find them, for example, in Chapter 188 of the *Mahābhārata*'s twelfth book (*Śānti-parvan*), where *viveka,* discrimination, is included as a third element. This *Mahābhārata* passage seems to draw on the early Buddhist theory of meditation, which also posits a sequence of four *dhyānas,* meditations. There, too, the first stage of meditation is characterised by *vitarka* and *vicāra,* but these are given up at higher levels.

What is apparent from the first two of the fourfold list is that *saṁprajñāta-samādhi* is achieved by properly utilising the conventional mental processes of deliberating and reflecting in order to understand the presence of our spiritual identity. When *viveka* is added, as in the *Mahābhārata,* it is more clearly apparent that the aim here is to realise the truth of the Sāṁkhya assertion *anyo 'ham,* 'I am different from the mental and physical embodiment with which I presently identify myself'. We will then naturally wonder why it is that *ānanda* and *asmitā* are added as two further means by which this realisation is attained. One might suggest that this is because of the deep sense of joy that arises when there is contact between the meditating mind and our spiritual nature, a joy referred to by the *Gītā* as *sukham ātyantikam,* endless delight (6.21). This sense of joy will inspire the practitioner towards a realisation of the spiritual source of that joy, whilst *asmitā,* the sense of selfhood, refers to the realisation of oneself as a transcendent individual being that is not a part of the material manifestation.

Vyāsa explains that there are four stages of *saṁprajñāta-samādhi,* all of which depend on some object. The first stage is characterised by all four attributes. In the second stage, *vitarka* is dropped, and in the third stage *vicāra* is dropped so that with the dropping of *ānanda* only *asmitā* remains in the fourth stage. When conscious deliberation is employed that is *vitarka,* but the *vicāra* stage is that in which one goes beyond such conscious deliberation. The terms *vitarka* and *vicāra* are explained by Vyāsa here and under other *sūtras* with reference to 'gross' and 'subtle' objects of contemplation (see *sūtras* 1.42-1.44 below). In the *ānanda* stage of pure spiritual joy, even *vicāra* is transcended, whilst *asmitā* is simply a changeless sense of 'I am'. Śaṅkara agrees with Vyāsa's reading by suggesting that the four are not so much stages towards attaining *saṁprajñāta-samādhi,* but rather the forms of consciousness that characterise *saṁprajñāta.* Vācaspati Miśra follows the same line by explaining that it is when *saṁprajñāta-samādhi* is attained that *vitarka, vicāra, ānanda,* and *asmitā* become manifest. Vijñāna Bhikṣu elaborates further on the meaning of the four terms, suggesting that *vitarka* means intense concentration on a particular object or form, such as the image of a deity, whilst *vicāra* is focusing the concentration on the subtle elements of which the mental faculty is comprised. Following Vyāsa more strictly, he then says that when one goes beyond *vicāra,* the concentration rests solely on the sense of pure bliss, *ānanda,* which is experienced by *yogins* in the higher stages of practice.

1.18 *virāma-pratyayābhyāsa-pūrvaḥ saṁskāra-śeṣo 'nyaḥ*

The other type of concentration is preceded by the practice that does not depend on any object so that only subconscious impressions (*saṁskāras*) remain.

Given the context of the discussion, we must presume that here the word *anyaḥ*, meaning 'the other', must refer to *asaṁprajñāta-samādhi*. This is confirmed by Vyāsa's commentary. In this alternative state of *samādhi*, there is no deliberation or reflection, for all mental processes are suppressed, and all that then remain are the *saṁskāras*, the subtle impressions left on the mind by previous mental states, by previous *vṛttis*. While the *saṁprajñāta-samādhi* depends on some object of meditation, Vyāsa explains that *asaṁprajñāta-samādhi* can only be reached by practice (*abhyāsa*) which does not have any object or support. Vyāsa adds that this highest state of *samādhi* can be achieved through the higher (*param*) type of *vairāgya*, which probably refers back to the renunciation of the three *guṇas* in *sūtra* 1.16. Vācaspati Miśra states that this highest state of yogic achievement is equivalent to the *nirbīja-samādhi* mentioned in later *sūtras*, whilst Vijñāna Bhikṣu asserts that *saṁprajñāta-* and *asaṁprajñāta-samādhi* are not to be regarded as alternative paths, for the *asaṁprajñāta* state involves the setting aside of all practices defined under the heading of *saṁprajñāta* that have previously been successfully undertaken.

1.19 *bhava-pratyayo videha-prakṛti-layānām*

For beings who do not have bodies, and those whose physical forms have merged back into *prakṛti*, it arises naturally.

Here we naturally ask the question as to who is being referred to by the term *videha*, meaning without a body, and this question is answered by Vyāsa who states these beings are the gods. Unlike ourselves, such beings do not inhabit forms composed of gross matter but have a more subtle form of existence. Vyāsa also distinguishes between two types of beings that are referred to here, the *videha* and the *prakṛti-laya*. He indicates that the *prakṛti-laya* are those who experience a transient state similar to liberation (*kaivalya*), but are ultimately born again.

Śaṅkara states that these two types of beings are those who have attained this state by birth, the gods, and those who have attained it by devotion to *īśvara* or *prakṛti*. Both appear to be approaching the state of liberation but they are not to be regarded as liberated because further progress is still required. Vācaspati Miśra offers a detailed and rather complex analysis of how it is possible to exist in this world whilst being *videha*, without a body, or *prakṛti-laya*, with one's existence merged back into primal *prakṛti*; unfortunately, we do not have the scope here to provide a detailed consideration of his ideas on this point.

This discussion of the *videha* and *prakṛti-laya* beings still leaves open the question of what is meant by *bhava-pratyaya*, which defines their state of existence, and on this point Vyāsa is not particularly forthcoming. Śaṅkara, however, glosses *bhava* as *janma*, 'birth', indicating that the state of *asamprajñāta samādhi* is natural for both the gods and those abosorbed in *prakṛti*.

1.20 *śraddhā-vīrya-smṛti-samādhi-prajñā-pūrvaka itareṣām*

> Others attain this state preceded by faith, vigorous endeavour, recollection, *samādhi*, and realised knowledge.

Here we are told that apart from the gods who are born into that state and those who have merged their individual existence into *prakṛti,* there are others who reach the state of *asaṁprajñāta-samādhi* through a series of attributes or practices, which precede its attainment. According to Vyāsa, this *sūtra* refers to yogins for whom *asaṁprajñāta-samādhi* does not arise naturally but rather through the means (*upāya*) listed in this *sūtra*. Vyāsa designates these as the means by which that goal is achieved and gives an informative outline of what each of them means. Perhaps unexpectedly, he defines *śraddhā,* faith, as serenity of mind, and from this serenity comes *vīrya,* which often means heroism or courage, but here probably indicates the intense endeavour that would be made on the basis of one's faith in the process. From *vīrya* then comes *smṛti,* which usually means memory. Perhaps the intended meaning of *smṛti* is close to the usage of the term in the Buddhist tradition where it is usually translated as 'mindfulness'. As noted by Gokhale, 'in the Buddhist theory of meditation, the same terms are used in the same order but are referred to as the five faculties (*indriya*)' (p. 37). The acquisition of *smṛti* allows one to reach *samādhi,* which Vyāsa defines in this context as meaning an undisturbed state of mind. The state of *samādhi* leads in turn to *prajñā,* defined by Vyāsa as *viveka-prajñā,* which, I propose, means a form of higher wisdom that allows discernment or discrimination in relation to *prakṛti* and *puruṣa*. Again, then, we find ourselves confronted by the Sāṁkhya idea of *anyo 'ham,* 'I am different from matter', which is the goal of the realisation sought through Yoga practice. Śaṅkara provides a summary of Vyāsa's analysis, whilst Vācaspati Miśra emphasises the role of faith in guarding practitioners against discouragement due to setbacks in their practice. Vijñāna Bhikṣu follows a similar line by emphasising the fact that faith is the basis of the necessarily intense yogic endeavours here referred to by the term *vīrya*. It is these endeavours that form the subject of the next two *sūtras*.

Sūtras 21 to 22: The Necessity of Endeavour

We now have a short passage in which Patañjali emphasises the need for deep commitment if one is to gain spiritual release, which has already been noted as the goal to be sought through the yogic endeavour.

1.21 *tīvra-saṁvegānām āsannaḥ*

> This state is very near for those who display ardent intensity in their practice.

This is one of the easiest *sūtras* to comprehend, as it simply makes the point that the more one commits oneself to Yoga practice, the sooner the desired results will be achieved. One point we might note, however, is that this short statement indicates the form of spirituality we are in contact with here. From the perspective of Yoga, spiritual perfection is achieved through one's own endeavours, a view that stands in contrast to the teachings of the *Bhagavad-gītā* in which divine grace is revealed as an alternative path to liberation. As the *sūtra* is quite straightforward, Vyāsa merely adds that it is referring to the acquisition and results of *samādhi*; our other three commentators have little further to add.

1.22 *mṛdu-madhyādhimātratvāt tato 'pi viśeṣaḥ*

> Even then, there is still a distinction between those who are leisurely, middling, or intense in their practice.

This is a slightly odd *sūtra* because it is still discussing those who are ardent in their practice and yet classifies some of these as *mṛdu*, which means mild, gentle, or leisurely in their yogic endeavours. One must presume that all serious practitioners are classified as *tīvra-saṁvega*, ardent in their endeavours, but that even amongst such ardent *yogins* some remain more committed than others. According to Vyāsa, there is in fact a ninefold classification of practitioners according to their means (*upāya*) and the intensity (*saṁvega*) of their practice. Each of these two attributes can be either leisurely, middling, or intense. Vyāsa makes the rather obvious point that those who adopt the most intense means and the most intense practice are closer to the goal than others who are *mṛdu* or *madhya,* mild or middling, with respect to either. Śaṅkara suggests that the intention of the *sūtra* is to encourage practitioners to give greater commitment to their endeavours. Vācaspati Miśra appears to recognise the apparent contradiction between this and the previous *sūtra,* but suggests that this is resolved in one's mind if one reads them aloud. Vijñāna Bhikṣu contends that this *sūtra* is referring to a special class of *tīvra yogins* who are most committed to succeeding in Yoga practice. Even amongst this class, however, there are still distinctions of endeavour and success to be noted.

Sūtras 1.23 to 1.28: Devotion to Īśvara

The final word of *sūtra* 1.23, *vā,* which means 'alternatively', indicates that a process different to *abhyāsa* or *vairāgya* can be adopted in order to attain the same desired outcome. This other process is designated as *īśvara-praṇidhāna,* devotion to God, and the commentators all make it clear that the efficacy of this alternative path to liberation is due to the divine grace that it invokes. Theism of this type is somewhat unusual in early Yoga treatises, such as those located within the *Mahābhārata,* although it is absolutely central to the ideas enunciated within the *Bhagavad-gītā.*

1.23 *īśvara-praṇidhānād vā*

Or it may be achieved by devoting oneself to the Lord.

In this and the following five *sūtras,* we can observe a marked change in the direction of the discourse, and one that is initially quite surprising. We can learn from Chapter 289 of the *Mahābhārata's Śānti-parvan* that the theism of the Yoga system was noted from earlier times as the distinguishing feature that set Yoga somewhat apart from Sāṁkhya, and this idea finds clear confirmation in this and the following *sūtras.* And although the Yoga treatises of the *Mahābhārata* rarely display a clearly theistic orientation, the same cannot be said for the *Bhagavad-gītā,* which combines teachings on the techniques of meditational yoga with a pronounced form of theism that includes the idea of liberation being gained through the love and grace of the Supreme Deity. I have earlier stated my suspicion that Patañjali had a knowledge of the *Gītā* which he made use of in compiling the *Yoga Sūtras,* and it is on the basis of this next group of *sūtras* that this suspicion is most particularly aroused, although it is to be noted that our text does not venture as far as Kṛṣṇa's revelation by referring to the love of God, or liberation being granted as a gift of divine grace.

The first one of this group of *sūtras* is fairly straightforward in its assertion that devotion to the Deity, *īśvara,* is an alternative form of spiritual practice that brings the same level of success as that achieved by *yogins* who are intense in their endeavours. The word *praṇidhāna* can mean either meditation or dedication, but if we take the *Gītā* as our guide we can see that it may well mean both; one's meditation is focused on *īśvara* who is also the object of one's devotion. It is often said that the *Bhagavad-gītā* offers alternative forms of spiritual practice, which include meditational yoga and *bhakti,* devotion to God, but a careful reading of its text reveals that these two apparently distinct paths are in fact inseparably intertwined, and it seems reasonable to suggest that here the *Yoga Sūtras* is adhering to that same position by recognising that the potency of devotion to God is equal to that of intense yogic endeavour.

Vyāsa here uses the word *anugṛhṇāti,* meaning 'he favours' or 'blesses' them, to indicate the divine grace invoked by the *praṇidhāna.* All the commentators follow Vyāsa and agree that what is being referred to here are expressions of devotion to *īśvara,* which invoke the grace of the Lord who then assists the *yogin* in his spiritual endeavours. Śaṅkara writes: 'the grace is effortless, by the mere omnipotence of the Supreme Lord. By that grace of the Lord, *samādhi* and its fruits are soon attainable' (Trans. Leggett). Vācaspati Miśra reminds us that *praṇidhāna,* acts of devotion, can be mental, verbal, or bodily, suggesting the usual forms of worship executed by Hindus.

Vijñāna Bhikṣu takes a slightly different approach by suggesting that *praṇidhāna* means fixed mental concentration on the Deity as a form of Yoga practice. He states that *sūtras* 1.21 and 1.22 are advocating meditation on the *jīvātman,* one's own spiritual identity, whilst here the focus is on *paramātman,* the manifestation of *īśvara* that is said to be present in each of us alongside the individual *ātman.* Such a suggestion notwithstanding, it is apparent that here we have a significant change of direction in the line of teaching, which again reminds us of the transition made in the *Bhagavad-gītā* between its sixth and seventh chapters. At the end of Chapter 6, after Kṛṣṇa has concluded his discourse on meditational yoga, Arjuna objects that the process described is impossibly difficult to follow, and then in the seventh chapter, we find the introduction of devotion to the Deity as an alternative path to spiritual perfection. It is perhaps the case that in these *sūtras* Patañjali is following the *Gītā*'s lead in structuring the course of his presentation.

1.24 *kleśa-karma-vipākāśayair aparāmṛṣṭaḥ puruṣa-viśeṣa īśvaraḥ*

> *Īśvara* is a special *puruṣa,* free from the influence of affliction, action, the ripening of accumulated karma, and latent impressions.

In this *sūtra*, Patañjali gives us more information about what he means by the term *īśvara* and it is not absolutely clear that this is to be equated with the idea of a Supreme Deity as found in overtly theistic texts such as the *Bhagavad-gītā*. First of all, *īśvara* is a special *puruṣa*, *puruṣa-viśeṣa*, that is free from all affliction, action, the results of action, and also from the subtle impressions left by earlier states of mind. This would suggest that *īśvara* is wholly transcendental to this world and its various fluctuations, but it does not indicate that *īśvara* is the creator and controller of the world as in more overtly theistic texts. And it might be argued that the definition offered here could equally apply to a previously non-special *puruṣa* that has gained liberation through Yoga practice. Given the previous *sūtra*'s reference to *praṇidhāna*, worship, however, that seems unlikely, and I think we must presume that the words here are offering a somewhat restrained version of theistic doctrine.

Vyāsa directly rejects any suggestion that *īśvara* is no more than a *puruṣa* that has gained liberation, stating, 'the earlier bondage known with reference to a liberated soul is not there with reference to *īśvara* (Trans. Rukmani)'. He further emphasises the monotheistic nature of the teachings in this passage by stating, 'he who has pre-eminence which is free from an equal or superior pre-eminence is that *īśvara*' (Trans. Rukmani). He also points to sacred texts as providing proof of the utterly transcendent nature of the Deity being referred to here. The other three commentators devote considerable attention to expanding on Vyāsa's interpretation of the *sūtra*, but, for the most part, construct their arguments along lines parallel to those followed by the primary commentator.

1.25 *tatra niratiśayaṁ sarva-jñatvabījam*

In *īśvara*, the seed of omniscience is unsurpassed.

The word *tatra,* meaning 'there' would most naturally refer back to *īśvara* mentioned in the previous *sūtra*. Here the use of the word *bīja,* meaning 'a seed', might suggest that *īśvara*'s knowledge of all things is something that has grown or developed from a previous state of non-knowingness, in the manner that it does for the *yogin* who attains liberation. Again, however, all the commentators follow Vyāsa's view in denying that there is any such intended meaning to be found here. Vyāsa points out that in this world *puruṣa* might move towards a state of omniscience through practices that lead to liberation and it is for this reason that the idea of a seed is referred to. *Īśvara,* however, is absolutely distinct, as in him the state of omniscience always exists in its ultimate form; it is not that he has at any time needed to cultivate that state.

Śaṅkara takes this opportunity to set forth a lengthy argument in favour of pure monotheism, debating with an imagined opponent who is attempting to disprove the possibility of any such idea. Vācaspati Miśra explains why the word *bīja,* seed, is used here. The *sūtra* refers to *sarva-jñatva,* omniscience, but this is to be understood as the ultimate point of a gradual process by which an individual's knowledge is expanded. For *īśvara,* however, there is no such gradual progression of knowing, for in his case *sarva-jñatva* is a permanent, unchanging attribute. Vijñāna Bhikṣu here provides a lengthy and complex discussion of different forms of knowledge, but also points out that the word *niratiśaya,* meaning 'unsurpassed', reveals again the absolute distinction between *īśvara* and any other *puruṣa,* whether liberated or not.

1.26 *sa pūrveṣām api guruḥ kālenānavacchedāt*

He was the *guru* of the ancient teachers, for he is unrestricted by time.

More information is given here about the nature of *īśvara* and an indication that he is active in this world as a teacher. One might feel that this *sūtra* thus tends to indicate that *īśvara* is in fact to be understood as an enlightened being of this world, the original *guru,* but we should also be aware of the widespread Śaivite view that it is Śiva himself who is the *ādi-guru,* who reveals knowledge of Yoga to sages of this world. Here one is perhaps more particularly reminded of the opening verses of the fourth chapter of the *Bhagavad-gītā.* In those verses, Kṛṣṇa, who is himself *īśvara,* reveals that at the beginning of creation he taught the science of yoga to Vivasvān, the sun god, who passed the knowledge on to others. It does not seem too improbable to suggest that it is these verses that Patañjali has in mind in presenting this *sūtra.*

Vyāsa here continues with the same line he has taken for previous *sūtras* by pointing out that the ancients to whom *īśvara* initially revealed the science of Yoga were themselves conditioned by time. The statement here that *īśvara* is unrestricted by time again demonstrates the clear distinction that is to be recognised between *īśvara* and all other living beings. Vijñāna Bhikṣu is of the view that the ancients referred to by the word *pūrveṣām* are in fact the triple deities, Brahmā, Viṣṇu, and Śiva, who are lesser manifestations of the absolute *īśvara.* He then takes the opportunity to present his own view of Vedānta, stating that *īśvara* exists within each one of us and can give guidance to us by acting as the inner *guru.*

1.27 *tasya vācakaḥ praṇavaḥ*

His sound form is *praṇava.*

In this and the following *sūtra,* a further technique is suggested, and it is one that has a clear relationship to the idea of *īśvara-praṇidhāna. Īśvara* is represented or embodied by the sound vibration of *oṁ*, which is here referred to by the accepted term of *praṇava*. This is a general term for a sacred vibration, but is used on almost all occasions to indicate the sound of *oṁ*. There are a number of references to *oṁ* in the Upaniṣads, and the *Māṇḍūkya Upaniṣad* in particular provides a detailed revelation of the significance of each of the letters of which it is comprised. Here we are simply told that *praṇava* is the *vācaka*, the verbal expression, of *īśvara*, although the degree of identity between them is not elaborated upon. A theistic meditation involving *oṁ* also appears in, for example, the eighth chapter of the *Bhagavad-gītā* and in the *Śvetāśvatara Upaniṣad*.

Vyāsa raises the question of whether *oṁ* is no more than a word that means *īśvara* by convention or whether the relationship between them is inherent and absolute. He answers by saying that the latter view is correct; it is like the relationship between father and son, which is unchanging, regardless of the words used to describe that relationship. So *oṁ* and *īśvara* have an eternal identification and it is this that gives spiritual potency to the vibration of *oṁ*. Śaṅkara takes the opportunity to embark on a fairly lengthy discussion of the relationship between words and the objects they denote, contending that because the Vedic usage of words is eternal, the relationship between the Vedic word and the object it denotes is also inherent and unchanging. This discussion is of great interest to followers of the Vedānta and Pūrva Mīmāṁsā systems of thought for whom the revelation of the Vedas is an absolute authority, and hence it is no surprise to find Vācaspati Miśra following that line of commentary. Vijñāna Bhikṣu refers to *oṁ* as a 'name' of *īśvara* but insists that this is not like the name of a person known as Devadatta. The name Devadatta is a temporary appellation for that living being, whereas the association of *oṁ* and *īśvara* is eternal.

1.28 *taj-japas tad-artha-bhāvanam*

The repetition (*japa*) and meditation on the object of that *japa* is the process *īśvara-praṇidhāna*.

This passage concludes with instruction as to one of the methods of *īśvara-praṇidhāna*. One might naturally think about the rituals of temple worship in that context, but we should bear in mind that at the time when the *Yoga Sūtras* was probably composed, the tantric rites of image and temple worship were not that widespread. Hence the method of worship or meditation focused on the Deity that is given here consists of the recitation of the mantra *oṁ*, which has been shown to have an intimate and inherent connection to the Deity. This practice of *japa* is still widespread amongst those Hindus whose religious orientation is primarily devotional, with a wide range of *mantras* being employed for that purpose, dependent on the particular deity who is the object of veneration and the particular devotional group to which the practitioner belongs. The word *japa* is attested in the Brāhmaṇa literature of the later Vedic period, but by the time of the Sanskrit epics it becomes associated with yogic currents; in the *Bhagavad-gītā* (10.25), Kṛṣṇa says *yajñānāṁ japa-yajño 'smi*, meaning, 'of all *yajñas* (sacrificial rites), I am the *japa-yajña*', whilst in Book 12 of the *Mahābhārata*, we have a lengthy passage entitled the *Jāpaka-upākhyāna* (Chapters 189–193), which tells of the fate of a resolute performer of *japa*, although we are not told whether or not it was *oṁ* that he recited. Pursuing what might appear to be a somewhat hackneyed theme, I would again suggest a link here to the ideas found in the *Bhagavad-gītā*, which states, *om ity ekākṣaraṁ brahma vyāharan mām anusmaran* (8.13), which means, 'reciting *oṁ*, the single syllable which is Brahman, and fixing his mind on me', thereby revealing a similar connection between meditation on *īśvara* and *japa* of *oṁ*.

Vyāsa then explains that the two practices of meditating on *īśvara* and reciting *oṁ* are effective in leading one to success in Yoga practice, which he refers to as *cittam ekāgram*, having a single-pointed mind. He then cites a verse confirming this idea, which appears to be taken from the *Viṣṇu Purāṇa*. Śaṅkara explains that *japa* can be either purely mental or enunciated in a quiet tone, though mental *japa* is better because it is closer to meditation. He also continues to emphasise the devotional orientation of these *sūtras*, stating that this practice is the way to attract the grace of the Lord. Vācaspati Miśra here merely summarises the points made by Vyāsa, but Vijñāna Bhikṣu comments at some length, providing quotations from various Purāṇas that show the relationship between *oṁ* and the Supreme Deity, who is represented in those citations as both Viṣṇu and Śiva.

At this point, it is worth pausing for a moment to recapitulate the main lines of discussion that Patañjali has presented in the first half of the *Samādhi-pāda*. We started off with a definition of Yoga as *citta-vṛtti-nirodha*, restraining the movements of the mind, which was said to allow the *puruṣa*, the true self, to come to exist in its full spiritual identity. This was followed by a discussion of the nature of the movements of the mind, the *vṛttis* that are to be restrained, presented in the form of a fivefold analysis. Then the consideration turned towards the process of restraint, the *nirodha*, which was explained in terms of two factors, *abhyāsa* and *vairāgya*, regular practice and renunciation. The best form of this *vairāgya* is not that achieved by a determined effort of the will, but rather through the achievement of spiritual awakening in the form of *samādhi*, which naturally draws one's mental faculties away from indulgence and worldliness. The best form of this *vairāgya* is not directed towards any particular object, but rather to the *guṇas* that pervade all material existence. And in providing further insight into the nature of *samādhi*, *sūtras* 1.17 to 1.20

then reveal that *samādhi* is achieved in two forms, designated *saṁprajñāta* and *asaṁprajñāta,* absorption of the mind in a single object of concentration, or else complete absorption devoid of any specific object of focus.

From *sūtra* 1.23, we then had an abrupt change of direction in the discourse heralded by the words *īśvara-praṇidhānād vā,* 'or else by devotion to the Lord', suggesting that the goal of liberation from worldly existence can be achieved either through detachment (*vairāgya*) and the meditational techniques (*abhyāsa*) or else by the practice of devotional religion. This dual emphasis can be recognised as inherent in the teachings of the *Bhagavad-gītā,* which repeatedly refers to both the techniques of meditational Yoga and devotional worship dedicated to the Supreme Deity. The passages on Yoga encountered elsewhere in the *Mahābhārata* do not generally manifest any devotional tendencies, but this is one of most noteworthy features of Kṛṣṇa's revelation to Arjuna.

From the verses of the *Bhagavad-gītā,* we can identify a dual approach to spiritual success defined as the *jñāna-mārga* and the *bhakti-mārga,* 'the way of knowledge' and 'the way of devotion' respectively. This division can be identified in 9.14–15 and 12.1–4 of the *Gītā,* although it is certainly the case that the two paths are at times closely interwoven, as is most evident in its eighth chapter. We have observed this same idea of a dual path emerging in the *Yoga Sūtras,* but we will have to be aware that, from this point on, it is the *jñāna-mārga* that remains almost constantly to the fore. This *jñāna-mārga* relies on the acquisition of the knowledge that can discriminate between *puruṣa* and *prakṛti,* the spiritual entity and its embodiment, and the means by which such knowledge is attained is through the techniques of meditational Yoga, which begin with the restraint of the external movements of the mind. *Īśvara-praṇidhāna* is referred to again later in the *Yoga Sūtras,* but the overwhelming emphasis now rests on the acquisition of awakened knowledge through the practice of Yoga. So let us now take up once more our review of the ways in which the remaining *sūtras* of the *Samādhi-pāda* pursue that line of instruction.

Sūtras 1.29 to 1.32: Obstacles to Progress

1.29 *tataḥ pratyak-cetanādhigamo 'py antarāyābhāvaś ca*

At that point, one realises the internal consciousness and the obstacles to practice cease to exist.

This *sūtra* begins with the word *tataḥ*, which means 'from that' or 'at that point', and must therefore refer to the result of the recitation of or meditation on *oṁ* that was the subject of *sūtra* 1.28 or to *īśvara-praṇidhāna* as a whole, as it is explained by Vyāsa. Now the result of this practice is considered and it is given as being twofold, *pratyak-cetana-adhigama* and *antarāya-abhāva*. Taking the first of these, *adhigama* means 'achievement', 'understanding' or 'acquisition', whilst *pratyak-cetana* means 'the internal consciousness', and is glossed by Vyāsa as *puruṣa*. He paraphrases this achievement as *svarūpa-darśana*, 'perception of one's own nature'. Hence we can see that the first result of the practice previously outlined is the ability to turn the mental faculties away from external perception and contemplation so that the focus is entirely inwards. In this way, one is able to discover the truth about one's own identity and realise the distinction, the *viveka*, between matter and spirit. In the second of the two phrases, *antarāya* means an obstacle or obstruction and *a-bhāva* means non-existence,[1] so the indication is that the same theistic practice also leads to the dwindling away of the

1 In the Sanskrit language, negative terms are formed by the addition of affix '*a*'.

obstacles to success in achieving liberation of *puruṣa* from *prakṛti*, which is the final and ultimate goal of Yoga. It is an explanation of these obstacles that is the subject of the three following *sūtras*.

Vyāsa goes beyond *sūtra* 1.28 in his explanation of the practice referred to by the word *tataḥ* and states that the results that are gained are in fact derived from the entire process of *īśvara-praṇidhāna* rather than just *japa* of *oṁ*. Vyāsa further explains that *īśvara-praṇidhāna* allows for the realisation of the identity of the individual *puruṣa* with the *puruṣa*, which is *īśvara* in so far as both are characterised by ultimately being distinct (*kevala*) from *prakṛti*. Śaṅkara expands on this point somewhat by expressing the view that realisation of the nature of *īśvara* as radiant and untouched by matter or evil leads to the understanding of oneself, *puruṣa*, as being possessed of those same qualities. *Īśvara* is a special *puruṣa*, but the spiritual attributes displayed by *īśvara* are shared by each individual *puruṣa* as well. Vācaspati Miśra makes a similar point. He again emphasises the distinction between *īśvara* and the living beings, but states that meditation on one object brings knowledge of a similar object and hence meditation on *īśvara* brings knowledge of *puruṣa*, which shares some of the spiritual attributes of *īśvara*. Following a similar line, Vijñāna Bhikṣu takes the opportunity to reassert his commitment to the idea that the individual *puruṣa* has only a limited degree of unity with *īśvara* and not the absolute unity taught by Śaṅkara's system of Advaita Vedānta.

1.30 *vyādhi-styāna-saṁśaya-pramādālasyāvirati-bhrānti-darśanālabdha-bhūmikatvānavasthitatvāni citta-vikṣepās te 'ntarāyāḥ*

These obstacles that distract the mind are disease, sloth, doubt, negligence, indolence, indulgence, misapprehension, failure to attain a level of concentration and retain it when it has been attained,

> failure to keep one's understanding firmly grounded,
> and a lack of consistency in one's practice.

What is set before us in this *sūtra* is a fairly straightforward list of things that prove to be obstructive to anyone who is attempting to gain success in achieving *citta-vṛtti-nirodha* and indeed gaining liberation from this world by reaching the state of *samādhi* or engaging in worship of the Deity. Essentially, these are afflictions that beset most people in their endeavours in this world and which sap our enthusiasm for what is a most difficult task in gaining mastery over the fluctuations of the mind. Anyone who has ever attempted to practise the meditational Yoga advocated by Patañjali or by the *Bhagavad-gītā* will surely find some resonance with personal experience when reading through this list.

Vyāsa notes that the list consists of nine obstacles and states that the removal of these will bring about restraint of the movements of the mind. In other words, *citta-vṛtti-nirodha* would be easily achieved were it not for the obstacles. Śaṅkara provides a brief definition of each of the terms used to describe the obstacles, but in doing so does not stray far from the obvious meaning. Vācaspati Miśra focuses in particular on ill health as an obstacle and draws on āyurvedic ideas to explain what this is and how it occurs. Vijñāna Bhikṣu also offers short definitions of what is meant by each of the obstacles, explaining in particular that *anavasthitatva* means failure to keep one's concentration fixed, as may occur for a *yogin* who has not yet achieved the fullness of *samādhi*.

1.31 *duḥkha-daurmanasyāṅgam-ejayatva-śvāsa-praśvāsā vikṣepa-saha-bhuvaḥ*

> The distractions are accompanied by distress,
> dejection, trembling of the body, and heavy inward
> and outward breathing.

Sūtra 1.30 described the obstacles to practice as being *citta-vikṣepa*, distracting to the mind, which means that they draw the *citta* away from the attempt to fix it on a single point in the state of *samādhi*. It is not immediately apparent why the distractions should be accompanied by the phenomena listed in this *sūtra* unless it be the case that intense disappointment arises when the mind is drawn away from the central focus of the practitioner. In that case, there might well be distress and dejection, which might in turn be accompanied by trembling and heavy breathing. Vyāsa simply gives brief and rather obvious definitions of the meaning of the terms and informs us that these are present for one whose mind is distracted but disappear when the mind is fixed on a single point. And perhaps, indeed, that is all that is intended by the *sūtra*, indicating that such signs of distress are an unavoidable part of life for one who cannot attain the state of *samādhi*. Śaṅkara's explanation is similarly limited in scope, but Vācaspati Miśra suggests that the involuntary inward breathing is in contrast to *recaka*, controlled exhalation, which is one of the forms of breath-control (*prāṇāyāma*) that aids concentration. Vijñāna Bhikṣu merely provides a further summarisation of Vyāsa's comments.

1.32 *tat-pratiṣedhārtham eka-tattvābhyāsaḥ*

In order to overcome the obstacles, one should engage in regular practice aimed at a single object.

This again is a fairly straightforward statement, which offers the means by which the obstacles can be overcome. It is nothing new, however, simply a further assertion of the efficacy of *abhyāsa*, strict and regular practice consisting of focusing the mind on a single point or entity (*tattva*), *eka-tattva-abhyāsa*. We may at times become discouraged by the apparent lack of progress we are making and begin to sympathise with Arjuna's view that regulating the mind is more difficult than controlling the wind. But here again Patañjali assures us that the means of progress is to be found in regulation and commitment to the practice over a long period of time without becoming deviated by any sense of disappointment. If we can retain our commitment and dedication, then we should have faith that eventually the obstacles will start to fade away and the light of *samādhi* will begin to emerge. It is accepted that this is no easy path to follow, but, at the same time, it is made clear that regular practice will eventually yield the result we seek.

Vyāsa does not see the need to provide any expansion on the words of the *sūtra* itself, but takes the opportunity to criticise the Buddhist idea of momentariness. The Buddhist view is that the mind can be fixed only on one point at any given moment because everything is in a constant state of transformation. Here, however, the phrase *eka-tattva-abhyāsa* indicates that this constant fluctuation can be arrested by the *yogin* who undertakes a consistent programme of regular practice. Following on from Vyāsa's relatively brief comments, Śaṅkara picks up on this point and presents a lengthy and thoroughgoing refutation of the Buddhist idea of momentariness; this is interesting in the context of Indian religious philosophy but takes us some distance away from the original *sūtra*. Vācaspati Miśra connects this *sūtra* to the previous group and states that the *eka-tattva*, the one object, on which the practice should be focused is in fact *īśvara*, the Deity who is the object of our devotion, thereby providing a restatement of the idea encountered in Chapter 8 of the *Bhagavad-gītā*. He then joins in with the general attack on Buddhist ideas. Vijñāna Bhikṣu is similarly drawn by Vyāsa's comments into a lengthy discussion and refutation of Buddhist doctrine, which again is rather interesting but not directly related to a study of the *Yoga Sūtras*.

Sūtras 1.33 to 1.40: Serenity of Mind and How to Achieve it

The previous four *sūtras* considered the obstacles to progress that cause an agitation of the mind, *citta-vikṣepa*. In the passage that follows these four, the opposite is considered, *citta-prasādana*, which means serenity or calmness of the mind. The word *prasāda* will be familiar to some as it also means grace or mercy, and is often applied to the food or other offerings made to the image in the temple and then distributed to the assembled congregation. Here, however, it is the yogic use of *prasāda* that is intended, as it is also encountered in the *Bhagavad-gītā*. In the *Gītā*'s second chapter (v64), it is said that one who can go beyond the duality of desire and loathing can attain that state of serenity, *prasādam adhigacchati*, and that when that state of serenity is reached, suffering comes to an end, *prasāde sarva-duḥkhānāṁ hānir asyopajāyate* (v65). It is surely that same meaning of *prasāda* that is intended here.

1.33 *maitrī-karuṇā-muditopekṣāṇāṁ sukha-duḥkha-puṇyāpuṇya-viṣayāṇāṁ bhāvanātaś citta-prasādanam*

> Serenity of mind is achieved when one shows friendship towards those who are happy, compassion for those who suffer, delight towards the righteous, and indifference towards the wicked.

This *sūtra* can be read as providing an insight not so much into the practice of Yoga techniques, but rather the proper manner in which a person should relate to the world and other living beings. This is important, for Yoga is not just about the practice of techniques, but is primarily concerned with the ideal state of consciousness that should be permanently present. One cannot have an aggressive, malicious, greedy, or selfish *yogin*; as long as such qualities remain embedded in the consciousness, then the practice will not be effective, and by the same token, when the practice is properly executed, then one's attitude towards the world is transformed into a mood that is utterly benign and filled with goodwill. Otherwise, what is being undertaken is not really Yoga. Hence one should be joyful to find oneself in the company of those who are joyful, without any envy for the good fortune of others; one should show compassion for those who are suffering by undertaking the *karma-yoga* that is focused on the wellbeing of the world; one should be delighted when others share in one's own virtuous way of living; and one should avoid the company of wicked-minded individuals, unless it be one's aim to soothe a vicious temperament. When one relates to the world in that manner, then the state of *citta-prasādana* will appear, and when the state of *citta-prasādana* becomes manifest, then one will instinctively relate to the world in the way described here. It is both the means and the end. Alternatively, the *sūtra* can be read as a reference to four techniques of meditation (*bhāvanā*) where, for example, the feeling of compassion (*karuṇā*) would not be applied in any particularly daily situation, but rather meditatively extended to all those who suffer as its object (*viṣaya*). The four meditations of *maitrī, karuṇā, muditā,* and *upekṣā* are found in the Buddhist tradition, where they are not limited to any specific beings and therefore known as *apramāṇa,* 'without measure'.

Vyāsa here repeats the ideas presented by the *sūtra,* and adds that the four practices or meditations (*bhāvanā*) described in the *sūtra* give rise to 'pure *dharma*' which in turn causes the *citta-prasādana*. When the mind is serene (*prasanna*) it also becomes single-pointed (*ekāgra*) and obtains the state of stability (*sthiti-pada*). The mention of 'pure *dharma*' reveals the moral dimension of the Yoga discourse.

Vācaspati Miśra asserts that one who has inimical feelings, such as jealousy towards others, will never be able to practise

Yoga successfully by fixing the mind in concentration, as there is an existential contradiction between these two opposing states of consciousness. Śaṅkara and Vijñāna Bhikṣu cite verse 65 of Chapter 2 of the *Gītā*. Vijñāna Bhikṣu also points out that the *prasādana*, the serenity referred to as being achieved by these modes of conduct, is an essential basis on which the steady fixation of the mind is dependent.

1.34 *pracchardana-vidhāraṇābhyāṁ vā prāṇasya*

Such serenity may also be achieved through
the exhaling and retention of the breath.

Here we are informed that in addition to the manner in which we conduct ourselves in relation to others or the four meditations, *citta-prasādana*, serenity of mind, may also be achieved by means of the process of *prāṇāyāma*, the regulation of the breathing that will be familiar to most Yoga practitioners. Here the terms used to define this practice are *pracchardana*, which means exhalation, and *vidhāraṇa*, meaning the retention of the breath. These can be equated with the terms *recaka* and *kumbhaka*, which are more commonly used for exhalation and retention respectively. In later Yoga treatises, formulated under tantric influences, we find that *prāṇāyāma* is advocated as a means of bodily transformation, as when the *kuṇḍalinī* is awakened and the *cakras* energised. The regulation of the breathing that is advocated here, however, is not referred to with the same end in mind. It is simply a process by which mental relaxation is achieved so that serenity of mind can be developed as an essential prerequisite for fixing the mind on a single point in the state of *samādhi*. The regulation of the breathing brings about a state of relaxation and calmness, a form of serenity from which one can begin the attempt to bring the mind under control, with its movements restrained, and then brought to the state of being focused on a single point.

Vyāsa suggests that the *pracchardana* is an act of exhalation of breath through the nostrils by means of a special effort (*prayatna-viśeṣāt*), whilst Śaṅkara confirms that the process being referred to here is that of *prāṇāyāma*. Vācaspati Miśra explains that retention of breath also involves holding back air from entering the nostrils. Vijñāna Bhikṣu, however, takes a different view and states that *prāṇāyāma* refers only to the processes of *pūraka* (inhalation), *kumbhaka* (holding of inhaled breath in the lungs), and *recaka* (exhalation), and not to holding back the breath from inhalation, which he says is not possible.

1.35 *viṣayavatī vā pravṛttir utpannā manasaḥ sthiti-nibandhinī*

Or by controlling the mind, and making it still when it becomes active in relation to an object. Or, when an activity based on a [supernatural] object arises, it fixes the mind in stability.

Each of these *sūtras* includes the word *vā*, which means 'or else', thereby indicating that each of the processes referred to is an alternative means of achieving a state of *citta-prasādana*, serenity of mind, although it may well be that the recommendation is for us to try to practise all of them conjointly. The first method was with regard to our dealings with the world or a meditation, the second was *prāṇāyāma*, and here there is a move back to the attempt to gain control over the fluctuating mind. The phrase *viṣayavatī pravṛttiḥ* indicates the movement of the mind, *manasaḥ*, towards a particular *viṣaya*, or object of perception. This movement of the mind is said to be *sthiti-nibandhinī*, which literally means 'binding the mind to that specific position'. This poses a problem of interpretation. The *sūtra* on its own seems to be saying that a movement of the mind will be the cause of steadiness, *sthiti*, of the mind, which may sound paradoxical.

Vyāsa, however, explains the paradox and gives a more elaborate interpretation of the *sūtra,* stating that the *viṣaya,* the objects of perception referred to here, are not the normal tastes, smells, etc. that we typically encounter through the action of the senses, but are in this case subtle, super-sensory perceptions that come to the *yogin* who is absorbed in meditation. The practice of Yoga techniques brings with it a heightened sense of perception by which the essence of aroma or taste awakens in the mind, beyond the aroma or taste of any specific object of perception. When this super-sensory perception enters the consciousness of the *yogin,* it binds the mind to steadiness (*sthiti*). This heightened sense of perception enhances the faith of the practitioner in the yogic process as the results of the practice can now be directly perceived. As is usually the case, our other three commentators follow Vyāsa's interpretation, with Śaṅkara relating the idea of heightened perception to the supernatural powers referred to in Chapter 3 of the *Yoga Sūtras.* Vācaspati Miśra reflects on Vyāsa's statement about faith, pointing out that faith in the revelation of sacred text may sometimes be lacking or partial, but can be fundamentality enhanced when one directly experiences the results of one's practice. Vijñāna Bhikṣu says that, despite the use of the word *vā* in the *sūtra,* this practice of fixing the mind on these higher perceptions is not an alternative but, is in fact, an essential element of the overall practice. He also notes the use of the word *manasaḥ* here in a series of *sūtras* that began with reference to *citta,* and concludes that *manas* and *citta* can therefore be taken as synonyms.

1.36 *viśokā vā jyotiṣmatī*

Or by remaining free of sorrow and filled with light.

If one does not regard Vyāsa and Patañjali as one and the same person, then one might feel that Vyāsa's commentary on the previous *sūtra* was something of an over-interpretation.

Most of these *sūtras* on the ways in which *citta-prasādana* can be achieved relate to what one might regard as preliminaries to the full practice of Yoga. Here the word *viśokā* provides a fairly straightforward assertion that such serenity comes when one is able to emotionally transcend the anxieties and problems that typically beset us in our journey through worldly life. The word *jyotiṣmatī* is less obvious in terms of its meaning, but one might take it as referring to a state of life in which one's consciousness is illuminated by wisdom, compassion, and a wholly benign outlook on the world. In this sense, we might equate *jyotiṣmatī* with the English word 'enlightened', as both are derived from the idea of intellectual and personal illumination.

Vyāsa begins by stating that the words *pravṛttir utpannā manasaḥ sthiti-nibandhanī* from the previous *sūtra* should be repeated here. This practice of not repeating the words from a former *sūtra* that are needed to complete the sentence of a later *sūtra* is known as *anuvṛtti* and is typical of the *sūtra* genre where each individual *sūtra* is ideally made as short as possible. Vyāsa again elaborates quite fully on what is meant here, suggesting that the activity, *pravṛtti*, qualified as free from sorrow, *viśokā*, arises by meditation on the lotus of the heart, the *hṛdaya-puṇḍarīka*, a phrase and an idea that is unusual in early Yoga treatises such as those found in the *Mahābhārata* and the *Bhagavad-gītā*, although it is probably based on a passage of the *Chāndogya Upaniṣad* (8.1.2). This meditation on the lotus in the heart also brings illumination and hence the arising activity is also described as being *jyotiṣmatī*. Repeating the phrase *sthiti-nibandhanī* from the previous *sūtra*, Vyāsa reveals that this sorrow-less and illuminated activity of the mind will also make the mind steady. Here again we are confronted by the question of whether or not to equate Vyāsa with Patañjali, particularly as Vyāsa's commentary moves us on a considerable distance from the wording of the original *sūtra*, which is itself somewhat obscure. The reference to the *hṛdaya-puṇḍarīka* might suggest a later date for the commentary and again, one feels that there may be something of an over-interpretation here.

Śaṅkara expresses the view that the illumination of the intellect, the *buddhi-sattva* spoken of by Vyāsa, comes as one begins to perceive the *ātman*, awareness of which frees one from the sorrows of this world and spreads illumination throughout one's mental processes. Vācaspati Miśra appears to adopt a more tantric understanding, explaining the nature of the lotus in the heart in relation to the *nāḍīs*, the channels of energy running throughout the body. He states that concentration should be fixed within the *suṣumnā nāḍī*, which is an interesting early reference to the tantric body, as such references are usually found only in later works on Yoga. Vijñāna Bhikṣu likewise discusses the nature of the heart-lotus, referring to the idea of the letters and *mantras* that are located on its petals; again an interesting line of discussion, but one that takes us well beyond the scope of the *sūtra* itself.

1.37 *vīta-rāga-viṣayaṁ vā cittam*

> Or when the mind has as its object something that is devoid of passion [it attains a state of stability].
> Or when the mind is free of longing for any object.

Again, the use of the word *vā* indicates to us that an alternative means of gaining *citta-prasādana* is being offered in this *sūtra*, and again it relates to our interactions with the world rather than any specifically yogic form of practice; and this in turn gives a further indication that these are preliminaries to be established before such practice can be successfully undertaken.

Vyāsa comments only briefly here but suggests that this *sūtra* is, in fact, defining an object for meditation, which is a mind free of longing or else a person whose mind is free of longing. This is certainly a possibility, although there is little in the *sūtra* itself or the context to suggest the addition of the instruction to meditate on such a state or person. The other commentators are equally brief, but Vācaspati Miśra puts forward the name of Vyāsa himself as one who has achieved a state of mind free of passion, whilst Vijñāna Bhikṣu similarly refers to the sage Sanaka and others.

As a technical note, it may be pointed out that it is not possible to grammatically link this and the following *sūtras* with the previous one's, although the word *vā*, meaning 'or', still links them thematically to what precedes. The commentary of Vyāsa provides a Sanskrit phrase necessary to complete the sentence: *yoginaś cittaṁ sthitipadaṁ labhate*, 'the mind of the *yogin* obtains the state of steadiness'.

1.38 *svapna-nidrā-jñānālambanaṁ vā*

> Or by focusing on the realisation acquired whilst dreaming or in a state of deep sleep.

Here again the word *vā* offers us another alternative means, this time defined by the compound *svapna-nidrā-jñāna-ālambana*. The word *svapna* can mean either sleeping or dreaming, but because *nidrā* also means sleeping, we must presume it is used here in the latter sense. As is well known, *jñāna* means knowledge or realisation, and hence we must take the phrase as a whole as referring to the insight that comes whilst one is dreaming or in a state of deep, dreamless sleep. It seems likely that Patañjali is here making reference to ideas found in the *Māṇḍūkya Upaniṣad*, which discusses four states of consciousness: waking, dreaming, deep sleep, and a fourth transcendent state, and equates them with progressive states of realised knowledge. The word *ālambanam* means a support or a basis and the likely meaning seems to be that the mind can attain serenity by using the realisation gained in the states of *svapna* and *nidrā* as a basis for contemplation. Exactly what the knowledge that comes in this way might be is not stated, but the indication of the *Māṇḍūkya Upaniṣad* is that this is the higher knowledge that leads ultimately to *turīya*, the fourth state that is perhaps equivalent to *kaivalya*, liberation from rebirth.

Vyāsa offers a simple recapitulation of the statement of the *sūtra* itself, but Śaṅkara explains that objects and ideas encountered in dreams have no physical substance, whilst in deep sleep there are no objects at all, and hence meditation on these provides an effective pathway to serenity of mind. Vācaspati Miśra is more specific about the type of dream one might fix the mind upon, referring to a dream in which one worships an image of *īśvara* in the forest, which is then made into a subject of subsequent meditation. In deep sleep there are no objects at all within the mind, and hence in this state, where all forms of external perception are suspended, knowledge of Brahman begins to appear. Vijñāna Bhikṣu branches out somewhat by suggesting that all the world we inhabit is a dream world, because all its objects are perishable like the objects created in a dream. And, similarly, deep sleep also indicates the nature of this world because the whole world is in a state of sleep, unaware of the grace of Viṣṇu that is available to them. Here one feels that Vijñāna Bhikṣu has moved some distance away from the more obvious meaning of both the *sūtra* and Vyāsa's brief recapitulation of it.

1.39 *yathābhimata-dhyānād vā*

Or by meditating on any object one likes.

This is the last of the '*vā*' *sūtras* that offer alternative means of developing *citta-prasādana*, and here for the first time we have direct rather than implied reference to the practice of meditation, in the form of the word *dhyānāt*, which means from or as a result of *dhyāna*. The object of the *dhyāna* is designated as *yathā-abhimata*, which means 'whatever one desires' or 'whatever is pleasing'. What this exactly means is not made clear, but one suspects that it refers to a particular *mantra* or object of worship, which is of importance in one's religious life. So, for example, one of a Vaiṣṇava persuasion might decide to meditate on the *mantra*, *namo nārāyaṇāya*, whilst one whose principal object of devotion is Śiva might use the *mantra*, *namaḥ śivāya*. This is pure speculation, however, as the brevity of *sūtra* leaves it open to a variety of viable interpretations.

Vyāsa is again very restrained in his comments, merely suggesting that if one starts out by meditating on a desirable object, one thereby attains the ability to fix the mind in the same way on any other object, desirable or otherwise. Śaṅkara qualifies the meaning of the *sūtra* by insisting that the object one desires should not be something that is pleasurable in a worldly sense, for that would run contrary to teachings given previously. Vācaspati Miśra confirms the idea that the object of meditation should reflect one's religious persuasion with the words, 'whichsoever particular deity it may be' (Trans. Woods), a view confirmed by Vijñāna Bhikṣu, who makes specific reference to images of Viṣṇu or Śiva as objects of meditation.

1.40 *paramāṇu-parama-mahattvānto 'sya vaśīkāraḥ*

> The result of this mental serenity is that one's control extends over that which is most minute, and up to that which is the largest thing.

The passage on gaining *citta-prasādana* is concluded in this fortieth *sūtra* with an assertion as to the power that comes to one who completes one or more of the prescribed methods outlined here. The word *vaśīkāra*, which means gaining control, reminds us again of the idea that Yoga is a means of personal empowerment. We can recognise this idea from the *Bhagavad-gītā*, which speaks of *yoga-balena*, using the power of Yoga in one's spiritual endeavours (8.10), whilst in the *Mahābhārata* we find these words: *nāsti yoga-samaṁ balam*, 'there is no power equal to that of Yoga' (12.304.2). Here it is stated that this control extends over objects that are *paramāṇu*, minutely small, as well as those that are *mahattva*, of huge proportions, by implication covering everything in between. Here we are certainly being given a hint of the ideas encountered in the *Vibhūti-pāda* of the *Yoga Sūtras* where the supernatural powers acquired through Yoga practice are expounded upon at some length. These far-reaching results said to be attained from the practices advocated in the previous *sūtras* might suggest that those practices are far more than preliminaries, but one might also regard the statement here as indicating that these are gateways to the full achievement of yogic accomplishment, which brings with it the extraordinary powers delineated in the *Vibhūti-pāda*.

Vyāsa's observations are particularly pertinent to the latter point as he states *yoginaś cittaṁ na punar abhyāsa-kṛtaṁ parikarmāpekṣate*, indicating that no further practice is required for the purpose of purification of the practitioner's mind. Here the word *parikarma*, meaning purification, certainly suggests that Vyāsa regards the practices outlined in these *sūtras* as purificatory preparations for the full undertaking of the techniques of Yoga. Vyāsa also suggests that the form of mastery mentioned here relates to the power of meditation, whereby the practitioner is able to fix the mind on any object, regardless of whether it is minute or vast. Śaṅkara confirms this view of Vyāsa, stating that what is being considered here is *dhāraṇā*, fixed concentration, which can be of three types: on things that are minute, on things that are vast, and on both of these. Vācaspati Miśra's brief commentary has little to add, but Vijñāna Bhikṣu focuses on another of Vyāsa's ideas by stating that the practices laid out in this passage are effective in removing the obstacles that normally inhibit the mind and prevent it from achieving fixed concentration on things that are minutely small or of gigantic proportions.

SŪTRAS 1.41 TO 1.46: THE STATE OF SAMĀPATTI

From *sūtra* 1.41, the discourse begins to move in a different direction by considering a state of yogic accomplishment that it refers to as *samāpatti*. *Sūtra* 1.41 defines *samāpatti* as the state of mind that appears when the *vṛttis*, the movements of the mind, fade away, so that the senses are withdrawn back into the mind. Four forms of *samāpatti* are delineated, two where the mind is absorbed in *vitarka* and *vicāra*, forms of reflective thought, and two where the mind stands completely still, bright, unwavering, and devoid of *vitarka* and *vicāra*. On this point, we are informed that this latter form of *samāpatti* is to be understood as the initial stage of *samādhi*, which is *sa-bīja samādhi*, *samādhi* that is based on a particular seed. These *sūtras* are often quite obscure in meaning and present the reader with a range of quite complex ideas, and I hope the discussions that are given here, along with the contributions of the commentators, will add some clarity to this next line of discourse.

1.41 *kṣīṇa-vṛtter abhijātasyeva maṇer grahītṛ-grahaṇa-grāhyeṣu tat-stha-tad-añjanatā samāpattiḥ*

Samāpatti, comparable to the colouring of a pure crystal, is the the colouring of the mind, whose *vṛttis* have diminished, when it rests in the preceiver, perception or perceptible objects.

Here then we have an explanation of what is meant by the term *samāpatti*. The point to note is that this state is achieved at a fairly advanced stage in the progression of a person's Yoga practice, for the opening compound, *kṣīṇa-vṛtteḥ*, indicates that the movements of the mind have been restrained and are diminishing. The state of *samāpatti* is then explained by comparison to a clear gemstone (*maṇi*), which, like the mind of the *yogin*, has no colouration of its own. It is pure, untouched, and crystal clear. The gemstone takes on the coloration of any object to which it becomes adjacent without becoming itself transformed by that colouration. And in the same way, the clear mind of the adept 'is coloured', namely, reflects the presence of the *grahītṛ*, the *grahaṇa*, and the *grāhya*. All of these nouns are derived from the verbal root *grah*, meaning to grasp, seize, or take hold of, and in this case all three words relate to the process of mental perception. The *grahītṛ* is that which perceives, which could be either the spiritual *puruṣa* or the facet of the mental processes known as *buddhi*, which receives perceptions and makes decisions based upon them. *Grahaṇa* is the means by which the objects of perception are grasped, and this term must therefore refer to the senses, not perhaps in their external form as the nose or ears, but as the internal process of perception, which we regard as a faculty of the mind. Then, finally, *grāhya* is that which is perceived, in other words, sense-datum such as aroma, flavour, or sound that the senses enable us to perceive. In our normal condition, the mind moves swiftly from one sensation to another in a state of constant transformation, as different sensations are perceived; such movements are the *vṛttis*, but now that these are wasting away, the mind becomes still and clear, simply reflecting what is proximate to it rather than moving constantly from one object to another. This state of serene stillness of the mind is *samāpatti*.

Vyāsa comments along similar lines to what has been said above, but uses the phrase *grahītṛ-puruṣa* to indicate that the perceiver referred to by the *sūtra* should be understood as the spiritual *puruṣa*, the true self of each living being. Hence the mind can reflect that spiritual identity due to the proximity of *puruṣa* to *citta* within a living being; this, of course, can only take place once the external *vṛttis* have been stilled and thus removed. Śaṅkara focuses his commentary on that point in particular, asserting that the mind does not have the ability to perceive *puruṣa*, which by its very nature as pure spirit is beyond the range of mental conception. What the *citta* can perceive when freed from the *vṛttis* is a reflection of *puruṣa*, as the colouration in the gemstone is a reflection of the true colour located within an object. Vācaspati Miśra offers a complex discussion of the relationship between the process of knowing and the object that is known, the *grahaṇa* and the *grāhya*, whilst Vijñāna Bhikṣu analyses *grahītṛ*, *grahaṇa*, and *grāhya* in line with the explanation above, considering the possibility that *grahītṛ* could refer to the *buddhi*, the intellectual faculty, but concluding that the meaning of the term in the present context is *puruṣa*, as Vyāsa has asserted.

The following three (1.42-44) *sūtras* introduce four types of *samāpatti*: *sa-vitarka*, *nir-vitarka*, *sa-vicāra*, and *nir-vicāra*.

1.42 *tatra śabdārtha-jñāna-vikalpaiḥ saṁkīrṇā sa-vitarkā samāpattiḥ*

When this state is adulterated by mental constructs relating to words, their meaning, and the idea they convey, it is to be known as *samāpatti* with *vitarka*, discursive thought.

This is another rather difficult *sūtra*, but its subject is clearly stated as *sa-vitarkā samāpatti*, which means the *samāpatti* that is accompanied by some form of *vitarka*, conscious reflection on a particular meaning. Given what was stated previously through the metaphor of the clear gemstone and the statement that the movements of the mind are diminished, one must presume that this is a less advanced form of *samāpatti* in which the process of *vitarka* remains present. In defining *sa-vitarkā samāpatti*, Patañjali qualifies this *samāpatti* itself as 'mixed' *saṁkīrṇa*. According to Vyāsa, the intermingling of a word, its meaning, and the idea it conveys, so that the purity of the *samāpatti* is adulterated. In the previous *sūtra*, the emphasis was on the clarity of the mind that is freed from the effects of *vṛtti*, but here it is said that the purity of the *samāpatti* can be affected by the intermminglings of the three components so that the clarity is diminished or to some extent clouded over. What this seems to mean is that there is a reversion to the conventional mental processes in which we hear a word, consider its meaning, and then form an idea of the object it refers to. *Samāpatti* takes us beyond that process, clearing all such mental configurations away, but when this process is adulterated, it is referred to as *sa-vitarka*, which indicates that the clarity is not entirely pure.

This is the meaning of the *sūtra* that Vyāsa confirms in his commentary, essentially saying that *sa-vitarka* means a reversion to the conventional mental processes that *samāpatti* transcends when it is fully developed. The word, its meaning, and the object it refers to are distinct from one another and are regarded in this light through the clarity of full *samāpatti*. But the intermingling of the three that characterises conventional thought processes stands in contrast to the purity of full *samāpatti*. Śaṅkara relates this understanding to the process of meditation in which the mind is to be fixed on a single object, as mentioned in *sūtra* 1.39, but the intrusion of *vitarka* into one's meditation is a disturbance, as one then begins to formulate thoughts and ideas about the object on which the mind is to be absorbed. What I think Śaṅkara is referring to here is a process of meditation in which one concentrates the mind on the form of a deity such as Śiva. Ideally, *samāpatti* would be unaffected by any thought processes, for it is pure, fixed, absorbed concentration, but when *vitarka* intrudes, one might start to draw in ideas about the nature of Śiva, about his relationship with Pārvatī, or about the actions of Śiva described in Purāṇic works. This would appear to be the adulteration of *samāpatti* that is being referred to here.

This understanding of what is being said here is confirmed by Vācaspati Miśra who again displays his interest in the nature of the association between words and their meaning. Vijñāna Bhikṣu follows a similar line of discussion in relation to words, objects, and meanings, but is quite clear about the nature of *sa-vitarkā samāpatti* when he concludes by saying, *iyaṁ ca samāpattir aparam*, this is an inferior form of *samāpatti*.

1.43 *smṛti-pariśuddhau svarūpa-śūnyevārtha-mātra-nirbhāsā nirvitarkā*

> But when memory is purified, the external form of the object disappears and it shines forth alone. This state is called *nir-vitarka*, non-discursive thought.

Here we are given an explanation of another form of *samāpatti*, which is designated as *nir-vitarka*, free of conscious deliberation. As with a number of *sūtras*, the precise meaning is hard to establish because the attempt is being made to formulate in words and concepts what is essentially an experiential process. The prerequisite for attaining *nir-vitarkā samāpatti* is defined as *smṛti-pariśuddha*, the purification of memory, or perhaps the purification of one's concentration. The word *smṛti* does usually mean memory or memorisation, but in Chapter 8 of the *Bhagavad-gītā*, we find it being used in a context that suggests a far more intense fixing of the mind than is the case in our conventional process of recollection. Hence my suspicion is that here the purification relates to the concentration undertaken, and is a form of purging of the *vitarka*, the conscious thought processes referred to in *sūtra* 1.42. When this purification is achieved, it appears that the mind is emptied of the external form of the object of concentration and there is total absorption in the essential nature of the object. Thoughts and reflections about that object are brought to an end and it is solely that essential nature that shines forth. This is what is meant by *nir-vitarkā samāpatti*.

Vyāsa begins his commentary with an explanation of *nir-vitarkā samāpatti* that shows that this is in fact identical to the definition of *samāpatti* given in *sūtra* 1.41. This is a higher level of *samāpatti*, whereas *sūtra* 1.42 gave us *sa-vitarkā samāpatti*, a less developed form of *samāpatti*. He then expresses the view that because our usual mode of perceiving objects is *sa-vitarka* we do not get a true perception of an object, which comes only through *nir-vitarka* concentration. Thus the world we perceive is not the real world, but a series of imperfect mental impressions. Vyāsa explains that the purification of memory (*smṛti-pariśuddhi*) refers to the forgetting of linguistic conventions (*śabdasaṁketa*), which presumably allows the meditator to overcome the confusion of the word, its meaning, and the thing it refers to. This allows the meditator to overcome mental constructions (*vikalpa*) that are fundamentally of a linguistic nature, and so come to realise the object of meditation or cognition in its true form. Śaṅkara takes the opportunity to again dismiss the Buddhist idea of momentariness, stating that the *sūtra* here and Vyāsa's commentary both demonstrate that objects do have a factual identity that is realised through *nir-vitarkā samāpatti*.

Vācaspati Miśra also comments at some length on this *sūtra*, again refuting the Buddhist notion of there being no permanent objects, and also considering the Vaiśeṣika view that all objects consist of a conglomeration of atoms. He does not wholly reject this latter idea but states that *samāpatti* on an object as it truly is does not mean perceiving its atomic structure. Vijñāna Bhikṣu makes the observation that the *sa-vitarkā samāpatti* that is regarded as inferior also includes reflection on the meaning of scriptural teachings, as these also consist of words, concepts, and meanings based on reflection, on *vitarka*. His point is not to deny the validity of scriptural authority, as the Buddhists and Jains might do, but just to show that intellectual knowledge of scripture does not amount to the highest form of realisation. All the commentators write at considerable length on this *sūtra* and it is not possible for our purposes to follow their individual lines of argumentation, particularly as they move the discussion some distance away from the primary meaning of the *sūtra* and of Vyāsa's *bhāṣya*.

1.44 *etayaiva sa-vicārā nir-vicārā ca sūkṣma-viṣayā vyākhyātā*

In this way, *samāpatti* focused on subtle objects, with and without reflective modes of thought, has now also been explained.

Here Patañjali says that the previous *sūtras* about *sa-vitarka* and *nir-vitarka samāpatti* should be used as a guide for understanding the other two types of *samāpatti* – *sa-vicāra* and *nir-vicāra*. In other words, the relationship between *sa-vicāra* and *nir-vicāra samāpatti* is the same as that between *sa-vitarka* and *nir-vitarka samāpatti*. Thus we can understand that *sa-vicāra samāpatti* involves a linguistic deliberation whereas, in *nir-vicāra samāpatti*, the object of meditation shines forth as it really is. The *sūtra* reveals the difference between the terms *vitarka* and *vicāra* by clarifying that *vicāra* meditation or reflection is based on a subtle (*sūkṣma*) object. *Vitarka*, however, is based on a gross (*sthūla*) object as explained by Vyāsa in his commentary to 1.17.

Here Patañjali brings one line of discussion almost to its conclusion with the first and final words of this *sūtra*. The word *etayā* means 'by this' or 'in this way' whilst *vyākhyāta* means 'declared' or 'explained'. Three words are used to describe what the author considers to have been explained in the previous few *sūtras*: *sa-vicāra, nir-vicāra,* and *sūkṣma-viṣaya*. The feminine form in which these appear, with the final *ā*, indicates that they are qualified as *samāpatti*, a feminine noun that is thus implied though not stated. What immediately strikes one here is the switch from the word *vitarka* to *vicāra*, which suggests a good degree of congruence between the meanings of these two terms. In the *Śānti-parvan* (Book 12) of the *Mahābhārata*, Chapter 188 forms a passage entitled *Dhyāna Yoga*, which provides a brief discussion of the techniques of meditation. Verse 15 of that chapter refers to *vicāra, vitarka,* and *viveka* as the preliminary stage of meditation, *dhyānam āditaḥ*, and I notice that there I translated *vicāra* as reflection and *vitarka* as deliberation, which reveals again that these two mental processes are not that dissimilar. In the *Yoga Sūtras* and most Sāṁkhya treatises, *viveka* is awarded a much higher status with the meaning of discrimination in relation to the recognition of the absolute distinction between *prakṛti* and *puruṣa*, matter and spirit, which brings liberation from rebirth. With regard to the *Mahābhārata*'s use of *viveka* in that passage, one suspects that it refers to a more mundane form of *viveka* that enables one to distinguish the true nature of an object.

Returning to the *sūtra* here, we can observe that Patañjali is simply reminding us of the ideas he has presented in the previous two *sūtras*. The compound *sūkṣma-viṣaya* means 'having subtle objects of perception', and this probably means the manner in which the perception engendered by *samāpatti* allows one to go beyond the external manifestation of an object and focus on the object in its pure, inherent identity; the object simply as it is without any specific context or associated processes of reflection. Our conventional mode of perception is flickering and is related to the external nature of an object as it exists within a specific location or context. *Samāpatti* enables the adept to go beyond conventional perceptions and to remain fixed on the object in its absolute, non-contextual form; this is probably what is meant here by *sūkṣma-viṣaya*, an object in its subtle identity.

Śaṅkara anticipates Vyāsa's comments on the next *sūtra* by stating that the subtle objects are in fact the primal states of the objects of our perception, colour/form, sound, flavour, aroma, and touch sensations. Until they become manifest as specific sensations, they have a primal, subtle identity that is perceived only when the mind penetrates beyond their overt manifestation, such as the aroma of a specific flower.

Vācaspati Miśra follows the same line as Śaṅkara, explaining that every time a perception enters our mind, it relates to a specific object that is spatially and temporally existent. Beyond these overt sensations, however, there is the primal, subtle object, known technically as a *tan-mātra,* of which all specific objects of perception are secondary manifestations. It is these subtle *tan-mātras* that are perceived through *samāpatti* which carries our mental perception beyond its normal range and scope. Vijñāna Bhikṣu also builds on Vyāsa's comments by pointing out that the type of perception being referred to here exists beyond the range of time. Our conventional sensory perceptions relate to a specific object present before us at a specific time, but this *sūtra* is speaking of perception of the primal, absolute source of such perceptions, which is not a perception relating to a particular time or place. Hence it is not associated with any specific movement of the mind. In line with the Sāṁkhya understanding of the origin of the world, he also explains that these subtle objects are the sources from which the elements of which this world is comprised evolve.

1.45 *sūkṣma-viṣayatvaṁ cāliṅga-paryavasānam*

And this subtle nature of objects extends as far as the *aliṅga*, that which has no defining marks.

Here Patañjali defines the subtle objects of *sa-vicāra* and *nir-vicāra samāpatti*, in contrast to our own conventional perception of their external, gross manifestations. Unfortunately, the definition only indicates the limit of a meditative object to be classified as 'subtle' without clarifying what other objects belong to this class. He states that this subtle nature extends up to that which is *a-liṅga*. The word *liṅga* means 'a defining or characteristic mark', just as it is sometimes said that non-violence, *ahiṁsā*, is the *liṅga* of *dharma*. So what is it that is *a-liṅga* in the sense of being undifferentiated and without any specific mark by which it can be identified? In understanding the meaning here, we must refer again to the Sāṁkhya ideas which provide Patañjali with the theoretical basis for his work. According to Sāṁkhya teachings, this world is a combination of *prakṛti* and *puruṣa*, *prakṛti* being the substance of matter, mental and physical, and *puruṣa* being the spiritual entities that give life to *prakṛti*, which is by nature lifeless and inert. In its primal, undifferentiated state, *prakṛti* is referred to as *pradhāna* and *avyakta*, primal and non-manifest.

Prakṛti exists in two forms. Initially, it is a non-variegated substance that has no defining characteristics because it is not existing as this world with all its diversity of objects and living beings. Due to the presence of *puruṣa*, the three *guṇas* that pervade *prakṛti* fall out of their state of equilibrium and, as a result, primal *prakṛti* begins to evolve into the various elements of which this variegated world is comprised. All the commentators agree that the term *aliṅga* used here refers to *prakṛti* in its primal form as *pradhāna*, which is *a-liṅga* because it has not evolved into the form of this world of variety, which displays a multiplicity of *liṅga* by which the objects we perceive in this world are defined. This primal state of *prakṛti* is subtle rather than gross because it has yet to manifest the *tan-mātras*, the subtle basis of the objects we perceive, and hence it is also known as *avyakta*, invisible or non-manifest. One significant point to note here is that if it be the case that *samāpatti* finds its limit in the most subtle form of *prakṛti*, and not in *puruṣa*, then we must conclude that *samāpatti* alone is not sufficient to provide the liberating *viveka-jñāna* that enables us to perceive the clear distinction between *prakṛti* and *puruṣa*, which is the means by which liberation is attained.

Vyāsa mentions that *puruṣa* is also subtle and raises the question of whether the most subtle object might in fact be *puruṣa*. Vyāsa dismisses that suggestion by arguing that the *aliṅga*, namely *prakṛti* in its unmanifest form, is more subtle than *puruṣa* because of the different roles they have in the production of the manifest world. While *puruṣa* acts as an instrumental cause (*hetu*) in the production of the manifest world, the unmanifest *prakṛti* is the material source or cause (*anvayi-kāraṇa*) of that manifest world and therefore it is more subtle. Śaṅkara takes up this discussion as to whether it is *puruṣa* that is being referred to as *aliṅga* and rejects the idea on the basis that the *sūtra* uses the word *paryavasāna*, meaning 'extending to'. There are varying degrees of subtlety and grossness in the evolutes that emerge from primal *prakṛti* and the word *paryavāsana* indicates that scale of subtlety from which *puruṣa* is entirely set apart.

Vācaspati Miśra applies the discussion of degrees of subtleness to the Sāṁkhya idea of the manner in which the manifest world is withdrawn back into the primal state of non-variegated *prakṛti*. The elements are withdrawn progressively, each one into its predecessor and, in the final stage of withdrawal, everything is absorbed into *buddhi*, the intellect in all beings, and this, in turn, then becomes non-manifest as it is withdrawn into primal *prakṛti*. Hence it is said that *prakṛti* in its *aliṅga* form is the ultimate state of subtlety in matter. Vijñāna Bhikṣu follows a similar line of commentary to the others, but adds a theistic element in line with his own particular doctrinal standpoint. According to Sāṁkhya teachings, the evolution of primal *prakṛti* into its variegated forms within this world is for the sake of *puruṣa* so that *puruṣa* can find a way to gain liberation from bondage. For Vijñāna Bhikṣu, this is not a blind process inherent in matter, but takes place under the control and direction of *īśvara*, the Deity, and in support of this view, he cites verse 10 of Chapter 9 of the *Gītā*, which makes precisely that point, thereby offering us a form of theistic Sāṁkhya.

1.46 *tā eva sa-bījaḥ samādhiḥ*

These are in fact *sa-bīja samādhi*, *samādhi* arising from a seed.

This *sūtra* provides a link that takes us from one topic of discussion to another, from *samāpatti* to *samādhi*. We will be aware that this opening chapter of the *Yoga Sūtras* is entitled the *Samādhi-pāda* and we might have noticed that so far not much has been said about *samādhi*. What seems apparent is that Patañjali's line of discourse has been building up to its crescendo, which comes in the final *sūtras* of the chapter where it is revealed how all the previous discussion has been a preparation for an understanding of the nature of *samādhi*. Now we are told that the four *samāpattis* described in the previous *sūtras* are in fact a form of *samādhi*; it is *sa-bīja samādhi*. And as the concluding *sūtras* of the chapter will demonstrate, we can now see that *samāpatti* is not the ultimate stage of yogic perfection, for beyond *samāpatti*, which is *sa-bīja samādhi*, there is also *nir-bīja samādhi*, which does indeed represent that ultimate stage. So what we can now recognise is the manner in which Patañjali has been offering us a progressive path from *citta-prasādana*, which is purificatory, to *samāpatti*, which is the preliminary state of *samādhi*, and finally through to *nir-bīja samādhi*, which is presented to us in the final *sūtra* of the chapter, indicating that this is the ultimate stage of yogic perfection.

Vyāsa here summarises the previous teachings by pointing out that *samāpatti* has been explained as fourfold: *sa-vitarka*, *nir-vitarka*, *sa-vicāra*, and *nir-vicāra*, with the distinction between *vitarka* and *vicāra* defined by whether the object of concentration is a gross manifestation as an individual object or the subtle ideal form respectively. Śaṅkara explains that *samāpatti* is *sa-bīja samādhi* because it has an object on which to focus, even where it is the subtle form of the object. The object on which the mind rests in absorbed concentration is the 'seed' indicated by the word *bīja*. Vācaspati Miśra adds that the four forms of *samāpatti* delineated by Vyāsa also indicate that there are four forms of perception and four identities of the knower who undertakes the *samāpatti*. Vijñāna Bhikṣu comments more fully here and reminds us of the term *saṁprajñāta* from *sūtra* 1.17, which he says is to be understood as equivalent to *samāpatti* and hence *sa-bīja samādhi*, debating at some length with an imagined opponent to demonstrate that this must be the case.

Sūtras 1.47 to 1.51: The Attainment of Nirbīja Samādhi

In these last five *sūtras* of the *Samādhi-pāda*, we have the final ascent to the ultimate stage of Yoga practice, referred to in *sūtra* 1.51 as *nir-bīja samādhi*. We are now moving beyond the concentration of *samāpatti*, which is *sa-bīja samādhi*, and which has as its highest stage *nir-vicārā samāpatti*, which is a focus on the primal form of a subtle object. In this final passage, *sūtras* 1.47 to 1.50 describe the elevated state of consciousness that is achieved as a result of *nir-vicārā samāpatti*, but then the conclusion of the chapter as a whole is given in the final *sūtra* with the statement that even this higher state must ultimately be transcended so that the adept can enter the form of yogic perfection designated as *nir-bīja samādhi*. This represents the ultimate triumph of the yogic endeavour and, looking ahead, it is this state of mental and emotional transcendence that brings *kaivalya*, the liberation of *puruṣa* from bondage and rebirth.

1.47 *nirvicāra-vaiśāradye 'dhyātma-prasādaḥ*

When one's mind becomes clear through *samāpatti* free of reflection *(nir-vicāra)*, one gains a serenity directly related to the ātman.

Here we have a reappearance of the word *prasāda*, in this context meaning tranquillity or serenity, but now in compound with the word *adhyātma*, so that what is being considered in this *sūtra* is the serenity of *adhyātma*. This of course raises the question as to what is meant by *adhyātma*, and although there are different definitions offered by different texts, the more usual understanding would be that *adhyātma* means 'in relation to the *ātman*', with *ātman* as an alternative term for *puruṣa*, the eternal spiritual entity that is the source of life in all of us.

In the *Bhagavad-gītā* (8.3), Kṛṣṇa defines *adhyātma* as *svabhāva*, the inherent nature with which we are born, but we should also note that one of the principal Sāṁkhya treatises of the *Mahābhārata* (*Śānti-parvan*, Chapter 187) is entitled the *Adhyātma Kathana*, the treatise on *adhyātma*, and the main focus of that passage is on seeking to establish a person's true spiritual identity. Hence I think what we can recognise here is a progression from the idea of focusing on the elements of *prakṛti* in their most subtle form towards the type of meditation on the *ātman* that is a dominant theme of the *Bhagavad-gītā*'s sixth chapter. This serenity comes not so much from stilling the mind by concentration on a single object, but from the realisation of *viveka*, discrimination between body and soul, which is the primary aim of Yoga practice. This *adhyātma-prasāda* comes as a result of what is referred to as *nirvicāra-vaiśāradya*. We have already learned that *nirvicāra* is to be understood as the most advanced stage of *samāpatti*, when the focus of the mind is on the subtle nature of objects rather than individual objects themselves, and the word *vaiśāradya* can mean either expertise or clarity. Either of these meanings could be applied here and Vyāsa does not give any indication of which of them he accepts. In either case, the meaning of the *sūtra* would be that proficiency in the highest form of *samāpatti* leads to a form of spiritual serenity related to the *ātman* rather than to the mind, body, or any material object.

Vyāsa indicates that the state of yogic proficiency being referred to here is one of purity in which all mental contaminations are removed and the quality of *sattva*, representing light, wisdom, and virtue, is unmixed with *rajas* or *tamas*. The *yogin* now looks upon the world without involvement in its transformations, just as a person looks down from a mountain top observing the world below. Vyāsa links *adhyātma-prasāda* with *sphuṭaḥ prajñālokaḥ*, 'a clear light of insight', which suggests that he understands *adhyātma* as that part of the mind in which the *prajñā* takes place. Śaṅkara makes a similar point regarding the purifying effects of *samāpatti*, which rids a *yogin* of the contamination of greed, selfishness, and hatred. When such impurity is thus washed away by the cleansing effect of yogic practice, then the light of true knowledge shines from within. This is knowledge of the *ātman*, as indicated by the phrase *adhyātma-prasāda*. Alternatively, the word *viveka* in Śaṅkara's commentary could be understood as 'capacity for insight', which would bring his commentary more in line with Vyāsa's and also avoid attributing to him the view that the highest goal of yoga is already achieved at this stage.

Vācaspati Miśra applies the meaning of clarity or cleansed to the word *vaiśāradya*, noting Vyāsa's reference to the impurity that is removed by yogic practice. This impurity is to be understood as the influence of the *guṇas* of *rajas* and *tamas*; Yoga removes the influence of these *guṇas* so that *sattva* shines forth alone, free from the taints of *rajas* and *tamas*. Vijñāna Bhikṣu states that the impurity Vyāsa discusses is *pāpa*, the wickedness that arises from self-centred involvement with the world. He does not accept the view that *adhyātma* refers to the innermost spiritual self, stating instead that it relates to the *buddhi,* the most refined of our intellectual faculties, although he also asserts that the clarity referred to brings the ability to distinguish *prakṛti* from *puruṣa*.

1.48 *ṛtaṁ-bharā tatra prajñā*

The realisation acquired in this way is laden with *ṛta,* absolute truth.

Now we have a short *sūtra* in which Patañjali describes the *prajñā,* the knowledge, wisdom, or realisation that comes as a consequence of this advanced state of *samāpatti*. This *prajñā* is said here to be *ṛtaṁ-bhara,* which means laden or filled with truth. This *ṛta,* this truth, is equivalent to the wisdom of Sāṁkhya, but here it is clear that it comes from within as a result of the realisation that comes through Yoga practice rather than from any external source, such as the words of a *guru* or sacred text. This is a vitally important point in the context of Indian religious thought where it is frequently asserted that the highest knowledge cannot be gained from any external source. In Śaivite teachings, we are told that all knowledge, all *prajñā,* is present within us, but is covered over by *mala,* contamination of the heart. When that covering is removed, then full knowledge shines forth without the need for any external teaching of doctrine. It would seem that it is this same idea that is being referred to here, and one is reminded of the life of Ramana Maharshi, who said that realisation came to him in a flash when he was a still a young man without his possessing any real knowledge of religious doctrine.

Vyāsa states that the knowledge that comes to the *yogin* is laden with truth because within it, there is no trace of error. The *pramāṇas,* the means by which knowledge is gained, were stated in *sūtra* 7 to be perception, inference, and tradition, but here Vyāsa cites a verse which adds the wisdom acquired through *dhyāna*, meditation, which is included along with scripture and inference whilst ignoring perception, either because the author of the verse regards normal perception as inadequate for perceiving the highest truth or because he takes the vision attained through Yoga as a special form of perception. Śaṅkara expands on the verse cited in Vyāsa's commentary by stating that learning from scripture or a teacher is the first stage of realisation; this is followed by logical analysis of such teachings so that they can be absorbed and properly understood; but the final stage of error-free knowledge is attained only through the inner realisation derived from meditation.

Interestingly, Vācaspati Miśra refers here to a famous path to knowledge outlined in a verse from Śaṅkarācārya's *Viveka Cūḍāmaṇi* (verse 364), which states that knowledge comes from, first, *śruti*, listening to scripture, then, *manana*, contemplating what has been heard, and, finally, *nididhyāsana*, deep meditation on that teaching. This is clearly relevant to what is being said here, which is why Vācaspati Miśra refers to it, but it is perhaps noteworthy that the commentary attributed to Śaṅkarācārya does not use these terms, perhaps because the commentary on the *Yoga Sūtras* was composed before the *Viveka Cūḍāmaṇi*. Vijñāna Bhikṣu relates the *sūtra* to the triple process of hearing, contemplation, and deep meditation, mentioned by Vācaspati Miśra, concluding that the *ṛtaṁ-bharā prajñā* is the result of the deep meditation, the *nididhyāsana*.

1.49 *śrutānumāna-prajñābhyām anya-viṣayā viśeṣārthatvāt*

This realisation has a different object to that acquired through the scriptures or through

> inference, because it is a particular object
> that is focused upon.

The key compound in this *sūtra* is *viśeṣa-arthatvāt,* which indicates that the object of knowledge gained through *nir-vicāra samāpatti* is *viśeṣa,* a word that means particularity or individuality. As an adjective, *viśeṣa* can also mean superior or special. This is contrasted with the *prajñā,* the wisdom or realisation, that is gained from scripture, or the logical reasoning of inference. The contention would seem to be that scripture and inference bring a form of knowledge that is general rather than specific, knowledge that offers truths about categories of things rather than about specific objects. *Samāpatti,* however, is fixed concentration on a specific object in a manner that absorbs absolute knowledge of that object into the consciousness of the practitioner. Hence it is said that this process has a different focus, *anya-viṣaya,* to the wide ranging, general conclusions that scripture and inference bring us. One might be tempted to regard the word *viśeṣa* as indicating that the knowledge derived from Yoga practice is hence superior to that gained from scripture and reasoning, but this may not be Patañjali's intention.

In relation to the sources of knowledge delineated in *sūtra* 1.7, it is interesting to note that of the three given there, scripture, inference, and perception, only two are mentioned here, with perception being omitted. One might therefore conclude that the intense concentration of *samāpatti* is a form of perception. In most of the Vedāntic systems, sensory perception is regarded as an inferior means of knowing because of the limited range of the senses in relation to spiritual truths, but what seems to be suggested here is that there is a non-sensory form of yogic perception, the *yogi-pratyakṣa* that is sometimes referred to in other texts, which brings a type of knowledge beyond even that offered through the revelation of scripture.

A word of caution is perhaps called for here. It is made clear that this type of yogic knowing comes only at the point of perfection in *nir-vicāra samāpatti,* which is in fact a form of *samādhi.* If we practice meditation, we may get a variety of ideas entering the mind during the course of meditation, but one must be cautious in presuming that this is the higher knowledge spoken of here. It is far more likely that such ideas are in fact *vṛttis* that move into the mind that is still as yet unrestrained.

Vyāsa makes the same point as that outlined above, pointing out that scripture and inference bring revelations of a general nature rather than relating to specific objects, as is the case with *samāpatti.* He also makes the point that this yogic means of knowing is not to be confused with the conventional mode of perception enacted through the five senses. Vyāsa insists that the knowledge gained by this means can be of *puruṣa* as well as the subtle form of material objects.

Śaṅkara reiterates the point that this is a form of knowledge through perception that is available only through *samāpatti* and is not to be confused with our normal sensory perception of the world. Vācaspati Miśra explores this difference further, explaining why it is that only this type of yogic perception is designated as *ṛtaṁ-bhara,* laden with truth. Our normal mode of perception through the senses and mind is affected by the *guṇas* of *rajas* and *tamas,* which prevent the absorption of the highest knowledge. Successful execution of *samāpatti* restricts the influence of *rajas* and *tamas* so that *sattva* shines through without admixture with these other two; thereby *samāpatti* brings knowledge that is laden with truth. Vijñāna Bhikṣu points out that the knowledge we acquire from scripture or from logical inference will be formulated in words, whereas the knowledge derived from *samādhi* does not take any such form. It goes beyond knowledge based on sequential reasoning and conceptualisation, and is simply a state of knowingness.

1.50 *taj-jaḥ saṁskāro 'nya-saṁskāra-pratibandhī*

The latent impression on the mind (*saṁskāra*) generated by this realisation serves to neutralise other saṁskāras.

Here the subject of discussion is *saṁskāra* and the effects of *prajñā*, the realisation obtained in *samāpatti*, which is *sa-bīja samādhi*, on the *saṁskāras*. So what is meant by *saṁskāra*? The idea is that every thought or idea that passes through the mind leaves an impression behind, and it is this process that underlies the progression of karma from one life to another as the subtle, mental embodiment transmigrates to another physical form along with the transmigrating *puruṣa*. As the *Bhagavad-gītā* repeatedly asserts, it is not physical actions that generate karma, but the state of consciousness that motivates the action. Hence constantly throughout life, we are reformulating our mental identity and, in a sense, recreating ourselves.

The accumulated *saṁskāras* left by thoughts and mental conditions bring us to another state of life; positive, wholesome, benign, and compassionate states of mind provoke corresponding actions and these lead us to a more elevated state of existence, whereas angry or malicious states of mind drag us downwards as karma unfolds. The idea is that the progression of rebirth is carried forward due to the accumulated *saṁskāras* with which our mental embodiment is marked. Here, however, Patañjali speaks of the *saṁskāras* left by *prajñā*, the realisation obtained during the practice of *samāpatti*, and states that these purifying *saṁskāras* have the effect of neutralising or impeding the *saṁskāras* arising from mundane states of consciousness, both good and bad, and thereby facilitate liberation from all karma, and hence from the cycle of action and rebirth.

Vyāsa suggests that the process being referred to here is about the *saṁskāras* produced from the *samādhi-prajñā*, the realisation in the state of *samādhi* preventing the awakening of the previously existing *saṁskāras* from their latent state. This understanding of the *sūtra* is certainly suggested by the word *pratibandhin*, which means blocking or impeding rather than destroying. Śaṅkara builds on this idea by stating that the *saṁskāra* generated by *samādhi* effectively seals off the previously existing *saṁskāras* that have been produced by the conventional movements of the mind and prevents them from having any future influence on the *yogin*. He also dismisses any suggestion that these *samādhi saṁskāras* might themselves come to fruition in the future, stating that their very nature is of '*saṁskāras* of inhibition' (Trans. Leggett), and therefore not sources of any unwanted movements of the mind.

Vācaspati Miśra reiterates this same idea, though one presumes without any knowledge of Śaṅkara's commentary, and states that the only movement of these *samādhi saṁskāras* is towards *viveka-jñāna*, the knowledge of the absolute distinction between *prakṛti* and *puruṣa* that brings liberation. Vijñāna Bhikṣu explains Vyāsa's comments as meaning that when the movements of the mind are wholly restrained through the attainment of *samādhi*, then the *saṁskāras* associated with such *vṛttis* are equally restrained and so can have no effect in giving rise to future karmic results. However, this suppression of *saṁskāras* applies only to those that are still in a latent state; *saṁskāras* that are awakened and active must run their course. Moreover, continual practice of Yoga is essential to ensure that *samādhi saṁskāras* are continually produced in order to prevent the awakening of the unwanted latent *saṁskāras*.

1.51 *tasyāpi nirodhe sarva-nirodhān nirbījaḥ samādhiḥ*

When even that *saṁskāra* is also restricted,
everything is restricted, and the state known as
nir-bīja samādhi, seedless *samādhi*, is attained.

This final *sūtra* of the *Samādhi-pāda* brings the discussion of the chapter to its logical conclusion. The previous group of *sūtras* has explained how it is that *sa-bīja samādhi* stills the movements of the mind and prevents the latent *saṁskāras* from becoming active and furthering the karmic bondage endured by *puruṣa*. And when that has been finally achieved through the triumph of the *yogin*'s practice, there is no longer any need for *sa-bīja samādhi*; its aim is fulfilled. The point is that *sa-bīja samādhi,* the fulfilment of *samāpatti,* also generates a *saṁskāra,* albeit one that has a positive, purifying effect, and as the ultimate aim is to be free of *saṁskāras,* the final stage of yogic progression means that this too must be set aside to leave a state of untrammelled clarity, designated as *nir-bīja samādhi, samādhi* that is the stillness of the mind devoid of any object.

Commenting on this *sūtra,* Vyāsa writes, '. . . the mind with its power exhausted, turns away (from its activity) together with the *saṁskāras* that lead to liberation' (Trans. Rukmani). He thereby indicates that what is being attained here is not just the cessation of the movements of the mind through fixed *samādhi,* but the liberation of *puruṣa* from its association with *prakṛti,* in other words *kaivalya.* Therefore, Vyāsa concludes his commentary on this chapter with the statement, 'When the mind turns away (from activity) the *puruṣa* stays in its own essence and is therefore called *śuddha, kevala, mukta,* pure, isolated, free' (Trans. Rukmani). This is the perfection of the yogic endeavour. Śaṅkara reiterates these observations, but adds that the existence of the purifying *saṁskāras* is demonstrated by the fact that one's ability to restrain the movements of the mind increases progressively along with practice; this heightened ability is due to the presence of these liberating *saṁskāras.*

Vācaspati Miśra builds upon this latter point, stating, 'according to the degree of perfection in passionlessness and in practice, perfection of restriction is experienced by the yogin' (Trans. Woods). In other words, one's success in cultivating *samādhi* will be marked by equivalent progression in the stilling of the movements of the mind. Vijñāna Bhikṣu draws a direct link between this *sūtra* and the ending of *punar-janma*, repeated births. He thus further asserts that as it is the *saṁskāras* that project *puruṣa* towards rebirth along with its mental embodiment, the removal of all *saṁskāras* terminates the progression of rebirth. Thus we can observe how this final passage of the opening chapter draws us towards the full conclusion of the Sāṁkhya and Yoga systems. Both are created and expounded with the sole aim of providing the embodied *puruṣa* with a means of breaking free from rebirth, suffering, and death, and it is on this particular conclusion that the *Samādhi-pāda* presents its final statement.

Conclusion

This study of the *Samādhi-pāda* has introduced us to a number of rather complex ideas, along with understandings of the path of meditation that might be unfamiliar. I have tried to cover these points in a manner that does justice to that complexity but at the same time renders the ideas interesting and accessible. Following on from the analysis of the obstacles that can inhibit one's ability to successfully undertake the practice of Yoga, we next encountered an outline of the progressive steps along the path to full yogic perfection. First of all, we had the preliminaries which have a purifying effect and create a mentality designated as *citta-prasādana,* serenity of mind. The next stage referred to was *samāpatti,* the intense concentration of the mind on a single object, which was shown to be of four types in a progression of successive achievement culminating in *nir-vicāra samāpatti* in which the mind is focused unwaveringly on the subtle, absolute identity of an object, beyond its own specific position in space and time. We were then informed that the four states of *samāpatti* were in fact a form of *samādhi, sa-bīja samādhi*. The purification of the mind in *nir-vicāra samāpatti* prepares the mind for a direct cognition of the object of meditation or contemplation. This cognition or realisation (*prajñā*) creates impressions on the mind, *saṁskāras,* which inhibit the fructification of the latent *saṁskāras* that generate karma and future rebirth. When that process of inhibition is complete, then even that highest level of *samāpatti* can be set aside as the progression of achievement proceeds to the final stage of *nir-bīja samādhi*. This represents the absolute cessation of the movements of the mind, as referred to in the second *sūtra,* and it is at this point that the adept attains the ultimate goal of Sāṁkhya and of Yoga, *kaivalya,* liberation from the bondage of rebirth.

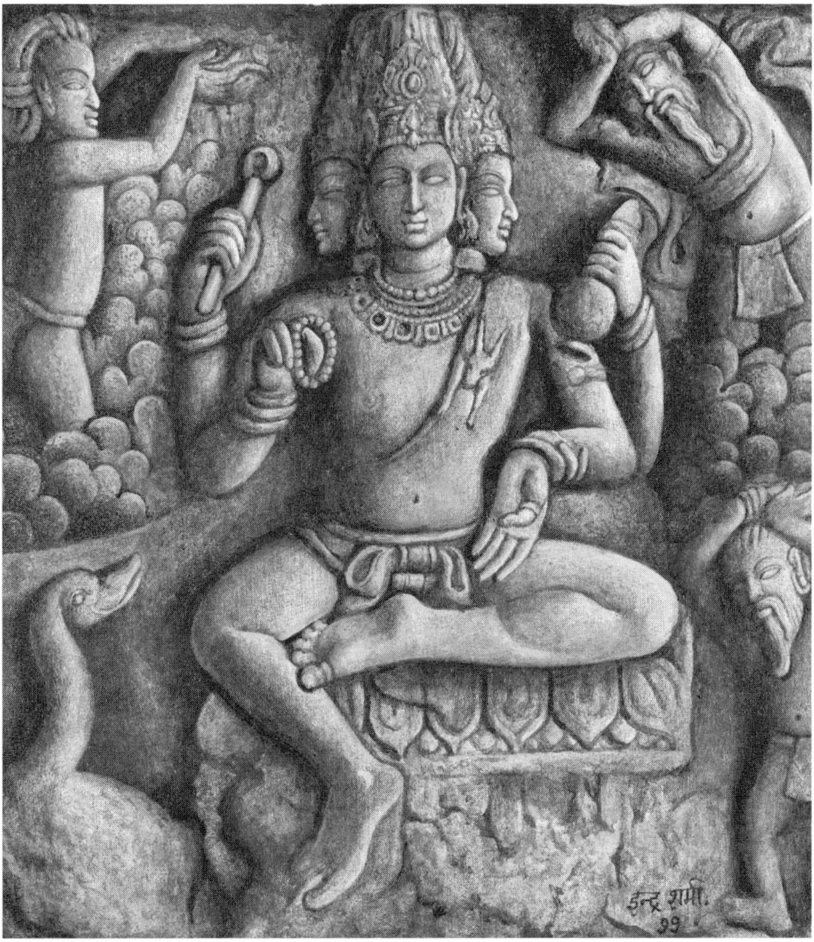

The true identity of the perceived world is that it exists solely for the sake of the seer.—2.21

II
THE *SĀDHANA-PĀDA*

The second chapter of the *Yoga Sūtras* is entitled the *Sādhana-pāda*. The word *sādhana* comes from the verbal root *sādh*, which literally means 'to travel straight towards a goal', hence, as you might expect, *sādhana* indicates the proper means to achieve the goal. The term is still commonly employed in contemporary Hinduism to indicate the regulated practices or rituals undertaken in religious life. Thus, whilst the *Samādhi-pāda* focused primarily on mental states, and the stilling of the mind, this second section deals with the practical steps by which this is achieved, and thereby introduces the eight limbs of Yoga. Before Patañjali moves his discussion directly on to the *sādhana*, however, there are extensive preliminaries to go through; the chapter is probably best understood as falling into three units of discourse.

The opening section, including *sūtras* 2.1 to 2.17, deals primarily with the problem of human existence, which is analysed in terms somewhat similar to Buddhist teaching. As the Buddha taught in his first noble truth, life according to Patañjali is predominated by affliction and suffering, which arises as karmic reactions come to fruition. This then is the problem faced by all living beings, but in the second section of the chapter (*sūtras* 2.18 to 2.27), it is revealed that the problem can be resolved, and that in fact the material manifestation exists solely for the purpose of enabling the *ātman* to liberate itself from affliction, a view that is also to be found in Īśvara Kṛṣṇa's *Sāṁkhya Kārikā* (60–68). Once these two preliminary points have been made, the second half of the chapter is given over to directly addressing the issue of *sādhana* as the eight limbs of Yoga practice are delineated and the first five discussed in more detail.

One might be tempted to suggest that a direct Buddhist influence can be detected in the division of the chapter into these three areas of discussion. These can certainly be equated with three of Buddha's four noble truths, and the fact that there are eight limbs of Yoga and an eightfold path prescribed by the Buddha may or may not be coincidental. It is also the case that, at the time when the *Yoga Sūtras* was probably composed, Buddhist thought had a position of great significance in Indian religion, and recent scholarship has showed that in many cases the *Yoga Sūtras* share terminology and ideas with Buddhist Abhidharma and Yogācāra in particular. Yet, it may not be helpful to think about the elements of the *Yoga Sūtras* as being exclusively 'Hindu' or 'Buddhist'. What seems likely is that there was a reservoir of ideas that were current in this period, which was dipped into at different times by those who followed the Buddha, and equally freely by Jains, Vedāntists, and others. One could even argue that the Buddha borrowed some of his ideas from the Yoga teachings he encountered on his travels, but again this type of assertion is probably too simplistic.

So let us now go forward to explore the ideas contained in the *Sādhana-pāda*, which offers the reader a presentation of the main forms of practice that bring the goals sought by the ancient practitioners of Yoga.

Sūtras 2.1–2.2: Kriyā-yoga

2.1 *tapaḥ-svādhyāyeśvara-praṇidhānāni kriyā-yogaḥ*

Kriyā-yoga consists of religious austerity (*tapas*), recitation (*svādhyāya*), and worship of the Lord (*īśvara-praṇidhāna*).

In its opening *sūtra*, the *Sādhana-pāda* commences with a brief discussion of what it refers to as *kriyā-yoga*, literally Yoga based on action. The definition it provides of this *kriyā-yoga*, of which we have heard nothing up till this point, is threefold, expressed by the terms *tapas*, *svādhyāya*, and *īśvara-praṇidhāna*. The idea of *tapas* is frequently encountered in Indian religious teachings and generally refers to acts of restraint, such as fasting or even harsher forms of austerity that are aimed at the deliberate mortification of the body in a manner that causes physical suffering. The *Bhagavad-gītā* is decidedly unenthusiastic about actions of this type and offers instead a more balanced form of *tapas* that consists largely of following a gentle, restrained lifestyle (17.14–16).

Svādhyāya can mean either study or recitation, or even the inward examination of oneself, but, as this is *kriyā-yoga*, I have chosen to regard it as meaning the recitation of sacred texts, a view that finds support from the *Gītā*, which includes *svādhyāya* as one of the means by which the *tapas* of the voice is undertaken. We have, of course, encountered *īśvara-praṇidhāna* before, in *sūtras* 1.23 to 1.28 of the *Samādhi-pāda*, but its inclusion here under the heading of *kriyā-yoga* indicates that it is to be understood as the physical actions of worship, such as are typically enacted in the temple or the home, rather than the internal meditation on the presence of the Deity that is described in Chapter Eight of the *Bhagavad-gītā*.

In his introduction to this *sūtra*, Vyāsa claims that it teaches yoga suitable for those whose mind is agited, whereas the previous teachings refer to a person whose mind is already concentrated (*samāhita*). In other words, the first chapter of the *Yoga Sūtras*, the *Samādhi-pāda*, mostly deals with advanced states of *samādhi*, but the *kriyā-yoga* of this *sūtra* is the means by which that state of concentration, *samādhi*, can be achieved. Vyāsa explains that *tapas* is necessary for a *yogin* as a means of ensuring that attraction for the pleasures of the world is reduced, though he implies that it should not be so harsh in its execution that it causes a disturbance to the tranquil mind. *Svādhyāya* is the recitation of a mantra such as *oṁ* or study of treatises on liberation (*mokṣa-śāstra*), whilst *īśvara-praṇidhāna* is explained in a way that reminds one of the *Gītā*'s understanding of *karma-yoga*. Action is to be performed without selfish desire as an offering to the Lord, as is asserted in 18.47 of the *Gītā*.

Śaṅkara states that *kriyā-yoga* is to be understood as an essential prerequisite for the practice of the meditational yoga that leads to *samādhi*, thereby seeking to integrate this passage into the wider scheme of Patañjali's teachings. Vācaspati Miśra also states that this *kriyā-yoga* is to be understood as providing the preliminary purification that reduces the effect of *saṁskāras* in order for the full techniques of Yoga practice to be successfully enacted. He also cites a verse (2.47) from the *Bhagavad-gītā* on *karma-yoga* as an explanation of what is meant here by *īśvara-praṇidhāna*. Vijñāna Bhikṣu comments at greater length than the others on this *sūtra*, but follows essentially the same line by explaining why the practice of *kriyā-yoga* is an essential prerequisite for undertaking the internal form of Yoga that will be outlined later on, citing verses from the *Mahābhārata* and Purāṇas to support his argument.

2.2 *samādhi-bhāvanārthaḥ kleśa-tanū-karaṇārthaś ca*

The purpose of *kriyā-yoga* is to achieve the state of *samādhi* and diminish afflictions.

This is another relatively simple *sūtra* to understand as it presents the *arthas*, the purposes or goals, of *kriyā-yoga* as being twofold: firstly, to assist in the attainment of the state of *samādhi* and, secondly, to diminish the *kleśas*, the obstructions, faults, or afflictions, that inhibit one's ability to achieve *samādhi*. This leads us progressively into the next group of *sūtras*, which offer an explanation of the nature of these *kleśas*.

Vyāsa comments only briefly here, stating that the diminishing of the *kleśas* allows for the development of the *viveka-jñāna* that distinguishes *puruṣa* from its material embodiment and thereby brings liberation from rebirth. Śaṅkara goes a little further and suggests that this discriminative spiritual wisdom comes through meditation, which is successful in the absence of *kleśas*. *Jñāna* of this type cannot be gained simply by reading sacred texts, but requires the higher realisation that comes only through inward meditation. Vācaspati Miśra states that *kriyā-yoga* can limit the effect of the *kleśas* but not destroy them completely; nonetheless, the weakening of their influence still allows discriminative knowledge to arise, so that one begins to experience the distinction between the true self and its embodiment. Vijñāna Bhikṣu makes a similar point, expressing the view that a weakening of the *kleśas* still prevents them from leaving behind *saṁskāras*, unwanted impressions on the mind and intellect.

Sūtras 2.3–2.9: The Afflictions that Kriyā-yoga Diminishes

This next group of *sūtras* focuses on the *kleśas* that the practice of *kriyā-yoga* can diminish. First of all, they are listed as ignorance, egotism, hankering, aversion, and attachment to life. It is then stated that *avidyā*, literally the absence of true knowledge, is the basis of the other four, and then each of them is defined in turn.

2.3 *avidyāsmitā-rāga-dveṣābhiniveśāḥ kleśāḥ*

The afflictions are ignorance, egotism, hankering, aversion, and attachment to life.

This is a simple enough *sūtra* that provides a list of the five *kleśas* referred to in *sūtra* 2.2 as the obstructions that prevent the development of *viveka-jñāna* and hence the attainment of liberation from rebirth. Vyāsa comments only briefly here, stating that the *kleśas* strengthen the effect of the *guṇas* and enhance the process of cause and effect by which the law of karma holds its predominance over each embodied being.

Śaṅkara elaborates further on the nature of these *kleśas,* stating that they should not be regarded as states of mind but rather as impurities that contaminate the mind. He cites a verse from the *Bhagavad-gītā* (3.38) that states that *kāma,* lust or desire, acts as a covering that obscures the true self and prevents knowledge of the self from arising. Vācaspati Miśra explains that all these *kleśas* are symptoms of *a-viveka-jñāna,* the false knowledge that fails to recognise the distinction between *puruṣa* and *prakṛti,* the true spiritual self and its material embodiment. It is because we identify ourselves with the body that egotism, hankering, and aversion are all present within our state of mind. Vijñāna Bhikṣu points out that the five *kleśas* should not be understood as acting independently. Rather, they are all closely related to each other and act on our limited state of mind in a concerted manner.

2.4 *avidyā kṣetram uttareṣāṁ prasupta-tanu-vicchinnodārāṇām*

Ignorance is the basis of the other *kleśas,* whether they be dormant, diminished occasional, or active.

This *sūtra* provides us with two significant indications about the nature of the *kleśas.* First of all, they can exist within us in a number of different forms; they may be in a dormant state awaiting certain stimuli that can awaken them; they may be manifest in our mental faculties but only to a slight degree due to being diminished; or they may be active and overtly present in the states of mind we manifest. Secondly, we are told that one of them, *avidyā,* ignorance, is the *kṣetra* of the other four.

The word *kṣetra* literally means 'a field', but we often find it being used metaphorically in philosophical works. Here the meaning would appear to be that ignorance is the fertile ground from which the other four *kleśas* sprout and blossom. In other words, ignorance is the basis on which egotism, hankering, aversion, and attachment to life are present within us.

Vyāsa explains that the dormant state is a pure potentiality in the mind. The *kleśa* becomes active when its object or 'support' (*ālambana*) is present. The diminshed state occurs when the *kleśa* begins to become manifest but is prevented from developing by the adoption of appropriate means. The occasional state is where the *kleśa* appears and is inhibited, but then appears again, latching on to some other stimulus. Hence it is not ever-present but continually reappears. The active state is that in which the *kleśa* is permanently present and exists without restriction or interruption. Vyāsa also discusses a fifth state, not mentioned in the *sūtra*, one in which the *kleśas* exist like burnt seeds. They are unable to sprout even when the objects that give rise to their development appear before them; in other words, even when a desirable object appears before the mind, the *kleśa* of hankering does not arise, and even when something revolting is present, no sense of aversion appears. A person whose *kleśas* have thus been destroyed (*kṣīṇa*) is called 'final-body' (*carama-deha*), which means that this person has taken on a body for the last time and will not be reborn again as there is no more karmic seed to bring about rebirth. Śaṅkara asserts that, although the other four *kleśas* may exist in a dormant state, this is not the case for *avidyā*, for that condition of ignorance is always present until the state of enlightenment is achieved through Yoga practice. He further comments at some length, exploring each of four states in which a *kleśa* may exist in a degree of detail that is beyond the present scope of discussion. Vācaspati Miśra further discusses the dormant state, explaining that this is different from a wholesale absence of the *kleśas* because they still exist in a potential form. He further reminds us that the means by which the *kleśas* are made dormant, diminished, or occasional is the practice of *kriyā-yoga* as set out in the first two *sūtras* of this chapter. Vijñāna Bhikṣu refers approvingly to the commentary of Vācaspati Miśra, confirming his view that it is true knowledge that counteracts *avidyā* and thereby inhibits the development of all five of the *kleśas* listed in the previous *sūtra*.

2.5 *anityāśuci-duḥkhānātmasu nitya-śuci-sukhātma-khyātir avidyā*

Avidyā, ignorance, is defined as regarding the temporary as permanent, the impure as pure, distress as pleasure, and thinking that which is not the self to be the self.

All of the points made here in the definition of *avidyā* relate to the absence of *viveka-jñāna*, the discriminating knowledge that enables us to see our true spiritual identity as something apart from the physical and mental embodiment. In the absence of this realised knowledge, we accept the present embodiment as our own true and permanent identity; we look upon the embodiment as our pure state of being when, in fact, it is an impure state that obscures the pure spiritual identity of the true self; we regard sensual delights as real pleasure rather than the spiritual joy that comes from within; and we regard that which is *anātman* as the *ātman*, in other words, we see this bodily form as the *ātman* without any awareness of the spiritual *ātman*, which is our true state of being. This is the condition of ignorance, the field in which the other *kleśas* grow and flourish, the great obstacle to the state of enlightenment sought by the *yogin*.

Vyāsa comments along the lines referred to above and, regarding the second item of the list, emphasises the impurity of the material body, with all its internal fluids such as blood and bile. Regarding the mistaken identification of the self (*ātman*), he mentions not just the body but also the mind (*manas*) as different from the *ātman*. Śaṅkara follows Vyāsa closely here in insisting on the impure nature of the material form, though he rejects an imagined opponent's view that there is therefore no point in washing the body. He also adds a lengthy discourse that builds further on Vyāsa's discussion of the nature of negative nouns like *avidyā*. Vācaspati Miśra is similarly preoccupied with this grammatical discussion, the main point being to determine whether *avidyā* is an actual entity with a power of its own or whether it is simply the absence of knowledge. Vijñāna Bhikṣu is particularly anxious to reject the view that this *sūtra* might indicate that the world is an unreal illusion, as is taught within the school of Advaita Vedānta, which follows the ideas of the original Śaṅkarācārya. He cites a verse of the *Bhagavad-gītā* (2.16) which he interprets in such a way as to demonstrate that the world is real as perceived and not the illusion emphasised by the system of Advaita. The body may be temporary, *a-nitya*, whilst the true self is eternal, *nitya*, but this is not the same as saying that the temporary embodiment is unreal.

2.6 *dṛg-darśana-śaktyor ekātmatevāsmitā*

> Egoism is when the seer and the power of seeing appear one and the same.

Here we see how it is that the four other *kleśas* grow out from the field of *avidyā*. It is because of ignorance of our higher, spiritual identity that *asmitā*, the sense of ego, is present. The *viveka-jñāna*, the power of discrimination sought through Yoga practice, establishes the principle of *anyo 'ham*, 'I am different', referred to in early Sāṁkhya treatises in the *Mahābhārata*. But in the absence of that discriminative knowledge, one fails to recognise the distinction between body and soul, and thus regards the seer of an object as identical to the power of perception by means of which the object is perceived. This is what is meant by *asmitā*, egoism, which is the first fruit that appears in the field of *avidyā*.

Vyāsa confirms that the seer mentioned here is *puruṣa*, the spiritual entity that is our true identity, and he relates the *darśana-śakti*, the power of seeing, to *buddhi*, the intellect that is supreme amongst our mental faculties. *Puruṣa* and *buddhi* are distinct, for *buddhi* is an element of *prakṛti*, but when *avidyā* gives rise to *asmitā*, this distinction is not recognised. Śaṅkara follows Vyāsa in recognising *buddhi* as being the power of seeing and points out that our mental faculties such as *buddhi* only have the appearance of sentience because of the presence of *puruṣa* in proximity to them. He also further emphasises the point that egoism is to be understood as a particular aspect of ignorance, the primary *kleśa*. Vācaspati Miśra elaborates on the idea of the utter distinction between *puruṣa* and its mental and physical embodiment, as is expressed in the *sūtra*. He writes: 'Immutability and other [qualities] are the properties of *puruṣa*; mutability and other [qualities] are the properties of *buddhi*' (Trans. Woods). *Avidyā* is the cause of the misidentification of the two and *asmitā* is the effect produced by *avidyā*. Vijñāna Bhikṣu speaks of this as a 'superimposition of identity', by which that which is utterly distinct from *buddhi* identifies itself with the experiences of *buddhi* that come to it through the senses. Only when this superimposition of a false identity is ended can *puruṣa* attain *kaivalya*, the state of liberation in which suffering and bondage are no longer experienced.

2.7 *sukhānuśayī rāgaḥ*

Hankering is the consequence that follows pleasure.

The point made here is a simple one. In this world, we experience pleasure in various forms, either through mental contemplation or through sensory perception. Once a form of pleasure has been experienced, then hankering arises as we long for a repeat of that pleasurable experience. Vyāsa comments only very briefly here, but includes the word *lobha*, meaning 'greed', under the heading of *rāga*, hankering. Śaṅkara merely suggests that this *sūtra* should be taken in conjunction with the one that follows, which relates to *dveṣa*, aversion, as these are two parts of the same mental condition. Vācaspati Miśra emphasises the role of memory in the development of hankering. It is the recollection of past pleasures that gives rise to a longing for their repeated experience. Vijñāna Bhikṣu makes the point that hankering for liberation is not to be included under the heading of *rāga*, for this moves one in the opposite direction away from the pleasures of the world that are enjoyed through the senses.

2.8 *duḥkhānuśayī dveṣaḥ*

Aversion is the consequence that follows suffering.

The form of this *sūtra* and the previous one are very similar, which is why Śaṅkara expressed the view that they should be taken together. *Rāga* is the *anuśayin*, consequence, of *sukha* and conversely, *dveṣa* is the *anuśayin* of *duḥkha*, giving us the very easy translations that we have. And again the meaning here is fairly straightforward. If we have an experience or encounter an object that leads to suffering, then we are naturally averse to any repeat of that event. The point being made here is that the state of transcendence of these *kleśas* is one in which one views the world dispassionately with a form of equal vision, very much in line with the teachings of the *Bhagavad-gītā*, which often uses phrases such as *sama-duḥkha-sukha* (2.15), meaning 'remaining equal and unmoved by one's encounters with suffering and pleasure'. Here the same point is being made with regard to the *kleśas*, and the method of *kriyā-yoga* is being prescribed as the means to reach that serene and transcendent state of mind. Vyāsa again comments only briefly, including anger and the desire to hurt others under the heading of *dveṣa*. Śaṅkara merely repeats Vyāsa's observations, whilst Vācaspati Miśra again refers to memory of past objects and events as the source of aversion. Vijñāna Bhikṣu also draws our attention to the link between this and the previous *sūtra*, stating that aversion is in fact a particular kind of hankering, presumably hankering for the absence of suffering.

2.9 *sva-rasa-vāhī viduṣo 'pi tathā rūḍho 'bhiniveśaḥ*

Even amongst men of wisdom, the longing for life flows of its own accord, and hence is firmly established.

The last of the five *kleśas* that are weakened by *kriyā-yoga* is the attachment for life that can be observed in ourselves and in almost every living being. One might feel that such attachment is entirely natural, and in one sense this *sūtra* agrees with that point, but still it is based on *avidyā*, the absence of higher knowledge. In a play, one might take the part of a character such as Julius Caesar who is murdered in the final act. One will not lament over the loss of that character's life because one knows that it is not oneself. Similarly, the highest realisation of spiritual truth brings a complete recognition of one's identity as *puruṣa*, which is entirely distinct from the present embodiment. Hence the longing for life to continue is classed as one of the four *kleśas* that arise from *avidyā*, even though that longing is present even amongst those who possess wisdom. It is a natural instinct; it flows instinctively without the need for reflection, but it is still a product of the existential ignorance of our true spiritual identity.

Vyāsa contends that this dread of death gives evidence to the fact that we have experienced the pain of death in previous lives. Without such prior experience, the instinctive dread of death would not arise in those who possess wisdom as well as in lowly creatures like worms. Śaṅkara contends that fear of death is logical for those who are ignorant of their true identity, but for those who have knowledge of that higher identity, it is wholly illogical. This is why the word *api*, meaning 'even', is added after *viduṣa*, which means 'one who possesses wisdom'. Hence we can conclude that this *abhiniveśa*, this longing for life, is instinctive rather than logical and, as Vyāsa states, must therefore be the result of the impressions on the mind left by experiences of death in past lives.

Vācaspati Miśra expands further on this same point, noting that even small children tremble at the sight of death without having any experience of what death is. This is due to the *saṁskāras*, the subtle impressions on the mind, which have been left by experiences undergone in past lives. Vijñāna Bhikṣu is similarly exercised by the question of why it is that even one who is wise should suffer from this particular *kleśa* but not the others. He discusses this point at some considerable length, countering hypothetical objections, but arrives at the same conclusion that this *kleśa* comes from the *saṁskāras* left by previous deaths to which all in this world are subject, whether they be wise or bereft of higher knowledge. Such mental impressions are overcome only when the full perfection of Yoga practice is achieved.

Sūtras 2.10–2.11: The Afflictions can be Overcome

Following on from the group of *sūtras* in which the specific natures of the *kleśas* are defined, Patañjali now reassures us that they can indeed be overcome by the determined aspirant. We learned earlier that *kriyā-yoga* consisted of forms of practice that have the effect of weakening the afflictions. If we follow Vyāsa's commentary on 2.11, the following two *sūtras* describe how the *kleśas* can be finally abandoned after being weakened by *kriyā-yoga*.

> 2.10 *te pratiprasava-heyāḥ sūkṣmāḥ*
>
> These afflictions in their subtle form are neutralised by turning them to their original source.

Two questions immediately come to mind on reading this *sūtra*: what is meant by the subtle state of the *kleśas*, and what is meant by turning them back to their original source. The first word, the pronoun *te*, meaning they, must refer to the *kleśas* and this is qualified by the word *sūkṣma* meaning 'subtle'. In the compound *pratiprasava-heya*, *pratiprasava* must refer to the reversal of creation (*prasava*) of the manifest world from *prakṛti*, whilst *heya* means 'to be avoided, shunned, or overcome'.

Vyāsa's short commentary certainly explains that this *sūtra* refers to the final abandonment of *kleśas* when they have become like roasted seeds, devoid of any effective potency. That is to say, the *kleśas* just naturally dissolve along with the mind of the *yogin* when it has fulfilled its purpose of achieving *kaivalya*. The word *pratiprasava* in the *sūtra* must refer to this returning of the mind to *prakṛti*, its original source. This process is the reversal of the emanation, *prasava*, of the material world from *prakṛti*, its source. As the very last *sūtra* 4.34 explains, the *pratiprasava* of the *guṇas* takes place when the final state of *kaivalya* is reached. Śaṅkara indicates that the returning to the original source of the mind and of the *kleśas* occur simultaneously because the latter are afflictions of the mind. Hence when the mind is absorbed back into *prakṛti* it must be the case that the *kleśas* afflicting the mind become sterile. Vācaspati Miśra explains that when the *kleśas* become manifest within the mind, then *kriyā-yoga* is the proper means of nullifying their effects, but when they are already in a subtle or latent form, we can no longer affect them directly through yogic practice. Expanding somewhat on Vyāsa's commentary, Vijñāna Bhikṣu suggests that *kriyā-yoga* acts to reduce the *kleśas* to a sterile state, like roasted seeds, but the teaching here refers to the removal of the *kleśas* when they are present in this sterile or latent state. This is what is meant by the idea of their existing in a subtle form, and, he suggests, it is still necessary to remove them because even from an inhibited form, the *kleśas* may begin to sprout again, just as it is sometimes seen that life may persist even in a burnt seed.

2.11 *dhyāna-heyās tad-vṛttayaḥ*

The movements of the mind they give rise to can be neutralised through meditation.

With its use of the plural form of the word *vṛtti*, this *sūtra* takes us back to the definition of Yoga given by Patañjali in the second *sūtra* (1.2) of this work: *citta-vṛtti-nirodha*, stilling the movements of the mind. In the phrase *tad-vṛttayaḥ* used here, we should probably take it that the word *tad* refers to the *kleśas*, which cause the mind to become restless. For example, hankering or aversion will give rise to all sorts of mental activity, which the practice of Yoga, as defined by the *Yoga Sūtras*, is designed to suppress. Another interpretation would be that the *vṛttis*, the movements, are the fluctuations of the *kleśas* themselves rather than movements within the mind caused by the *kleśas*. The difference, however, is quite minor, as the *kleśas* are very closely connected to our mental states. How can such movements be inhibited? The answer given here is that it is through the practice of *dhyāna*, meditation, which we will find later on included as the seventh of the eight limbs of Yoga. That though is a separate discussion, and here we are being presented with *dhyāna* as one of the means by which the disruptive influence of the *kleśas* can be neutralised.

Vyāsa refers here to a progressive process by which *kleśas* can be removed. The gross, overt, active manifestation of the *kleśas* is repressed by means of *kriyā-yoga*, so that they can then be more fully suppressed through the practice of meditation, which is what is referred to in this *sūtra*. They then exist only in their subtle form, the removal of which requires more intense forms of yogic endeavour, as described in the previous *sūtra*. Śaṅkara adds that the process of neutralising the *kleśas* becomes even more difficult after they are reduced by *kriyā-yoga* to a subtle state like burnt seeds. The final goal is to remove such seeds altogether.

Vācaspati Miśra expresses the view that one's progress in the practice of Yoga is directly related to the capacity one displays with regard to the suppression of *kleśas*. Vijñāna Bhikṣu provides us with a clear assertion that the word *tad* used here should be taken as meaning the *kleśas*, and hence the compound *tad-vṛttayaḥ* means 'the mental fluctuations invoked by the presence of the *kleśas*'. These are weakened by *kriyā-yoga* and finally removed by *asamprajñāta samādhi*, the final form of *samādhi* taught in the *Yoga Sūtras*.

Sūtras 2.12–2.14: The Kleśas as Giving Rise to Karmic Reactions

These next three *sūtras* continue the discussion of the influence of the *kleśas* over our lives and indeed our whole state of existence. Here the focus is on the Indian doctrine of karma, the law of causation by which actions give rise to future results, and the influence of the *kleśas* over the constant progression of action and reaction. This is significant in relation to the primary aim of the teachings of the *Yoga Sūtras*, which is to provide the means by which liberation from rebirth, *kaivalya*, may be attained. For this to be achieved, the cycle of karma must be brought to an end, and here we are shown why it is that the *kleśas* are such formidable obstacles to the pursuit of the highest spiritual goals of life.

2.12 *kleśa-mūlaḥ karmāśayo dṛṣṭādṛṣṭa-janma-vedanīyaḥ*

The accumulation of karma is based on these afflictions, and are experienced in seen and unseen births.

This *sūtra* considers the *karma-āśaya*, 'the accumulation of karma' that we progressively store up as we proceed through life. This is a well-known doctrine that is common to almost all strands of Indian religious thought and in the Hindu tradition is first presented in the Upaniṣads. The *sūtra* tells us two things about the *karmāśaya*. First of all, its 'root', its *mūla*, is the *kleśas* that have been discussed in the previous *sūtras*. Ignorance, egoism, hankering, aversion, and longing for life all provide an impetus for the performance of righteous and iniquitous deeds, which in turn create a *saṁskāra* on the mind out of which the results of action become manifest. Secondly, we are told that karmic results are *dṛṣṭa-adṛṣta-janma-vedanīya*, they are experienced in seen and unseen births; in other words, the results of our actions are experienced both in the present life, in which the deeds were performed, or else in a future incarnation. One might feel that the results of righteous deeds are desirable, but from the perspective of Sāṁkhya and Yoga, all karma is to be transcended, good or bad, so that one can escape completely from the endless cycle.

Vyāsa comments at some length here, discussing the ways and means by which positive and negative karma are accumulated. He classifies the causes of karma as *lobha*, *moha*, and *krodha*, greed, illusion, and anger. These states of mind arise due to the presence of the *kleśas* in an intense form, and they cause us to act with neglect towards those who are anxious, sick, or distressed, towards those who look to us for help, and towards those who are superior persons, or are undertaking acts of austerity. All of this leads to the accumulation of negative karma, and one presumes that actions of the opposite type lead to the accumulation of positive karma. With regard to positive karma, Vyāsa actually refers to intense meditation, acts of austerity, chanting *mantras*, and the worship of *īśvara*, lesser deities, and persons of high spiritual standing.

Śaṅkara, commenting on Vyāsa, explains how it is that *lobha*, 'greed' or, in this case, 'hankering' more generally, can give rise to both positive and negative forms of action, *puṇya* and *pāpa*. Hankering for existence in the realm of the gods may prompt us to perform righteous acts or sacred rituals, but hankering for other forms of pleasure may lead to sinful deeds, as in the *Mahābhārata* when Karṇa's longing for knowledge of weapons led to him telling his *guru* a lie. Vācaspati Miśra refers back to the idea that the other four *kleśas* all sprout from *avidyā*; it is that ignorance of our true identity that gives rise to feelings of hankering and aversion, which lead in turn to the performance of deeds such as theft or other harmful acts. Vijñāna Bhikṣu sees these three *sūtras* as providing an explanation of why it is that the *kleśas* must be neutralised. Life in this world is inherently beset by suffering, and the continuation of this existence is the result of the ongoing ripening of the results of karma, which is based on the *kleśas*. Therefore, the sufferings of this existence can only be brought to an end when the *kleśas* are counteracted.

2.13 *sati mūle tad-vipāko jāty-āyur-bhogāḥ*

As long as this basis exists, karma will come to fruition as the type of birth one takes, lifespan, and the fortune one experiences.

In this *sūtra*, Patañjali moves on from his previous statement by defining the precise manner in which the results of action appear in an individual's existence. This takes place as long as the 'root', the *mūla*, of karma exists, and, as we have been told, the root or basis of karma is the prevalence of the *kleśas*. Karma is defined as appearing in three forms: first of all, it relates to *jāti*, the type of birth one assumes, as one who is rich or poor, or even in divine or animal form; then there is *āyus*, the length of one's life, long life being the result of positive karma and an early death a consequence of negative karma; and finally there is *bhoga*, the variegated forms of experience. Even if we are born into a state of relative poverty, there are still many forms of pleasure to be experienced, and even a person of high status may find little pleasure in life. These three jointly comprise the ways in which our karma unfolds.

Vyāsa comments at some length here, discussing whether or not it is a single action or an accumulation of actions that gives rise to a particular birth and whether the results of an action are experienced in one birth or in a series of future incarnations. His conclusion is that one's future life is shaped by the total actions performed and that the actions performed in the present life will affect only one future birth. Nonetheless, the latent impressions, the *saṁskāras*, present within the mind of an individual remain influential over a series of incarnations. He also points out that because the actions performed by most people are a mixture of righteous and wicked deeds, the experiences we undergo contain an admixture of pleasure and suffering. Śaṅkara follows Vyāsa in commenting at length on this *sūtra*, generating in the process a fairly substantial treatise on the subject of karma and rebirth. Both Vācaspati Miśra and Vijñāna Bhikṣu also take the opportunity to provide detailed explanations of their own understandings of the progression of karmic results, but unfortunately we do not have the scope here to discuss the topic in that same level of detail.

2.14 *te hlāda-paritāpa-phalāḥ puṇyāpuṇya-hetutvāt*

These fruits then take the form of joy and misery, dependent on whether the karma is shaped by virtue or iniquity.

The meaning behind this *sūtra* appears quite straightforward, as it presents the widely understood doctrine of karma. *Hlāda* is 'pleasure', *paritāpa* is 'suffering', whilst *phala* means 'the fruits'; hence the meaning of the first phrase is that the results or fruits of action come in the form of pleasure and suffering. The second phrase indicates the causal factors that give rise to those differing results; these are *puṇya*, which means virtuous or righteous acts, and *a-puṇya*, which is exactly the opposite. Vyāsa merely paraphrases the obvious meaning of the *sūtra* and Śaṅkara follows that same pattern. Vācaspati Miśra expands slightly on the points made, stating that *jāti*, *āyus*, and *bhoga*, birth, lifespan, and experience, are in varying degrees the direct results of action, and it is these that in turn give rise to pleasure and misery. Vijñāna Bhikṣu comments at greater length, setting forth the view that pleasure and pain never exist in isolation from one another, for there will be some suffering even at times of enjoyment and, similarly, even when we are predominantly in a state of suffering, there will be some experience of happiness.

Sūtras 2.15–2.17: Suffering is an Inherent Feature of Existence

At the beginning of the *Sāṁkhya Kārikā*, Īśvara Kṛṣṇa states that the reason he has written this work is so that the suffering endured by living beings in this world can be brought to an end, and it is clear that Patañjali has a similar goal in mind when he presents his *Yoga Sūtras*. In the previous *sūtras*, it has been shown that the five *kleśas* are the causal factors underlying the continuous progression of karma, repeated action and reaction. Now the point will be made that even though some pleasure may be gained from virtuous acts, this will never put an end to the suffering that arises from negative karma. Suffering is an inherent feature of existence in this world, and the practice of Yoga is therefore prescribed as the means by which suffering can be finally brought to an end when *kaivalya* is achieved.

2.15 *pariṇāma-tāpa-saṁskāra-duḥkhair guṇa-vṛtti-virodhāc ca duḥkham eva sarvaṁ vivekinaḥ*

> Because of the misery caused by transformations, because of the suffering due to latent impressions, and because of the way in which one attribute of the world conflicts with another, discriminating persons see all life as suffering.

If we break this *sūtra* down into its component parts, it talks about the *vivekins,* those with the power of discernment, and their vision of the world is *duḥkham eva sarvam,* 'everything is just suffering', a phrase that resonates with the first of the Buddha's noble truths. The preceding words provide us with a threefold explanation for why this is the case. First of all, there is *pariṇāma-tāpa,* the misery that comes from change and transformation, the point being that all the things we achieve and gather, and the relationships we form, are eventually brought to an end due to the changes wrought by the irresistible progression of time. The second cause is *saṁskāra-duḥkha,* the suffering that arises due to the presence of *saṁskāras,* latent impressions on the mind left by previous thoughts and deeds. It is these *saṁskāras* that cause karma to fructify into the varied results previously mentioned in terms of birth, longevity, and varying experiences of pleasure. Our karma cannot be avoided and all of us have been guilty of unrighteous acts either in this or a previous life; this is another reason why suffering is inevitable. And finally, there is *guṇa-vṛtti-nirodha,* which means the inevitable conflict of one aim or attribute with another. Whatever we attempt to achieve in life, the path is rarely a smooth one, as a contrary factor arises that thwarts or inhibits our endeavours. At a most basic level, we can see how our aim of gaining good health is thwarted by the contrary progression of disease. This view of the world as a place of inevitable suffering is found in many works of Indian religion or philosophy. The *Mahābhārata* contains a series of treatises on frustrated ambitions (*Śānti-parvan,* Chapters 168 to 173), whilst the *Bhagavad-gītā* (13.8) speaks of one of the attributes of knowledge as perceiving the misery inherent in birth, death, old age, and disease. This constitutes a recognition of the existential problem of our lives; the next stage is to identify the solution.

Vyāsa again offers a substantial commentary on this *sūtra,* analysing in detail why it is that the embodied being's existence in this world is always beset by suffering of one form or another. The *vivekin* who sees the world as it truly exists is a practitioner of Yoga who thereby gains a superior understanding of the nature of the world. Such a person recognises the *kleśa* of *avidyā,* ignorance of one's true spiritual identity, as the root cause of the suffering referred to in this *sūtra*. Vyāsa interprets the first compound of the *sūtra* differently, and posits that there are three kinds of suffering (*duḥkha*). He takes *tāpa* as a third kind of suffering in addition to *pariṇāma* and *saṁskāra*. *Tāpa* appears to be suffering in a straightforward sense, being associated with *dveṣa,* as opposed to *pariṇāma,* transformation, where an initial pleasure or happiness is necessarily frustrated with the course of time. Śaṅkara also provides a detailed commentary in which he considers the nature of our existence and the inherency of suffering in our present condition of life. He explains why *duḥkham eva sarvam,* 'everything is suffering', is a valid assertion in light of the fact that people are seen to enjoy pleasure as well experience suffering. The answer is that the experience of pleasure depends on the acquisition of wealth and our schemes for prosperity inevitably bring suffering to another, and this in turn brings suffering to ourselves as the law of karma unfolds. The thought arises that this view of Śaṅkara could readily be applied to the exploitative nature of modern global capitalism. Of course, the statement could be taken as more broadly applicable to the inequality of all known human societies, including Ancient India, where kings commonly exercised violence to accumulate *artha*.

Vācaspati Miśra also provides a detailed commentary on this *sūtra*, discussing the intricacies of the process by which suffering arises and the impossibility of avoiding suffering by material means. He cites a verse from the *Bhagavad-gītā* (18.38) in which it is said that pleasure related to passion and desire is like nectar at the beginning but in the end is like poison for the suffering it brings. Our desires for pleasure remain always frustrated, for however much we experience pleasure, our desire is never satiated. It is like putting fuel on a fire; the more we fulfil our cravings, the greater those cravings become, and this in turn leads to suffering. Vijñāna Bhikṣu is similarly expansive in his discussion of this point, further entering the debate over why it is that our experience of pleasure does not prove that the assertion that 'all is just suffering' must be false. He accepts that pleasure can be experienced in this world, but contends that the experience of misery is always greater, to the extent that the inherent nature of this world is defined by the suffering we must inevitably undergo.

2.16 *heyaṁ duḥkham anāgatam*

It is, however, necessary to prevent future suffering.

Swami Vivekānanda once remarked, 'the Vedānta system begins with tremendous pessimism, and ends with real optimism', and we can observe this same point in this and the previous *sūtra*. We may be plunged into despair by the idea of *duḥkham eva sarvam*, but here the voice of optimism is heard as we are told that this situation can be remedied, and in this, we can detect an introduction to the *sādhana*, the eightfold practice that will be outlined in the second half of this chapter. There is a means of escaping the endless cycle of suffering and the means is the techniques of Yoga practice that bring the adept to the beatific state of *kaivalya*. The wording here is quite simple: *heya* means 'to be avoided, shunned, or overcome', *duḥkha* is 'suffering', and *anāgata* means 'that which has not yet arrived', giving us the optimistic rendition of the *sūtra*.

Vyāsa is quite brief here, pointing out that present suffering cannot be alleviated because we are feeling it in the here and now, but future suffering can be prevented by the adoption of suitable means; Śaṅkara here does little more than expand slightly on Vyāsa's comments. Vācaspati Miśra is equally brief, but Vijñāna Bhikṣu is a little more expansive. He raises a possible objection that suffering yet to come does not exist and so cannot be removed, and responds by making the point that it is the causes of future suffering that are to be neutralised. That is the clear meaning of the *sūtra* and, furthermore, liberation means that state in which there is no further suffering. He refers to the philosophical systems of Nyāya and Sāṁkhya on that point, quoting *Sāṁkya Sūtra* 1.1: 'The absolute aim of man is the total annihilation of the threefold pain' (Trans. Rukmani).

2.17 *draṣṭṛ-dṛśyayoḥ saṁyogo heya-hetuḥ*

The contact between the seer and the objects that are seen is the cause of the suffering which is to be prevented.

In essence, this *sūtra* is about *kaivalya,* the state of existence in which *puruṣa* becomes entirely free from its association with *prakṛti* and stands alone in its true spiritual nature. Whilst existing in this present state of being, we must endure different forms of suffering, but in the previous *sūtra,* we were informed that this suffering can be brought to an end. Here the word *hetu* means the root cause, and *heya* means 'to be avoided, shunned, or overcome' , but this term was defined as 'future suffering' in the previous *sūtra.* The phrase *draṣṭṛ-dṛśyayoḥ saṁyoga,* means the union or conjunction of the seer, *draṣṭṛ,* and that which is seen, *dṛśya.* The seer is *puruṣa* and that which is seen is the world formed from *prakṛti,* and it is the present state of union between them that is the cause of suffering, a causal factor that must be inhibited by bringing about a disjunction of that state of unity. This state of separation is *kaivalya,* liberation from the world and from the suffering that is an inherent feature of existence in this world.

Vyāsa is even more specific and explains that the nature of that *saṁyoga,* that conjunction, is between *puruṣa* and *buddhi,* the intellectual faculty of the mind. This conjunction brings sentience to *buddhi,* but also engenders within *puruṣa* a sense of identity with the perceptions and experiences of which *buddhi* is the repository. Hence although *puruṣa* is utterly transcendent, it still experiences suffering. If it be asked when and how this conjunction occurred, then according to Vyāsa it is without a beginning, *an-ādi.* There is, however, a remedy and one can now see how all of this discussion is leading us towards a detailed analysis of that remedy, which is the *sādhana,* the practice of Yoga. Śaṅkara explains that objects perceived within the *buddhi* via the senses are then presented to *puruṣa,* which thereby becomes the *draṣṭṛ,* the seer of the world. He re-emphasises Vyāsa's observation that the union of seer and seen is *an-ādi,* without any temporal beginning point, and also makes the point that *puruṣa* itself, being immutable, does not actually experience suffering. That experience is confined to *buddhi,* but because of the unwanted state of union, the suffering of *buddhi* is presented before *puruṣa* and reflected in the existence of *puruṣa*.

At this point, Vācaspati Miśra offers a lengthy discussion of the manner in which thoughts and perceptions enter the *buddhi* and are then transmitted to *puruṣa* so that it becomes the seer. This complex analysis is interesting but takes us some distance beyond the statement of the *sūtra* itself. Vijñāna Bhikṣu follows a similar line and is equally expansive in commenting on this *sūtra,* his main line of discussion being to establish how it is that *puruṣa,* which is non-material, can be subject to the suffering that pertains only to the material domain. Again the response is that this is due to the close association between *puruṣa* and *buddhi,* which is the cause of suffering and which must be broken if liberation from suffering is to be attained.

Sūtras 2.18–2.27: Liberation from Suffering

Now the *Sādhana-pāda* starts to bring us to the point where the progression of *sādhana* can be delineated via its eight constituent parts. First we heard about *kriyā-yoga* as a means of weakening the *kleśas;* the nature of these *kleśas* was then analysed; then it was explained that the *kleśas* are the basis of karma, which fills our existence with suffering; then it was said that the suffering can be ended when the causes of suffering are neutralised. The next ten *sūtras* will now tell us more about the state of existence in which there is no suffering, *kaivalya,* along with the process of removing suffering, and the assertion that this whole world of *prakṛti* exists solely for the purpose of allowing *puruṣa* to reach the state of *kaivalya*. We are thus presented with the ultimate goal of *sādhana* as a preface to an analysis of the nature of the *sādhana* itself.

2.18 *prakāśa-kriyā-sthiti-śīlaṁ bhūtendriyātmakaṁ bhogāpavargārthaṁ dṛśyam*

The world we perceive can havc a nature that is illuminated, active, or still, and it consists of the material elements and the senses of perception. It can be used either for experience or to achieve liberation from rebirth.

As is often the case, the subject of this *sūtra* is given as its final word, *dṛśya,* which means the world that is perceived, in other words the domain of *prakṛti.* Three items of information relating to the visible world are given here. First of all, it is *prakāśa-kriyā-sthiti-śīla,* which means that its nature can be *prakāśa,* illumination, *kriyā,* activity, or *sthiti,* stillness, terms which must relate to the three *guṇas, sattva, rajas,* and *tamas,* which Sāṁkhya doctrine asserts are pervasive qualities of *prakṛti* in both its manifest and non-manifest states. Secondly, the visible world is composed of the great elements, the *bhūtas,* which are space, air, fire, water, and earth, and of the five senses, *indriya,* which are sight, touch, smell, hearing, and taste. And finally we learn that the purpose, the *artha,* of the world is both experience, *bhoga,* and liberation, *apavarga.* This latter point will be expanded upon in later *sūtras.*

Vyāsa first discusses the *guṇas,* pointing out that in all persons in all situations of life, their threefold presence fluctuates constantly. He then refers to the existence of the elements, the *bhūtas,* and the five senses, the *indriyas,* noting that these can be used either for experience or for the spiritual pursuit of liberation. But we are here told that the existence of this world enables us to gain realisation of the true nature of *puruṣa;* in this world, *puruṣa* has the chance to free itself from illusion and to come to know itself as it truly is. Śaṅkara offers a lengthy and detailed discussion of the nature and influence of the *guṇas* before turning again to consider how it is that the perceptions of the senses, which are material, can be received by *puruṣa*, which is wholly distinct from them. In response, he notes Vyāsa's use of the metaphor of the king and his soldiers; the king resides in his palace and does not act, but his soldiers go forth and fight. The king only experiences the result of the fight just as the *puruṣa* remains inactive and merely experiences.

Vācaspati Miśra also provides a detailed analysis of the changing influence of the three *guṇas* in the lives of all persons, so that they may at times be wise and illuminated, at other times passionate and active, and then again lazy, stupid, and uncaring. Vijñāna Bhikṣu comments at some length on this and the following *sūtra*, taking the opportunity to explain the relationship between the *guṇas* and *prakṛti*, and the manner in which the *guṇas* can exert an influence over the transcendent *puruṣa*. Interesting as his presentation is, it is more to do with Vijñāna Bhikṣu's personal philosophy than with the overt meaning of Patañjali's *sūtras*.

2.19 *viśeṣāviśeṣa-liṅga-mātrāliṅgāni guṇa-parvāṇi*

> The divisions of the *guṇas* can be designated as being specific or non-specific, as marked by observable characteristics, or as being free of such characteristics.

This is not an easy *sūtra* to comprehend and is related to some of the complexities of Sāṁkhya doctrine. The subject is *guṇa-parvāṇi*, a slightly awkward phrase. The word *parvan* means a section, a division, or a phase, and the indication here would seem to be that presence of the *guṇas* is manifest in different ways. These phases of the *guṇas* are said to be *viśeṣa* or *a-viśeṣa*, specific or non-specific, and *liṅga* or *a-liṅga*, with or without identifiable characteristics. So we can be sure that the *sūtra* is discussing the three *guṇas*, but what it is saying about them is somewhat obscure.

Turning to the commentaries for an explanation, we can note that Vyāsa indicates that the *sūtra* is discussing the nature of *prakṛti* and in particular the process by which it evolves from a non-manifest, non-variegated substance, into the variegated form composed of twenty-four elements that can be identified in the world as we experience it. This is a complex line of discussion that is not fundamental to an understanding of the *Yoga Sūtras* as a whole; hence one can try to grasp the main points being made, but if it seems overly confusing there is no need to be too concerned, and there is no harm in moving on to the next *sūtra*.

But for those who wish to explore this *sūtra* in more detail, we can note that in Sāṁkhya teachings, *prakṛti* evolves from its undifferentiated state by a specific process. According to Vyāsa, the *a-viśeṣa*, the non-specific, are those elements that evolve further and are transformed into other elements. These are the *tan-mātras* that are the essence of perceivable objects: aroma, flavour, colour/form, touch sensations, and sound; to these five is added the general sense of egoism, *asmitā* (more usually *ahaṁkāra*), so that the total for *a-viśeṣa* is six. The *viśeṣa*, the specific, are the five great elements of earth, water, fire, air, and space, the five senses of perception, sight, hearing, touch, smell, and taste, the five organs of action, voice, hands, feet, anus, and genitals, and the *manas* that identifies perceptions, making a total of sixteen in the category of *viśeṣa*. The first five of these, the elements, are related to the five *tan-mātras* as their *a-viśeṣa*, the non-specific, counterparts, whereas the remaining elements in this list have *asmitā* as their *a-viśeṣa*, the non-specific, counterpart. To these twenty-two we can add *prakṛti* in its prior unevolved form and then the primal element, named as *mahat*, which is also identified as *buddhi*, to give us the conventional Sāṁkhya total of twenty-four. Vyāsa further explains that the term *a-liṅga*, devoid of characteristics, refers to *prakṛti* in its primal, unevolved state, whilst *liṅga* is used to refer to *prakṛti* in its evolved state as the diverse world we experience. The phrase *guṇa-parvāṇi* is used in this context because *prakṛti* is pervaded by the *guṇas*, and hence the transformations and states of *prakṛti* are transformations and states of the *guṇas*.

As mentioned above, you may decide that this whole line of discussion is not that helpful in understanding the *Yoga Sūtras* as a whole, and this is by no means an unreasonable position to take. What we should note, however, is the extent to which Patañjali relies on the intricacies of Sāṁkhya thought in formulating his discourse on Yoga. Śaṅkara, Vācaspati Miśra, and Vijñāna Bhikṣu all comment at some length on the manner in which Vyāsa relates the *sūtra* to Sāṁkhya teachings, but I think enough has been said on this subject already and we can safely move on now in our discussion of the *sūtras*.

2.20 *draṣṭā dṛśi-mātraḥ śuddho 'pi pratyayānupaśyaḥ*

> Although the seer is entirely pure, and does nothing but observe, it still perceives the world in relation to this form of conceptualisation.

This *sūtra* provides a definition of the term *draṣṭṛ*, the seer, from 2.17 and refers to the difficult question of how it is that *puruṣa* remains untouched and unchanging whilst at the same time utilising *buddhi* and other mental faculties in order to become the seer of the world. It might be objected that the process of perception entails a degree of transformation as one object after another is perceived and recognised, but here any direct association between *puruṣa* and the visible world is rejected. Whereas *buddhi*, the intellect, is touched and at times rendered impure by its absorption of perceptions, *puruṣa* is always *śuddha*, untouched by any such impurity, and is nothing more than an observer, without undergoing any of the transformations experienced by *buddhi* as a result of its changing perceptions. *Buddhi* is involved, *puruṣa* is detached. Nonetheless, because all perceptions are presented to *puruṣa* by *buddhi*, its position as a seer is still mediated through the mental processes. As in the metaphor of the king and his ministers, the knowledge of the kingdom gained by the king is mediated through the words of the ministers; so it is with the knowledge that comes to *puruṣa* through the perception of the mind and senses.

Vyāsa comments on the exact nature of the relationship between *puruṣa* and *buddhi*, stating that they are neither similar nor entirely distinct in this process of perception. The main distinction is that within *buddhi*, knowledge of the perceived objects fluctuates constantly and is sometimes present and sometimes absent, but the knowledge existing within *puruṣa* is constant and unchanging because the real object of *puruṣa*'s perception is *buddhi*, which is always available to it. Thus, *puruṣa* is distinct from *buddhi*, but not entirely distinct because the knowledge of *puruṣa* as seer is knowledge of *buddhi* as it absorbs the various perceptions. *Puruṣa* does not perceive the world directly; it perceives the image of the world present within the *buddhi*, which is the object of *puruṣa*'s own perception. Śaṅkara places an emphasis on the word *dṛśi-mātra*, meaning being only a seer, recognising that the use of the word *mātra* only gives a clear indication that *puruṣa* has no greater interaction with the world and is thus entirely distinct from the domain of *prakṛti*.

Vācaspati Miśra carries on the same discussion, noting that *buddhi* takes on the form of any object that is subject to perception. It thus falls under the influence of the *guṇas* that pervade all aspects of the world of manifest *prakṛti*. *Puruṣa*, by contrast, just observes these fluctuations in *buddhi* without adopting their form, as is the case for *buddhi*. Vijñāna Bhikṣu provides another lengthy commentary in which he considers each part of Vyāsa's commentary in close detail. He also focuses on the words *mātra* and *śuddha* in the *sūtra,* stating that *mātra,* only, indicates that as a mere observer, *puruṣa* is untouched by the *guṇas,* whilst the purity indicated by the word *śuddha* confirms that *puruṣa* is not composed of the material elements such as the *bhūtas* of earth, fire, air, water, and space, or of the five senses. These are all potential sources of mundane impurity from which *puruṣa* remains detached in a state of eternal purity.

2.21 *tad-artha eva dṛśyasyātmā*

The true identity of the perceived world is that it exists solely for the sake of the seer.

The subject of this *sūtra* is the *ātman* of the *drśya,* the *ātman* of the visible world. Here one should probably avoid the temptation to take the word *ātman* in its usual sense as a synonym for *puruṣa,* and understand it in the sense of 'the true identity', meaning the whole reason for its existence. That true identity is defined as *tad-artha eva,* meaning 'for the sake of that alone'. Here the word *tat,* meaning 'that', must refer to *puruṣa* (*draṣṭṛ*), the seer that was the subject of the previous *sūtra,* and so here we have a clear indication that the existence of the physical world is for the sake of *puruṣa,* presumably with the dual purpose of experience, *bhoga,* and liberation, *apavarga,* as mentioned in *sūtra* 2.18 and explained by Vyāsa in his commentary to this *sūtra.*

Naturally enough, the question then arises as to whether this does not imply that the world is created by an intelligent being, by *īśvara,* with that purpose in mind. On this question, differing opinions are encountered in different texts. The *Sāṁkhya Kārikā* shares the view that the world becomes manifest to allow *puruṣa* to gain liberation, but it makes no reference at all to this being the intention of any deity. The *Bhagavad-gītā,* by contrast, asserts that the expansion of *prakṛti* into the variegated forms of life takes place under the control and direction of the Deity, Kṛṣṇa himself (9.10). It really depends on the way one reads the *sūtra*; it could mean that the visible world is used as a tool for liberation, or it could equally mean that the visible world is designed by a creator with that specific purpose in mind. Different individuals will have differing views on that point.

Vyāsa's short commentary offers no resolution on this debate, as it simply looks ahead to the next *sūtra*, which discusses the disappearance of the world once liberation is attained by *puruṣa*. Śaṅkara expands slightly on that point by explaining that since the sole purpose of the world is the liberation of *puruṣa*, it is to be understood that when liberation is attained that purpose is complete and there is no longer any need for the existence of the world. Vācaspati Miśra goes still further on that same point. He notes that without the presence of *puruṣa*, all the elements of *prakṛti*, including the mental faculties, are inert and lifeless. Hence when *puruṣa* is liberated and disappears from the material domain, it is impossible for the world to continue, as *prakṛti* must resume its previous state of inertia and non-manifestation. Vijñāna Bhikṣu focuses on the word *dṛśya*, that which is perceived, and takes up the literal meaning. Being perceived depends on the presence of perception, and once *puruṣa* renounces its association with *buddhi*, then perception disappears, as *buddhi* is only an organ of perception because of the proximity of *puruṣa*. Liberation of *puruṣa* puts an end to the perception of the *dṛśya*, the perceived world, which at that point must therefore cease to be.

2.22 *kṛtārthaṁ prati naṣṭam apy anaṣṭaṁ tad-anya-sādhāraṇatvāt*

Although the perceived world ceases to exist when that purpose is achieved, it does not cease to exist entirely, for it continues to exist in relation to others.

Here we get what might appear to be a rather obvious point regarding the disappearance of the world once liberation is achieved. As the commentators have pointed out, the world of *prakṛti* must cease to exist in the absence *puruṣa*, but this does not mean the wholesale dissolution of the world because it relates only to the individual *puruṣa* that has achieved liberation. For all the other *puruṣas* which remain in a state of bondage, the world will certainly continue. The argument here is relevant in relation to one of the arguments frequently levelled by opponents against the Advaita Vedānta system of thought. The philosophies of *advaita*, non-dualism, set forth the idea that Brahman alone is real, and hence our perception of ourselves as individuals is an illusion. The question then raised is that if one spiritual aspirant achieves liberation, why is it that others remain in bondage if there is no distinction between one individual and another? The Sāṁkhya-Yoga system insists that each *puruṣa* is an eternally individual entity, even after liberation, and hence that tricky question does not arise, as the present *sūtra* makes clear.

Here Vyāsa does little more than restate the overt meaning of the *sūtra*, pointing out that the earlier statement that the relationship between *prakṛti* and *puruṣa* is *anādi*, beginningless, is now explained because the ending of that conjunction takes place only for a single individual. Interestingly, the commentary attributed to Śaṅkara does not try to assert the advaitic rejection of individuality. He writes: 'But from the distinction of body and senses (*kārya-karaṇa*) it is certain there is a variety of *puruṣas*, and the difference between *puruṣas* is also established from the fact of variety of happiness and suffering' (Trans. Leggett). This statement seems somewhat at variance from the usual teachings of Advaita Vedānta and raises questions about the true identity of the author.

Vācaspati Miśra, another adherent of the school of Advaita Vedānta, similarly makes no attempt to impose his own views onto the direct meaning of the *sūtra* and Vyāsa's commentary. He simply explains the meaning of both, and cites a verse from the *Śvetāśvatara Upaniṣad* (4.5), the most obviously dualist of all the major Upaniṣads, in support of that meaning. Vijñāna Bhikṣu is an ardent opponent of Advaita Vedānta and does not miss this opportunity to draw out the full significance of the *sūtra*. He cites the same verse of the *Śvetāśvatara Upaniṣad* as Vācaspati Miśra, and creates an imagined opponent who raises the question of why there are numerous statements in the Upaniṣads that refer to the unity of all beings. His response is that these statements mean that each *puruṣa* is identical to others, in the sense that they are all of the same spiritual nature, but this does not mean that there is no distinction between them.

2.23 *sva-svāmi-śaktyoḥ svarūpopalabdhi-hetuḥ saṁyogaḥ*

> The state of union between the seer and the perceived world exists in order to allow the seer to understand the true nature of the energies of the owner and the owned.

Here again the subject of the *sūtra* is given in its final word, in this case *saṁyoga*, the state of union. Thus, this *sūtra* provides the definition of the term *saṁyoga* from *sūtra* 2.17. Essentially, the *sūtra* is again asserting the point that the existence of *puruṣa* in this world provides it with a means of gaining the knowledge that brings liberation. *Puruṣa* exists in a state of semi-unity with *buddhi* and the other elements of its embodiment, and whilst this state of *saṁyoga* is symptomatic of its condition of bondage, it also presents it with the means of gaining release. The world is both our prison and our means of escape. The state of union is a *hetu*, a causal factor, which facilitates the *upalabdhi*, the recognition, of the *svarūpa*, the true nature of *sva-svāmi-śaktyoḥ*. Here the word *śaktyoḥ* is the dual form of *śakti,* which means energies, powers, or potentialities, whilst *svāmin* is the master or owner and *sva* refers to that which is owned. Thus the knowledge to be gained is of the distinct nature and potentialities of *puruṣa,* the *svāmin,* and *prakṛti,* the bodily form it possesses.

Vyāsa makes it clear that the *sūtra* is really about *upalabdhi,* understanding or perceiving, which carries forward the theme of liberation in this passage. The perceiving (*upalabdhi*) of the material world (*dṛśya*) is experience (*bhoga*). *Saṁyoga* is also the cause of the comprehension of the truth, which in turn banishes ignorance and brings *puruṣa* towards the state of liberation. He then provides a complicated analysis of the process by which this knowledge is gained, presenting eight distinct theories on the nature and origins of ignorance and the awakening of spiritual enlightenment. Śaṅkara closely follows this analysis, taking the opportunity to explain the various ideas on the nature of *avidyā,* ignorance, which is characterised by a failure to see the distinction between *prakṛti* and *puruṣa,* and of the manner in which seeing that difference, as referred to in this *sūtra,* destroys *avidyā* and brings *kaivalya* as its direct consequence.

Vācaspati Miśra explains the use of the terms owner and owned, *svāmin* and *sva,* by reminding us of the previous statement that the perceived world exists only for the sake of *puruṣa* in the manner of its property. He then presents his own substantial analysis of the eight theories of knowing and ignorance set forth by Vyāsa. Vijñāna Bhikṣu is similarly expansive in his comments, first of all asserting that the *saṁyoga* specifically means the close relationship that exists between *puruṣa* and *buddhi,* as has been explained previously. He notes the question posed by Vyāsa, *kiṁ cedam adarśanam,* 'what is this ignorance?', and then, like the other commentators, proceeds through the eight possibilities suggested by Vyāsa as potential answers to this question. Vijñāna Bhikṣu also makes the point that the cultivation of *viveka-jñāna,* recognition of the distinction between *puruṣa* and *prakṛti*, is the same as the removal of *avidyā*. As *vidyā* develops, *avidyā* disappears to the same degree.

2.24 *tasya hetur avidyā*

It is ignorance that is the cause of this state of union.

This is a simple enough *sūtra* to translate, consisting as it does of only three words. The first of these, *tasya*, means 'of that' and must refer to the subject of the previous *sūtra*, which was *saṁyoga*, the state of union between the seer and the seen, *puruṣa* and *buddhi* or *prakṛti*. Thus the meaning is that the cause (*hetu*) of the state of unity (*saṁyoga*) is ignorance (*avidyā*), which must be ignorance of the truth of the ultimate distinction between matter and spirit. This is easy enough to understand, but the previous *sūtra* suggested that this unity might be a positive thing as it facilitated the cultivation of discriminative knowledge. Hence we can understand that whilst the existence of this world provides a means by which *puruṣa* can attain liberation, that same existence is in fact a result of the *avidyā* that keeps *puruṣa* in a state of bondage. A paradox perhaps, but a relatively minor one, and here the example of using a thorn to remove a thorn is appropriate. When one has a thorn in one's foot, one may use another thorn to remove it, and then discard that thorn as well. The *avidyā* that afflicts *puruṣa* causes it to exist in a state of semi-unity with *buddhi*, but it is by the appropriate application of *buddhi* through the techniques of Yoga that this *avidyā* is ultimately removed and complete separation from *buddhi* is achieved.

It is this exact point that Vyāsa makes in his commentary. When affected by the latent impressions of the past life, *buddhi* becomes subject to *avidyā*, and thus *puruṣa* remains in its state of bondage, but when *buddhi* is shaped by *viveka-jñāna*, true knowledge, then *puruṣa* is liberated and *buddhi* has fulfilled its primary function. At that point, when *avidyā* is no longer present, the existence of *buddhi* fades away and *puruṣa* stands alone; this is *kaivalya*. Śaṅkara here discusses the *saṁskāras*, the latent impressions left on the mind by previous mental states that are gathered into groups known as *vāsanā*. It is these that are inextricably linked to ignorance, and cause the persistence of ignorance, lifetime after lifetime. Vācaspati Miśra makes the point that ignorance only perpetuates the bondage of *puruṣa* because of the state of association that exists between *puruṣa* and *buddhi*, as the latter is the actual location of *avidyā*. Vijñāna Bhikṣu offers a longer commentary in which he expands on the understanding of *saṁyoga*, the idea of the connection between *puruṣa* and the world. He puts forward the view that there is the more general *saṁyoga* that exists between *prakṛti* in general and *puruṣa*, and then there is the specific *saṁyoga* referred to in this *sūtra*, which is the proximate position of *puruṣa* and *buddhi*, because of which the *avidyā* present within *buddhi* is expanded so that it appears to affect *puruṣa* as well.

2.25 *tad-abhāvāt saṁyogābhāvo hānaṁ tad dṛśeḥ kaivalyam*

> When that ignorance ceases, the state of union also ceases, and there is escape from suffering. For the seer, this is the state known as *kaivalya*, liberation from the world.

This *sūtra* can be taken in three parts. Firstly, a cause, then the effect of that cause, and then an explanation of the significance of that effect. The causal factor is *tad-abhāva*, the ceasing to be of that, where 'that' must refer to *avidyā* as that was the subject of the previous *sūtra*. The effect or consequence of the non-existence of *avidyā* is *saṁyoga-abhāva*, the non-existence of *saṁyoga*; in other words, when *avidyā* ceases, the connection between *puruṣa* and *prakṛti*, or between *puruṣa* and *buddhi*, also ceases. This consequence is then further explained as *hāna,* escape. The thing to be escaped from or prevented (*heya*) was defined in 2.16 as suffering, and, as Vyāsa points out, *hāna* therefore means 'cessation of suffering'. This *sūtra* consists of two sentences. The second sentence begins with the pronoun *tad,* that, which most naturally refers to the word *hāna,* escape from suffering, from the first sentence, as is also explained by Śaṅkara. This happens to the *dṛśi,* the seer which is *puruṣa,* which escapes from its state of *saṁyoga,* its connection with the mundane existence brought about by its embodiment. The final word extends this idea by defining it as *kaivalya,* separation from this world, literally 'aloneness', which is the state of liberation.

Vyāsa is quite brief in his comments here, expanding on the term *kaivalya* to explain it as a complete ending of *bandhana,* of bondage, freedom from the effect of the *guṇas,* and release from the state of suffering that is inherent in the condition of *saṁyoga*. Śaṅkara responds to an imagined critic who argues that there can be no liberation because there is still karma in a form yet to mature, and this must be experienced within a bodily existence. This view is rejected on the basis of what has been said before, namely the idea that the *saṁskāras* that generate karmic reactions are reduced to a sterile state by the practices that neutralise the *kleśas*. Hence liberation is possible as soon as *avidyā* is brought to a state of *a-bhāva,* non-existence. Vācaspati Miśra suggests another way of reading the *sūtra* in which *kaivalya* is taken in an adjectival sense, meaning 'complete' or 'absolute', that qualifies *hāna,* the escape or release. This is certainly a valid alternative reading of the *sūtra,* although the meaning is not that dissimilar. Vijñāna Bhikṣu takes the same line in reading the *sūtra,* taking the meaning to be *hānaṁ kaivalyam,* absolute escape from this existence rather than *kaivalya* being the state that *puruṣa* escapes into. And this is not just escape from the state of being associated with *prakṛti,* the real significance is that it is escape from all the suffering we must otherwise continue to undergo lifetime after lifetime.

> 2.26 *viveka-khyātir aviplavā hānopāyaḥ*
>
> The continuous application of discriminative understanding is the means by which that escape from suffering is achieved.

Again the subject of the *sūtra* is given in its final phrase, which is *hāna-upāya,* the means, the *upāya,* by which the release or escape, the *hāna,* is achieved. And that means is defined by the phrase *viveka-khyātir aviplavā*. Here *viveka* means 'distinction', as between *puruṣa* and *prakṛti,* whilst *khyāti* means 'perception' or 'cognisance' of that distinction. Then *aviplava* means 'without going astray'. In other words, the prescribed means by which release from this world is obtained is an undeviating awareness of one's true spiritual identity as *puruṣa,* which is wholly distinct from the physical and mental embodiment. Of course, the attaining of this state is a gradual process and, similarly, the state of liberation is attained slowly, step by step. As Kṛṣṇa says at the end of Chapter 6 of the *Gītā*, there is no question of failure in this endeavour, only degrees of success, and whatever success is achieved is never lost as it serves as the platform for future progression.

Vyāsa points out that initially any perception of distinction is likely to be wavering until such time as the false understanding of *saṁyoga,* of unity, is dispelled and reduced to a state like the burnt seed which cannot sprout again. At that point, the *guṇa* of *sattva* exists in a state untainted by association with *rajas* or *tamas;* and in that state the pure knowledge of enlightenment becomes clear. Śaṅkara likewise asserts that the path to enlightenment is one of uneven progression, as materialistic perceptions and desires present constant interruptions. Vācaspati Miśra again emphasises the fact that this *viveka-khyāti* does not mean the type of theoretical understanding that can be gained by study of philosophy or texts; knowledge of that type will never be *aviplava*, unwavering, and cannot prevent the *saṁskāras* from continuing to exert their influence. Vijñāna Bhikṣu states that the disturbances which cause *plava*, wavering, are the *kleśas* and *malas*, contaminations such as hankering, aversion, and greed. When these are suppressed and controlled, then *sattva-guṇa* stands unblemished, and pure discriminative knowledge becomes manifest. Reminding us of the previous lines of discussion, he further points out that it is *asaṁprajñāta-samādhi* that is the source of *viveka-khyāti* and is therefore to be included in this analysis of the means by which *viveka-khyāti* is to be achieved.

2.27 *tasya saptadhā prānta-bhūmiḥ prajñā*

The realisation derived from that discriminative understanding is sevenfold, and reaches the ultimate point.

Here the subject of the *sūtra* is the final word, *prajñā*, which means 'knowledge', 'realisation', 'understanding', or 'wisdom', and the other words and phrases offer us information about that *prajñā*. First of all, we have the word *tasya*, meaning 'of him' or 'of that'. We are next informed that the realisation (*prajñā*) gained from *viveka-khyāti* by the practitioner is sevenfold, a statement that is impossible to understand without reference to the commentary, which in turn provides some confirmation for the view that Vyāsa's commentary is the work of Patañjali himself because the seven aspects of *prajñā* are not mentioned in the subsequent *sūtras*. An alternative view would be that Patañjali expected his *sūtras* to be used by a *guru* giving instruction to disciples, and that the *guru* would explain the idea behind the word *saptadhā*. Moreover, that realisation is *prānta-bhūmi*. The word *bhūmi* usually means the element earth or the earth itself, but in this case, it refers to a point, position, or level of attainment, whilst *prānta*, or *pra-anta*, means the conclusion, the end, or the final limit. So the indication is that this level of realisation, attained through discriminative knowledge, is the ultimate stage of spiritual enlightenment.

We are indebted to Vyāsa for providing us with a breakdown of the seven subjects or realisations referred to in the *sūtra*. These seven are statements that the realised practitioner of Yoga understands. They are divided in two groups of four and three respectively. They first four resemble the four Noble Truths of Buddhism, especially if we keep in mind that *heya*, which appears in all four in one form or another, was defined as suffering in 2.16. The last three statements, however, use Sāṁkhya categories, such as *guṇa*. The first quartet are called 'release of wisdom', *vimuktiḥ prajñāyāḥ*. The latter triad are known as 'release of the mind', *cittavimukti*:

1. *parijñātaṁ heyam* that [suffering] which is to be broken free from has been completely understood;
2. *kṣīṇā heya-hetavaḥ*, the causes of that [suffering] which is to be broken free from have been destroyed;
3. *sākṣāt-kṛtaṁ nirodha-samādhinā hānam*, the escape [from suffering] through the *samādhi* of the cessation [of the mind] has been personally realised by me;
4. *bhāvito vivekakhyātirūpo hānopāyaḥ*, the means of escape [from suffering] in the form of discriminative knowledge has been cultivated;
5. *caritādhikārā buddhiḥ*, *buddhi* has fulfilled its purpose;
6. *guṇā . . . svakāraṇe pralayābhimukhāḥ saha tenāstaṁ gacchanti*, the *guṇas* (...) moving towards merging back into their original state disappear along with that [*buddhi*];
7. (...) *kevalī puruṣaḥ*, *puruṣa* stands alone in a liberated state.

Śaṅkara, Vācaspati Miśra, and Vijñāna Bhikṣu all provide further discussion of the meaning and significance of the seven stages of *prajñā* as delineated by Vyāsa, but as our primary focus is on the *sūtras* themselves, I think that whilst acknowledging Vyāsa's contribution to our understanding of the meaning of Patañjali's *sūtras,* we can pause and draw breath at this point in order to review the principal ideas presented in the first half of the *Sādhana-pāda*. Certainly this passage of the *Yoga Sūtras* represents one of the more taxing parts of the work as a whole, as it contains passages of detailed analysis as well as close reference to some of the more complex features of Sāṁkhya doctrine. Nonetheless, I think we can recognise the manner in which these *sūtras* provide a basis for the presentation of the *sādhana* itself, which occupies the second half of this second chapter, and indeed extends into the first part of Chapter Three.

The chapter begins with a statement regarding the practice of *kriyā-yoga,* a Yoga based on physical actions that is effective in weakening the five *kleśas,* afflictions that are obstacles on the path to success in the yogic endeavour. These are then delineated and it is explained that the *kleśas* are the cause of the continual engendering of karma in the form of action and reaction; and for those beings of this world who are subject to the influence of karma, suffering is an inevitable concomitant of that existence. The final phase of the pattern of instruction we have been exploring so far in this chapter then reveals that there is a solution to the seemingly insoluble problem of karma and suffering. That solution is the cultivation of *viveka-khyāti,* the realisation that one's true identity is as *puruṣa,* a spiritual entity that is wholly distinct from both the mind it occupies and the world of *prakṛti* that it currently experiences. And it is on this point of revealing how the existential problem of life in this world can be solved that the *Yoga Sūtras* turns to providing a more detailed outline of the *sādhana* itself, which is the means by which this discriminative realisation can be achieved through Yoga practice.

What seems to be the case is that the discussion encountered so far in this chapter is to be seen as a philosophical preparation that explains the reasons why the practice should be undertaken. This pattern of first giving the Sāṁkhya theory and then following on with a presentation of the concomitant forms of practice is a constant feature of the Sāṁkhya and Yoga passages found in the *Śānti-parvan* of the *Mahābhārata*. And as an aside, we might notice here that Patañjali does not refer to sacred text as a source of this enlightenment, as is the case for Vedānta, but rather proceeds to offer a means by which knowledge of that distinction is achieved through direct perception. So as we go forward now to the end of this second chapter, the focus of the discussion switches to the means by which the liberating *viveka-khyāti* can be cultivated. It is at this point that the idea of a Yoga of eight limbs is introduced, providing a progressive path forward towards ultimate enlightenment in the state of *samādhi*.

The remainder of the *Samādhi-pāda* provides an outline of the first five of these eight stages and one has to say that for the most part this discussion is rather more straightforward than that which has confronted us so far. The philosophising is now more or less complete and we can move on to the practices based on the philosophical truths thus far revealed to us.

Sūtras 2.28–2.29: The Eight Limbs of Yoga Outlined

2.28 *yogāṅgānuṣṭhānād aśuddhi-kṣaye jñāna-dīptir āviveka-khyāteḥ*

When impurities dwindle due to the practice of the eight limbs of yoga, the light of true knowledge

> emerges, reaching as far as discriminative understanding of the difference between *puruṣa* and *buddhi*.

The subject of this *sūtra* is *jñāna-dīpti*, the light of knowledge, and the three other phrases all provide further information about that inner illumination. The first of these is *yoga-aṅga-anuṣṭhānāt*, which indicates that the *jñāna-dīpti* appears as a result of one's being committed to the practice, the *anuṣṭhāna*, of the *yogāṅga*, the limbs of Yoga. Here the word *aṅga*, literally meaning 'a limb', is particularly significant and it is usually taken in the sense of a 'component part'. Some, however, have pointed to a group of texts known as the *Vedāṅgas*, which deal with additional subjects not central to the Vedic revelation as a whole, such as grammar, astrology, and forms of poetry. Because these are ancillary works outside the central theme, it has been suggested that the *yogāṅgas* should be understood in the same way as ancillaries to the central practice of Yoga. Given the wider context of the *Yoga Sūtras*, however, in which the eight *aṅgas* play a central role, it seems far more likely that here the word *aṅga* is used in the more literal sense of a component part.

The next phrase is *aśuddhi-kṣaye* and this describes the point at which the *jñāna-dīpti* starts to become manifest. It is when impurities, *aśuddhi*, start to diminish or dwindle away, as indicated by the word *kṣaye*. Here we encounter a principal theme of several strands of Indian religious thought, notably the Śaivism of the Śaiva Siddhānta tradition, but also the ideas encountered within the *Bhagavad-gītā*. The idea is that in our pure identity each of us contains the inner light of higher, spiritual knowledge, but this is not fully manifest because it is covered over by *mala*, contamination, such as greed, self-absorption, and an absence of compassion. The spiritual endeavour is aimed at gradually removing this *mala* so that the ever-present inner light increasingly shines forth. From this perspective, it is seen that the highest knowledge comes not from any external source, but from within where it is always present as a part of our true spiritual identity. The process is one of cleansing away the coverings so that this inner light can shine forth and fill our whole being. In both the Śaivite and the *Gītā*'s teachings (10.11), it is stated that the Deity present within each being acts to bring about this purification, but despite its theistic tendencies, the *Yoga Sūtras* does not go that far.

The third of the three qualifying phrases is *āviveka-khyāteḥ*, which is a reassertion of the idea of *viveka-khyāti*, discriminative understanding, that we have heard of in previous *sūtras*. Here the more usual form of *viveka-khyāti* is changed to *āviveka-khyāti* with the prefix *ā* indicating progression in the sense of 'up to the point of'. The idea is that the *jñāna-dīpti* brings higher knowledge up to its ultimate stage of realisation, which is the *viveka-khyāti* by which the absolute distinction between *puruṣa* and *prakṛti* is identified and fully known.

Vyāsa explains that the limbs of Yoga bring about the dwindling of impurity, which in turn gives rise to the manifestation of spiritual knowledge. The enlightenment gained is not absolute in an all or nothing sense, but is a gradual emergence of the light of knowledge proportionate to the diminution of impurity. One does not need to await absolute perfection in the disciplines of Yoga, for even a small amount of progress brings a commensurate removal of impurity, and from that a commensurate emergence of spiritual awakening. As the light of knowledge expands, it finally reaches the ultimate object of knowledge and liberating insight occurs. Vyāsa then proceeds to give a complex nine-fold analysis of the precise stages by which the discriminative knowledge emerges, which goes beyond our requirements for this study. Śaṅkara reviews this nine-fold analysis in some detail, stating that it is taken from the teachings of Manu, and Vācaspati Miśra has a similar focus in his commentary. Both of them note, however, that the impurity referred to in the *sūtra* will also include the deposits of latent karma present in the mind that adherence to the limbs of Yoga may prevent from maturing into tangible results. Vijñāna Bhikṣu also offers a lengthy discussion of the nine processes by which *viveka-khyāti* comes to the fore, but prior to that, he points out that *kṣaya* means diminution rather than destruction; hence, if the practice of the limbs of Yoga is interrupted, the impurities are likely to expand once more.

2.29 *yama-niyamāsana-prāṇāyāma-pratyāhāra-dhāraṇā-dhyāna-samādhayo 'ṣṭāv aṅgāni*

Yama, niyama, āsana, prāṇāyāma, pratyāhāra, dhāraṇā, dhyāna, and *samādhi* are the eight limbs of Yoga.

In an earlier translation I made of the *Yoga Sūtras*, I translated the terms used for the eight limbs as restraints (*yama*), observances (*niyama*), sitting postures (*āsana*), breath control (*prāṇāyāma*), withdrawal of the senses (*pratyāhāra*), concentration of the mind (*dhāraṇā*), meditation (*dhyāna*), and complete absorption (*samādhi*). On reflection, however, I think it is better to retain the original Sanskrit terms, partly because they are quite widely known today, and partly because any English equivalents are inevitably somewhat imprecise. Moreover, as we go through the following *sūtras*, an explanation of the meaning of the terms becomes quite readily apparent. This *sūtra* is in fact one of the simplest we encounter, as it is a straightforward list of the limbs of Yoga, which are said here to be eight in number, and the next groups of *sūtras* provide the explanation of what is meant by each of them.

Vyāsa merely states that each limb should be followed in succession, and the other commentators follow his lead in terms of brevity, although Śaṅkara does emphasise the point that *yama* and *niyama* are integral to Yoga practice and not mere preliminaries. Vijñāna Bhikṣu explains that where other elements of Yoga such as *vairāgya*, renunciation, have been mentioned, these are to be understood as being included in the eight limbs established here.

Sūtras 2.30–2.32: The Yamas and Niyamas Listed

In these next three *sūtras*, Patañjali provides two further lists, one of the five *yamas* and the other of the five *niyamas*. Similar lists are quite often encountered in other early texts on Yoga, such as those found in the *Mahābhārata* and Purāṇas, although the number and names on the lists quite often vary. Again this group of *sūtras* is relatively simple to follow, as the vocabulary used to designate them is not at all obscure.

2.30 *ahiṁsā-satyāsteya-brahmacaryāparigrahā yamāḥ*

> The yamas are not harming (*ahiṁsā*), truthfulness (*satya*), never stealing (*asteya*), celibacy (*brahmacarya*), and not seeking ownership (*aparigraha*).

Here I have opted to translate the terms included in the list of five *yamas* mainly because these have a more general meaning in Sanskrit literature and are not technical terms employed in Yoga discourse. *Yama* means a restraint and hence it is not surprising that three of the five are negatives formed by adding the prefix *a* to a noun, *hiṁsā* being harm, *steya* being theft, and *parigraha* being grasping or acquisition. *Ahiṁsā* is a frequently encountered word, and was popularised in the speeches and writings of Mahatma Gandhi. It is sometimes translated as non-violence, but it has the wider meaning of not causing any harm, and this applies to our thoughts and words as well as our deeds. *Satya* has the literal meaning of truth, although elsewhere it is sometimes asserted that the test of *satya* rests on the consequences of our words as well as their veracity. Hence a speech may be literally true, but if its intent and consequences are harmful, then it is not *satya*. *Brahmacarya* is often translated as sexual restraint, but it actually means celibacy and its inclusion in this list of *yamas* clearly suggests that fully devoting oneself to the path of Yoga is only for renouncers of the world. *Asteya* is a fairly straightforward prohibition, but *aparigraha* again suggests a withdrawal from materialistic aspirations, which frequently focus on the acquisition of money, property, power, and desirable goods. Clearly, Yoga is for those who are moving away from the conventional preoccupations of modern society with its constant emphasis on consumption.

Vyāsa asserts that *ahiṁsā* is central to the practice of *yama*, as the other four all rest on that fundamental precept. He also expounds at some length on the principle of *satya* in line with what was said above regarding the consequences of one's speech. He writes of speech that is factually true but harmful, 'In so far as there would be a false kind of merit, a resemblance of merit, it would be the worst of evils. Therefore, let a *yogin* first consider what is good for all creatures, and speak only then' (Trans. Woods). Śaṅkara confirms this point by insisting that truthful words should never be uttered if they contravene the higher precept of *ahiṁsā*; he also suggests that *brahmacarya* means restraint of all the senses that are used to gain sensual pleasure and not just physical sexuality.

Following a similar line to the others, Vācaspati Miśra points out how it is that contravening the four other *yamas* will inevitably involve a contravention of the precept of *ahiṁsā*, although he does not fully explain how this applies to *brahmacarya*. He also provides a series of examples to demonstrate that strict adherence to *satya* can contravene the ideal of *ahiṁsā*; hence a rigid vow to speak only words that are truthful is not always a true acceptance of that element of *yama*. Vijñāna Bhikṣu refers to the story of the killing of Droṇa in the *Mahābhārata*; when Yudhiṣṭhira made the announcement that Aśvatthāman had been slain, Droṇa stopped fighted, assuming that this statement referred to his son Aśvatthāman, but in fact only an elephant bearing the same name had been killed. Yudhiṣṭhira's words were true in a literal sense, but because the motive behind his speech was deception, then it was not *satya*.

2.3 *jāti-deśa-kāla-samayānavacchinnāḥ sārva-bhaumā mahā-vratam*

> These principles are not dependent on birth, place, time, or custom, but are equally applicable to all. Together, they constitute the great vow.

In this *sūtra*, Patañjali is anxious to place the discussion of *yamas* beyond the more conventional teachings on conduct, which are generally contingent on factors such as caste or gender. In particular, this *sūtra* makes the point that the *yogāṅga* are open to all persons and are not confined to those born as Brahmin males. The *yamas* that have been outlined are very similar in nature to the mode of conduct that is widely asserted to be the *dharma* of a Brahmin, but this apparent correspondence of lifestyle is not to be misconstrued as an indication that Yoga practice is for Brahmins alone. An interesting point is made here about ethics and morality in general. It is often said that moral principles are relative to the particular time or place in which they are presented, so that we cannot judge the conduct of people in the past by our contemporary standards. Here this view is rejected, and we might also note the term *sanātana-dharma*, universal *dharma*, which indicates that the fundamental principles of ethical conduct exist at all times in all locations. And the fundamental precept on which all subsequent systems of morality are to be based is *ahiṁsā*; furthermore, although *ahiṁsā* is a negative term, it is elsewhere asserted that *ahiṁsā* also involves taking positive action for the welfare of others. This view is clearly asserted in the *Liṅga Purāṇa* (8.12), which provides a discussion and commentary on the Yoga system of Patañjali.

Hence although this *sūtra* itself makes a fairly simple point, its wider significance is not to be underestimated. *Anavacchinna* means 'not dependent upon', or 'not conditional on', and the factors listed in relation to that term are *jāti, deśa, kāla,* and *samaya,* birth, place, time, and custom. The *yamas* listed in the previous *sūtra* are in fact *sārva-bhauma,* universally applicable for the entire world, and hence they jointly comprise the *mahā-vrata,* the great vow. This phrase *mahā-vrata* is quite frequently encountered elsewhere, and it is sometimes used to refer to the vow of atonement for one who has killed a Brahmin, as was performed by Śiva after his beheading of Brahmā, but here it is applied to the definition of moral conduct that is universal and absolute rather than relative to time, place, and circumstance. The term *mahā-vrata* is also used in the Jaina tradition to refer to the same group of five observances that are here called *yamas*.

Vyāsa emphasises the absolute nature of these five precepts, pointing out that there can be no exceptions, such as that of a fisherman who vows only to kill fish, or a soldier who vows only to kill in battle. This is not the *mahā-vrata*. This implies that there is also 'the small vow' such as that practised by Vyāsa's fisherman whose non-violence is limited by species (*jāti*). Following Vyāsa's line of reasoning, Śaṅkara then concludes that the path of Yoga being laid out in this chapter can only be followed by renunciants and not those whose means of livelihood leads them to contravene the precepts. Vācaspati Miśra comments only briefly, summarising Vyāsa's observations, but Vijñāna Bhikṣu considers whether the acts of violence in sacrificing animals in the Vedic ritual are also forbidden by the precept of *ahiṁsā*. He argues unequivocally that this type of ritual is incompatible with this first limb of Yoga, noting that in the *Gītā*, Kṛṣṇa refers to a *jñāna-yajña*, the internal ritual of knowledge, which should be adopted in place of the external Vedic ritual in which animals are killed as an offering into the fire.

2.32 *śauca-santoṣa-tapaḥ-svādhyāyeśvara-praṇidhānāni niyamāḥ*

The observances are purity (*śauca*), contentment (*santoṣa*), austerity (*tapas*), recitation (*svādhyāya*), and worship of the Lord (*īśvara-praṇidhāna*).

Here Patañjali provides a five-fold list of the *niyamas*, the observances that should be undertaken as the second element in the progressive path of Yoga practice. *Śauca* generally refers to both inward and outward purity, as confirmed by Vyāsa. As inward purity, *śauca* probably relates to purity of the mind in the sense of avoiding angry, aggressive, envious, or malicious forms of thinking. *Santoṣa* is the state of contentment in which one is satisfied with the position in life one has reached, and is no longer troubled by aspirations for further material aggrandisement. Most people have a desire for greater wealth, fame, or power, but the *yogin* should avoid such tendencies and remain content with his or her lot. *Tapas* usually refers to the acceptance of an austere lifestyle, adhering to vows such as fasts or else more severe mortifications of the body in order to gain mastery over its demands. The *Bhagavad-gītā* (17.5–6 and 17.14–16), however, is very critical of the practice of such severe acts of austerity, and proposes an alternative form of *tapas* which is based on respectful, gentle conduct with body, words, and mind.

Svādhyāya is sometimes taken to mean the study of sacred texts, or even the study of one's own nature, but it is possibly better understood as the verbal recital of *mantras*, verses, or hymns of the Veda. This finds confirmation in the fact that the *Gītā* includes *svādhyāya* as one element in its definition of the *tapas* of speech. We have encountered *īśvara-praṇidhāna*, worship of the Lord, a couple of times already, first of all in the *Samādhi-pāda* (*sūtra* 1.23) as an alternative means of reaching *samādhi*, and then in the *Sādhana-pāda* (*sūtra* 2.1) as one of the elements of *kriyā-yoga*. Here, as one of the *niyamas*, it probably means performing the daily acts of worship that are a common feature of contemporary Hindu religious practice.

Vyāsa states that *śauca* means maintaining a good standard of bodily hygiene as well as purity of the mind, and expresses the view that *tapas* does indeed refer to harsh acts of bodily austerity, such as exposing oneself to extremes of heat and cold, or undergoing extended periods of fasting from food and water. In his view, *svādhyāya* means recital of writings on spiritual topics or else the mantra *oṁ*, whilst *īśvara-praṇidhāna* means the offering of all one's actions to the Lord as a form of devotional *karma-yoga*. Śaṅkara elaborates on the various forms of austere vows that should be undertaken under the heading of *tapas*, whilst Vācaspati Miśra suggests that *śauca*, purity, also refers to the consumption only of pure foods, such as the offerings made in ritual worship. He also provides a citation from the *Viṣṇu Purāṇa*, which gives a fuller explanation of the *niyamas* listed here. In line with his own devotional ideals, Vijñāna Bhikṣu here places the greatest emphasis on *īśvara-praṇidhāna*, stating that it is the most important of these five observances. He also cites the same verses from the *Viṣṇu Purāṇa*, which suggests that he might have been making use of Vācaspati Miśra's commentary, despite the differences of religious orientation between them.

Sūtras 2.33–2.34: Advice on How to Observe Yama and Niyama

The mind, as we have heard, is fickle, and as a result, it may be difficult to adhere strictly to the *yamas* and *niyamas* delineated in the previous *sūtras*. Hence in these next two *sūtras*, Patañjali offers words of advice on how one may become better able to adhere strictly to these principles. This will then be followed by ten *sūtras* in which the results obtained from the observance of each of them are specifically outlined.

2.33 *vitarka-bādhane pratipakṣa-bhāvanam*

When afflicted by perverse tendencies, one should adopt an opposing mode of thought.

It may well strike the reader that the *yamas* and *niyamas* will be very difficult to fully observe, simply because the materialistic tendencies of the heart, which afflict all of us, will tend to drag us in the opposite direction. When this occurs, Patañjali's advice is that we should direct the mind towards a contrary line of thought. For example, if we feel a longing for some item of pleasure, we should turn our minds to consider how little true satisfaction is to be derived from such forms of acquisition. Or if we feel aggressive towards someone, we should develop a sense of benign compassion that will dilute the unwanted sense of anger and ill-will. This point is explained more fully in the following *sūtra*.

Vyāsa offers a slightly different perspective by suggesting that when perverse tendencies contrary to the *yamas* arise in the mind, one should think of the negative karma such thoughts engender and of the cycle of death and rebirth one has been forced to previously undergo. Śaṅkara gives examples of the perverse tendencies referred to in the *sūtra* and adds that one should counter these by considering the negative effect they have on one's ability to practise Yoga. Vācaspati Miśra merely states that there is nothing here that requires further explanation, but Vijñāna Bhikṣu draws our attention to the particular use of the word *vitarka* in this *sūtra*. Previously (1.17) we have seen the word *vitarka* used to refer to one of the mental processes that lead to *saṁprajñāta-samādhi*, but here the meaning is quite different. Here it is used in the sense of *vi-tarka*, meaning contrary ideas, or thought processes, which afflict the mind. These are to be countered by *pratipakṣa*, the opposite mode of thought. This is the meaning.

2.34 *vitarkā hiṁsādayaḥ kṛta-kāritānumoditā lobha-krodha-moha-pūrvakā mṛdu-madhyādhimātrā duḥkhājñānānanta-phalā iti pratipakṣa-bhāvanam*

Such an opposing mode of thought consists of regarding perverse tendencies such as harming others as producing unlimited misery and ignorance. This applies to all such tendencies, whether they are performed directly, through others, or simply approved of, whether they are based on greed, anger, or delusion, or whether they are adopted slightly, moderately, or with intensity.

This is one of the longest *sūtras* included by Patañjali in his *Yoga Sūtras* and it is devoted to providing a fuller explanation of what he means by the notion of *pratipakṣa-bhāvana*, the opposing mode of thought by means of which tendencies contrary to the *yamas* can be nullified. The basis of the *pratipakṣa* is a consideration of the unlimited *duḥkha* and *ajñāna*, sorrow and ignorance, which are the fruits, the *phala*, that are experienced when the *yamas* are not adhered to. This could be the sorrow and ignorance brought upon the victims of perverse acts, but it is more likely that what is being referred to here are the karmic results of perverse actions, which take the form of sorrow and ignorance. One is essentially being asked to consider the effects such actions will have on one's own future existence.

Further insight is also given here into the nature of the perverse tendencies that inhibit our ability to adhere to the *yamas*. Such *vi-tarkas* are first defined as '*hiṁsā* and the rest' (*hiṁsādayaḥ*), *hiṁsā* being the opposite of *ahiṁsā*, and hence meaning causing harm to others. Furthermore, these harmful acts may be performed by oneself directly, *kṛta*, or by someone else whom one engages to perform them, *kārita*; and the pernicious effect remains even if one merely gives approval for such actions, *anumodita*. Hence one may accept the services of a sacrificing priest or of a slaughterhouse to avoid a direct act of violence, but this does not free one from the negative karma of such an action. Then we are told of the states of mind that exist prior to such perverse acts being performed, which are the root causes of such acts; these are *lobha*, *krodha*, and *moha*, greed, anger, and delusion. And finally, the *sūtra* stresses that whether it be the case that such deviations from *yama* are performed in a manner which is *mṛdu*, *madhya*, or *adhimātra*, mild, moderate, or intense, still the attempt must be made to counteract these tendencies by the means advocated here. Thus a careful reading reveals that although the *sūtra* is quite lengthy, the precise meaning is relatively easy to determine.

Vyāsa comments at some length here but adds little to the above discussion, except perhaps to confirm that the unlimited suffering and ignorance caused by perverse acts is that which befalls the performer of the acts as a result of the negative karma thereby accrued. Śaṅkara expands a little on Vyāsa's words by examining the different ways in which karma is experienced in future lives, but Vācaspati Miśra considers why ignorance should be seen as a karmic consequence of perverse acts alongside suffering. It is because acts that harm others lead to a predominance of the *guṇa* of *tamas* in the next life, and, as is well known, where *tamas* prevails in a person's mentality, ignorance is a certain consequence. Vijñāna Bhikṣu explains that the suffering one experiences as a karmic consequence of harmful acts is exactly commensurate with the amount of suffering caused by those acts. He also adds a theistic dimension to the discussion by arguing that pain caused to another living being is also painful to *īśvara*, as the Deity is present within each being.

SŪTRAS 2.35–2.39: THE FIVE PRINCIPLES OF YAMA

This next group of *sūtras* expands on what has been said before by providing more detail about the five principles designated as *yama*, with a specific focus on the results that come to the practitioner as a result of their strict observance. In some cases, the designated results seem to be mystical or magical in nature, in a manner that appears to be a precursor to the central theme of the third chapter, the *Vibhūti-pāda*. Again, these *sūtras* are fairly straightforward and, in each case, their meaning can be quite readily understood.

2.35 *ahiṁsā-pratiṣṭhāyāṁ tat-saṁnidhau vaira-tyāgaḥ*

> When the principle of *ahiṁsā* is firmly established,
> any sense of enmity is given up in his presence.

Each of the first four of these five *sūtras* begins with one of the five *yamas* followed by the word *pratiṣṭhāyām*, which means 'when firmly established'. Here it is the principle of *ahiṁsā* that is considered and the consequence of its being established is said to be *vaira-tyāga*, the abandonment of all sense of enmity, in his presence, *tat-saṁnidhau*. The meaning would therefore appear to be quite simple. When one absorbs the precept of *ahiṁsā* so as to make it an integral part of one's consciousness, the sense of enmity towards others will never arise, however great the provocation. A Christian priest once said to Gandhi, 'I think my religion is superior because it teaches me to love my enemies', to which Gandhi replied, 'Yes that would be impossible for me, because my religion teaches me to have no enemies' – which is what is being taught here.

Vyāsa has virtually nothing to say here, presumably because he regards the meaning of the *sūtra* to be self-evident. Śaṅkara merely says that in the presence of a *yogin* of perfect *ahiṁsā*, even the snake and mongoose would give up their enmity, and Vācaspati Miśra adds the horse and buffalo and the mouse and cat to the list of existential foes whose outlook would be thus transformed. Thus, the effect of *ahiṁsā* appears to be supernatural. Vijñāna Bhikṣu is similarly brief on this *sūtra*, noting that this is the beginning point from which the yogic endeavour must begin.

2.36 *satya-pratiṣṭhāyāṁ kriyā-phalāśrayatvam*

When the principle of truthfulness is firmly established the results of action are rendered certain.

This *sūtra* pertains to the firm establishment of the second of the five *yamas*, *satya*, truthfulness, within the mind of the practitioner of Yoga, but the meaning here is slightly less obvious. *Kriyā-phala* means the fruits of action and can be taken in the sense of both the unfolding of karma and also in a more conventional sense of achieving what is sought through the performance of a particular action. *Āśrayatva* means a state of dependence, here in the sense of causality; Vyāsa interprets this in a somewhat supernatural sense, or at least the sense of particular empowerment. He gives two examples to illustrate what is meant. If the adept who is fixed in *satya* says to another person 'become dedicated to *dharma*', then the recipient of this instruction will indeed become *dhārmika*, and if he says to another, 'achieve the domain of the gods', then the recipient of this instruction does attain *svarga-loka*. Thus the meaning of the *sūtra* is that when *satya-pratiṣṭhā* is achieved, a person's words become empowered so that they guarantee the successful result of any instruction given. And as the following *sūtras* also have a supernatural dimension to them, it seems likely that the intended meaning is that this empowerment goes beyond the usual laws that govern life in this world.

Śaṅkara gives examples from various Purāṇas in support of Vyāsa's assertion regarding the empowerment of words, repeating Vyāsa's final statement that, 'His word is infallible' (Trans. Leggett). This would seem to take the idea of *satya* some way beyond just honesty and truthfulness. Vācaspati Miśra further confirms this idea by stating that actions and their results depend on the words spoken by the *yogin*. Vijñāna Bhikṣu adds that this applies to the *yogin*'s thoughts as well as his words, for he only has to focus his mind on a particular outcome and it will come to pass.

2.37 *asteya-pratiṣṭhāyāṁ sarva-ratnopasthānam*

When the principle of not stealing is firmly established, every type of gemstone approaches him.

Here we are quite clearly encountering a statement about the supernatural results gained as a result of establishing a principle of *yama* within the consciousness. When one utterly renounces any tendency towards unrighteous acquisition, then riches will come to him without any further endeavour. This is a quite simple statement, although one that is perhaps rather difficult to accept. Neither Vyāsa nor Śaṅkara have anything further to add here, simply accepting the statement of the *sūtra* as factually the case, and Vācaspati Miśra merely repeats the *sūtra* and concludes with the words, 'Easily understood'

(Trans. Woods). Vijñāna Bhikṣu is similarly reticent in adding any further explanation at this point.

2.38 *brahmacarya-pratiṣṭhāyāṁ vīrya-lābhaḥ*

When the principle of celibacy is firmly established, great potency is acquired.

We move on now to the fourth of the five principles of *yama, brahmacarya,* sexual restraint or celibacy, and here we make contact with the idea that the discharge of semen reduces a man's potency, whilst retention and reabsorption of semen enhances a man's potency. This idea becomes more prominent as tantric ideas gain wider currency in Indian thought, but from an early time the view of semen as an empowered substance appears to have been widespread. Here the phrase used is *vīrya-lābha,* in which *lābha* means 'to gain' or 'obtain', whilst *vīrya* means 'strength', 'heroism', 'vigour', and 'potency'. In this context, it could mean either physical strength undiminished by the emission of semen, or else the spiritual potency that is a central theme of tantric teachings. *Vīrya* was also mentioned in *sūtra* 1.20 as one of the elements of the yogic path.

Vyāsa seems to imply that the *vīrya* referred to relates to the practitioner's mental and intellectual capacity, as he states that this enables him to impart teachings to others. The celibate teacher is possessed of a vigorous mental capacity that enables the mind to grasp ideas and to impart them to students. Śaṅkara gives his understanding of the *sūtra* by stating, 'The sense is that he cannot be thwarted by any obstacle' (Trans. Leggett), whilst Vācaspati Miśra goes further and suggests that it is the *vīrya* attained through *brahmacarya* that brings various *siddhis,* the mystical and magical abilities outlined in the *Vibhūti-pāda.* Vijñāna Bhikṣu is more restrained in his views here, simply stating that *brahmacarya* brings knowledge without obstruction and the ability to perform actions without being thwarted by any external hindrance.

2.39 *aparigraha-sthairye janma-kathantā-saṁbodhaḥ*

When the principle of not seeking ownership becomes fixed, the understanding of previous births is awakened.

Here the final word of the opening phrase is changed from *pratiṣṭhāyām* to *sthairye,* although the reason for that change is not clear and the meaning remains the same: being fixed in dedication to the principle of the *yama* under consideration. In this case, that principle is *aparigraha,* which means an absence of grasping tendencies in the sense of a desire for personal gain and acquisition. It really means to become free of materialistic desires. When that state of mind becomes firmly fixed in the practitioner, then there arises what is described as *janma-kathantā-saṁbodha*. Here *saṁbodha* means 'knowledge', 'understanding', or 'awakening', *janman* means 'birth', and *kathantā* literally means 'the how'. In other words, the internalisation of this precept brings an understanding of how birth comes about. This could refer to a knowledge of one's own previous births, such as was achieved by the Buddha as a part of his own enlightenment, or it could mean a more general understanding of how and why birth, death, and rebirth occur. Either reading is perfectly valid.

Vyāsa seems to accept both readings at the same time, as he claims that the power acquired here brings an understanding of past, present, and future births, and of how and why such births took place, although he is clear that this knowledge is specific to one's own cycle of rebirth. Śaṅkara provides the explanation that it is because the *yogin* is no longer preoccupied with external matters that the understanding of his inner identity naturally comes to the fore, bringing with it the knowledge of past births that is normally latent and concealed within the consciousness of one whose mind is absorbed in thoughts of the external world. Vācaspati Miśra adds that knowledge of one's birth also entails a knowledge of the nature of the embodiment and the elements out of which that mental and physical embodiment is formed. Vijñāna Bhikṣu suggests that it is because the *yogin* gains knowledge of the *ātman*, the true self, that knowledge of past, present, and future births is understood. The thought does come to mind that if the *yogin* gains complete success in his or her practice, then there will be no future births, but this point is not addressed by the commentators.

Sūtras 2.40–2.45: The Five Principles of Niyama

These next six *sūtras* follow a similar pattern to that encountered in the previous five, as the results gained from adhering to each of the five *niyamas* are delineated. Six *sūtras* are devoted to this discussion, as the first two of them focus on a single *niyama, śauca*. Here the results outlined have far less of a supernatural dimension, and are for the most part related to the manner in which one lives one's life and interacts with the world, although the point is reiterated that the *niyama* of *īśvara-praṇidhāna* is an effective way of obtaining the yogic perfection of *samādhi*.

2.40 *śaucāt svāṅga-jugupsā parair asaṁsargaḥ*

> As a result of practising purity, one develops distaste for one's own body, and avoids intimate contact with others.

Here we are given the consequence of the observance of the principle of *śauca*, purity, which is first in the list of the five *niyamas*, and this consequence is perhaps a little surprising. The point here reflects, I think, the dualism inherent in the Sāṁkhya view of personal identity, which emphasises the distinction between the pure, changeless *puruṣa* and the material embodiment with all its contaminations, material and spiritual. Striving for purity, one becomes increasingly aware of the unpleasant nature of the embodiment, which is filled with substances such as flesh, blood, stool, urine, and bile. As the *yogin* becomes ever more focused on the pure spiritual identity that is the true self, there is concomitant distaste for the elements of his embodiment, as well as a reluctance to make contact with those same elements in the bodies of others. It is interesting to note that, in this *sūtra*, the word *aṅga* is used to indicate the body as a whole, and one might therefore more literally translate the *sūtra* as meaning a distaste for the limbs of the body.

Vyāsa comments only briefly, but makes the connection between the endeavour of the spiritual aspirant for a higher identity and the distaste that arises for the lower identity in the form of his embodiment. Realisation of *puruṣa* entails casting aside attachment for the body formed of *prakṛti*. Neither Śaṅkara nor Vācaspati Miśra sees the need for any further explanation here, whilst Vijñāna Bhikṣu merely makes the point that this *jugupsā*, this distaste for the body, appears only gradually as one progresses slowly towards spiritual enlightenment.

2.41 *sattva-śuddhi-saumanasyaikāgryendriya-jayātma-darśana-yogyatvāni ca*

> Through the principle of purity one also acquires purification of one's existence, a genteel disposition, the ability to focus on a single object, mastery over the senses, and the ability to perceive the *ātman*.

In this second *sūtra* on the results of practising *śauca*, we are given a further list to be added to the distaste for the bodies of oneself and others. This list consists of *sattva-śuddhi*, purity of one's existence or perhaps the mind, *saumanasya*, gentility, *ekāgra*, one-pointedness, *indriya-jaya*, mastery over the senses, and *ātma-darśana-yogyatva*, the ability to perceive the *ātman*. We will observe that the items on this list are in fact fundamental to the yogic endeavour as a whole that Patañjali is setting forth in his *Yoga Sūtras*. If we take *sattva-śuddhi* to refer to purity of the mind and *saumanasya* to indicate a complete absence of malice in all one's mental processes, then we can observe that restricting the outward movement of the senses and the ability to fix the mind constantly on a single point are the means typically prescribed in the early Yoga teachings by which the adept gains *ātma-darśana*, perception of the true self. And it is this higher form of perception that represents the enlightened knowledge, the *viveka-khyāti*, which brings liberation from rebirth. So there can be little doubt as to the significance of this principle of *niyama* in Patañjali's wider perception of the means by which Yoga practice is undertaken.

Vyāsa here merely summarises the *sūtra* itself, and Śaṅkara sees no need to offer any further elaborations on its statement. Vācaspati Miśra explains that the significant results referred to here with regard to perfection in Yoga practice are gained through the purification of the mind, which thereby becomes a suitable tool to be used in achieving the spiritual goals of Yoga. Vijñāna Bhikṣu takes the word *sattva* in the sense of the *sattva-guṇa* and states that when the mind is predominated by this quality, gentility and friendliness towards others are a natural consequence, and the sattvic mind can also be employed in the task of gaining realisation of the *ātman*.

2.42 *santoṣād anuttamaḥ sukha-lābhaḥ*

As a result of contentment, the acquisition of happiness is unsurpassed.

This is another fairly straightforward *sūtra* in which Patañjali presents the result that comes from the *niyama* of *santoṣa*, contentment. In these *sūtras*, the ending of *āt*, or in this case *ād*, added as a suffix, gives the sense of 'due to', 'from', or 'as a result of'. Here the result of *santoṣa* is given as *sukha-lābha*, the acquisition of happiness or joy, and this phrase is in turn qualified by the word *anuttama*, which means 'unsurpassed'. It is not too difficult to see the meaning here, for quite obviously one who is absolutely content with his lot is one who is perfectly happy. It is said that the wealthiest person in the world is one who has no desires at all.

Vyāsa is brief here again, merely citing a verse from the *Mahābhārata* which states that all the pleasures of this world do not amount to a sixteenth part of the joy that arises when hankering comes to an end. Neither Śaṅkara nor Vācaspati Miśra has anything further to add here, the latter citing a verse spoken by Yayāti in the *Viṣṇu Purāṇa* that makes a similar point regarding the joy that comes when all desires are set aside. Vijñāna Bhikṣu, however, is somewhat more forthcoming, continuing his theme of discussing the influence of the *sattva-guṇa*, which, he says, puts an end to the greed that destroys contentment. He further points out that *īśvara* is by nature free of all cravings, and hence *ānanda*, pure joy, is one of the attributes of the divine nature of *īśvara*.

2.43 *kāyendriya-siddhir aśuddhi-kṣayāt tapasaḥ*

As a result of the dwindling of impurities due to acts of austerity, the body and senses attain higher powers.

Here we are informed of the results gained from the practice of *tapas*, acts of austerity, and the result is here given in stages. First of all, there is *aśuddhi-kṣaya,* the wasting away of impurities, and then, from that removal of impurity, there is *kāya-indriya-siddhi.* The word *siddhi,* meaning 'success' or 'perfection', is quite frequently encountered in treatises on Yoga where it has the specific meaning of magical powers that defy the conventional laws of nature. Here the idea of *siddhi* is related specifically to the body, *kāya,* and to the senses, *indriya,* suggesting that the execution of *tapas* brings superhuman attributes of the body and abnormal powers of sensory perception. The idea of severe *tapas* being performed to gain individual empowerment of a superhuman type is one that we often find in Indian texts, sometimes being undertaken by evil individuals who thereby gain the power to triumph over the gods and disturb the *dharma* of the world. Hence it is not surprising to find Patañjali following that line by stating that the result of the *niyama* of *tapas* is *kāya-indriya-siddhi,* higher powers of the body and senses. We will hear much more about this type of *siddhi* in the next chapter, the *Vibhūti-pāda.*

Vyāsa is once again restrained in his comments but does confirm that the *siddhis* referred to here are supernatural powers, giving the example of the ability to become minutely small in the case of *siddhis* of the body, and the ability to hear sounds from a great distance away in the case of *siddhis* of the senses. Śaṅkara adds that it is wrongdoing that veils the senses and so, when this is removed by *tapas,* the full power of the senses is unveiled. Neither Vācaspati Miśra nor Vijñāna Bhikṣu sees the need for further comment on this *sūtra.*

2.44 *svādhyāyād iṣṭa-devatā-saṁprayogaḥ*

> As a result of recitation, there is contact with the chosen deity.

Here then is the result that arises from practising the *niyama* of *svādhyāya,* recitation of a *mantra* or of a sacred text.

This is said to be *iṣṭa-devatā-saṁprayoga*, being united with one's own particular deity. In Indian religion, worship is offered to a number of different deities, although it is generally understood that these are diverse manifestations of *īśvara*, the one Supreme Deity. The deity an individual is particularly drawn towards for devotional practices is the *iṣṭa-devatā*, one's own chosen deity. Here it is said that *svādhyāya* brings one into contact, *saṁprayoga*, with that deity, a phrase which calls to mind the idea that the deity and the *mantra* of that deity are one and the same. Hence, by chanting that particular *mantra*, contact is made with the deity who is the particular object of one's devotion. It is not clear whether or not this is the idea underlying this *sūtra*, but it may be that this is what Patañjali has in mind. Vyāsa comments that *svādhyāya* brings *darśana*, direct vision, of gods, sages (*ṛṣi*), and perfected beings, *siddhas*, who provide assistance in his work, but does not explain how or why this is so. Śaṅkara, Vācaspati Miśra, and Vijñāna Bhikṣu are all similarly reticent.

2.45 *samādhi-siddhir īśvara-praṇidhānāt*

As a result of worshipping the Lord, there is success in attaining the state of *samādhi*.

With this *sūtra*, Patañjali completes his discussion of the results that are gained from practising the five *niyamas*, here referring to *īśvara-praṇidhāna*, worship of the Lord. We have already seen in *sūtra* 1.23 of the *Samādhi-pāda* that such adherence to the way of *bhakti* is an alternative means of reaching the state of *samādhi*, and, as we noticed at that point, this offering of an alternative devotional path mirrors the teachings of the *Bhagavad-gītā* in which *jñāna* and *bhakti*, knowledge and devotion, are both advocated as means by which liberation from rebirth is achieved. In the *Yoga Sūtras*, the main emphasis is on the path of *jñāna*, the *viveka-khyāti* that has previously been emphasised, but it is interesting to note this acknowledgement that the *samādhi-siddhi*, the perfection of *samādhi*, is also arrived at through devotion to the Supreme Deity. In the *Gītā* (18.66, 12.7), this is said to be due to the idea of grace by which the Lord himself acts to grant the gift of liberation due to his compassion (10.11) and love (12.14); it is not clear whether or not Patañjali has any such doctrine of divine grace in mind.

Vyāsa is again brief in his comments, just adding that the *samādhi-siddhi* achieved through devotion enables the devotee to understand everything he wishes to know. He does not explain why or how this is so. Śaṅkara has nothing to add at this point, but Vācaspati Miśra contends that *īśvara-praṇidhāna* should not be taken as an alternative path that obviates the need for all other elements of Yoga practice. It does not bring the full perfection sought by the *yogin*, and is only a partial step on the full path of Yoga. This assertion would appear to be more reflective of Vācaspati Miśra's own ideas and beliefs, rather than the overt statement of the *sūtra*. As might be anticipated, Vijñāna Bhikṣu holds to a different view, and suggests that the other limbs of yoga, the *yogāṅga*, are to be understood as being devotional practices dedicated to *īśvara*. It is for this reason that *īśvara-praṇidhāna* is said to bring the full perfection of the yogic endeavour in the form of *samādhi*.

Sūtras 2.46–2.48: The Practice of Āsana

Āsana is central to much of contemporary Yoga practice and is considered as a part of the *yoga-sādhana*, as the third of the eight *yogāṅga*. In contrast to contemporary practice, however, *āsana* is dealt with here relatively briefly and none of the more well-known non-seated *āsanas* are referred to. As has been mentioned before, the *Yoga Sūtras* and other early

Yoga treatises are primarily about a Yoga of the mind rather than a Yoga of the body, and this being the case, it appears that *āsana* is referred to here only in as far as it enables one to adopt a comfortable posture in which the mental components of Yoga can be undertaken. This is not about awakening latent energies within the body, not about *cakras*, and not about enhancing the body's physical abilities. It is just about finding the best practical means by which the refocussing of the mind from external to internal perception can be achieved.

2.46 *sthira-sukham āsanam*

A sitting posture should be steady and comfortable.

The meaning of this first *sūtra* on *āsana* is quite clear, as it merely states that the *āsana* should be *sthira* and *sukha*. *Sthira* means firm, steady, or fixed; *sukha* means happy, pleasurable, or easy, and in this context 'comfortable' probably best reflects the intended meaning. The point is that if one is to undertake extended periods of concentration or meditation, then it is essential that one's posture can be maintained for such periods of time without bodily discomfort that would distract the mind from its yogic endeavour.

Commenting on this *sūtra*, Vyāsa does in fact give a list of eleven *āsanas*, some of which will be readily recognised by contemporary practitioners. These are:

1. The Padmāsana
2. The Vīrāsana
3. The Bhadrāsana
4. The Svastika
5. The Daṇḍāsana
6. The Sopāśraya
7. The Paryaṅka
8. The Krauñca-niṣadana

9. The Hasti-niṣadana
10. The Uṣṭra-niṣadana
11. The Sama-saṁsthāna

Given the fact that lists of this type in relation to *āsana* are virtually unknown elsewhere in the early period when the *Yoga Sūtras* is believed to have been composed, the list presented here does raise doubts over the contention that Vyāsa's commentary is the work of Patañjali himself. On the other hand, all of these appear to be seated postures and are different from the more complex *āsanas* that are listed in later medieval Yoga texts. Śaṅkara says very little about the *sūtra* itself, but provides details of how the *āsanas* included in Vyāsa's list are to be adopted. Vācaspati Miśra states that the lotus position, the *padmāsana*, is widely known, and then provides similar details to those given by Śaṅkara, with some slight variations. Vijñāna Bhikṣu also describes these *āsanas*, referring to the writing of Vasiṣṭha and to another Yoga text he names as the *Yoga-pradīpa*.

2.47 *prayatna-śaithilyānanta-samāpattibhyām*

This is achieved through the relaxation of exertion, and absorption in the unlimited.

In this *sūtra*, Patañjali explains how an *āsana* can be made steady and comfortable, and he gives two methods between which the conjunctions 'or' or 'and' can be inserted. Again the idea here seems to be finding a specific posture in which one is able to withdraw the mind from external circumstances and turn its focus inwards without the distraction caused by any physical discomfort. The first method is *prayatna-śaithilya*, which means 'the relaxation of exertion or endeavour', indicating that the sitting posture should be adopted without any strain being put on any part of the body. This idea clearly ties in with the previous recommendation that the posture should be steady and comfortable.

The second method is *ananta-samāpatti,* and here we will recall our previous encounter with the term *samāpatti* in *sūtras* 1.41 to 1.44 of the *Samādhi-pāda* where it was used to designate a state of intense concentration achieved prior to the state of *samādhi.* Here it is said that this *samāpatti* must be applied to that which is *ananta,* without limit, and one must presume that this refers to the part of our identity that is entirely spiritual, the *ātman* or *puruṣa.* The idea in this case would seem to be that when the consciousness is entirely absorbed in experiencing this unlimited, purely spiritual identity, all concerns over the material dimension of our existence are set aside, and the *āsana* then naturally becomes steady and comfortable. It is so because the mind has entirely transcended its usual material preoccupations.

Śaṅkara states that this relaxation occurs once the posture is 'locked into position, or (when it is familiar) by not exerting effort at all' (Trans. Leggett). He further adds that the word *ananta* refers to that which pervades the universe, although he refrains from philosophising on what is meant by that. Vācaspati Miśra contends that *āsana,* as referred to in these *sūtras,* cannot be a conventional sitting position, but must be a special posture that is to be taught to the practitioner; otherwise there would be no need to refer to *āsana* at all. He also suggests that the word *ananta* here refers to the serpent Ananta that is the bed of Viṣṇu as the Deity lies sleeping on the vast ocean. This seems a little fanciful, although it is a view shared by Vijñāna Bhikṣu.

2.48 *tato dvandvānabhighātaḥ*

Then there is no further affliction from the dualities of existence.

This again is a fairly straightforward *sūtra* consisting of just two words (the second being a compound of two members), *tataḥ*, meaning thereupon, *dvandva*, meaning duality, and *an-abhighātaḥ*, meaning without affliction. The idea is that in conventional life we are beset by constant fluctuations or dualities of existence: happiness and misery, heat and cold, good health and sickness; but in the condition being referred to here, one transcends these dualities by entering a state of aloof serenity of mind. It would seem to be most likely that this is not a reference to *āsana per se*, but to the state of *ananta-samāpatti* introduced in the previous *sūtra*: absorption of the mind in the unlimited, spiritual dimension of existence enables us to transcend conventional dualities.

Vyāsa takes a rather different line in his short commentary and states that it is the mastering of *āsanas* that brings this relief from duality, and here he must be going beyond the *sūtras* themselves and considering the eleven specific postures mentioned earlier in his commentary. Vyāsa explains that the dualities mentioned in this *sūtra* are the likes of heat and cold. This suggests that he understands the perfection of *āsana* to overcome physical sensations that might prevent success in meditation. Neither Śaṅkara nor Vācaspati Miśra sees the need to comment further, and Vijñāna Bhikṣu merely observes that, 'the commentary is easy here'.

Sūtras 2.49–2.53: The Practice of Prāṇāyāma

In these next five *sūtras*, Patañjali moves on to consider the fourth of the eight limbs of Yoga listed previously: *prāṇāyāma*, the regulation of the breathing process. He refers specifically to *prāṇāyāma* as the *viccheda* of the breath, a word that literally means 'cutting off', and one must presume that this indicates that conscious restrictions are to be imposed on the inward and outward flow of the breath. This is said to be of four types: inward, external, retention, and a form of *prāṇāyāma* that goes beyond both the internal and external movements of the breath. Almost certainly, the first three of these are the *pūraka, kumbhaka,* and *recaka* that will be familiar to most practitioners, but the identity of the fourth type is less certain. It is also said here that the primary function of *prāṇāyāma* is to provide a basis from which one can move on to the practice of concentration, *dhāraṇā,* indicating again that Patañjali's primary focus is on a Yoga of the mind rather than a Yoga of the body, and serving to distance the *Yoga Sūtras* from the understanding of *prāṇāyāma* encountered in later texts on Yoga in which the influence of *tantra* is to the fore.

2.49 *tasmin sati śvāsa-praśvāsayor gati-vicchedaḥ prāṇāyāmaḥ*

> When this is achieved, the movements of the
> inhaled and exhaled breaths can be restricted.
> This is *prāṇāyāma.*

In this first *sūtra* on *prāṇāyāma,* Patañjali offers us a straightforward definition of what he means by that term. First of all, he says *tasmin sati,* when that is achieved, meaning when *āsana* is established, there is *gati-viccheda.* Derived from the verb 'to go', *gati* means 'the goal', 'the path', 'the progression', or 'the movement', and here it is the last of these that is clearly most appropriate. *Viccheda* means cutting off or restriction, and the object of that restriction is said to be twofold, *śvāsa* and *praśvāsa,* meaning the inhaled and exhaled breaths. *Prāṇāyāma* is thus defined as taking place when *āsana* is mastered, and there is then a progression towards the restriction of the inhaled and exhaled breaths.

Here Vyāsa merely summarises the *sūtra.* Śaṅkara is only slightly more forthcoming, but notices the connection between the process of inhalation with the internal bodily airs known as *prāṇa* and *apāna*. Vācaspati Miśra refers to a different, lengthier version of Vyāsa's commentary on this *sūtra,* and provides a more detailed explanation of how *prāṇāyāma* should be properly performed based on counting the duration of inhalation and exhalation, and involving the whole body in the process. Vijñāna Bhikṣu follows the shorter version of Vyāsa's commentary, but makes the point that despite the words *tasmin sati,* one should understand that the first six limbs of yoga are not to be practised one after the other, but simultaneously, as they are mutually reinforcing.

2.50 *bāhyābhyantara-stambha-vṛttir deśa-kāla-saṁkhyābhiḥ paridṛṣṭo dīrgha-sūkṣmaḥ*

> The movement of the breath is internal, external, and then held steady. *Prāṇāyāma* can be observed in accordance with place, time, and number, and it can be either extended or subtle.

Here we are given more information about the practice of *prāṇāyāma,* and the three elements of which it consists, designated as *bāhya,* outward or external, *ābhyantara,* inward or internal, and *stambha,* steady, in relation to its *vṛtti,* its movements. As the commentators make clear, this is to be understood as a means of undertaking the *pūraka,* where the breath is drawn in to the lungs, the *kumbhaka,* where the breath is held within the lungs, and the *recaka* where the breath is exhaled from the body. We are then informed that the practice of this threefold *prāṇāyāma* can be *dīrgha,* meaning 'deep' or 'extended', or it can be *sūkṣma,* meaning 'subtle', or more likely 'shallow' in this context, and it can be practised in relation to the place, the time, and the number of repetitions. The exact meaning of this is not entirely clear, but what is probably meant is that there are varying degrees of intensity in the manner in which the practitioner performs *prāṇāyāma*. There may be deep or light inhalations and the threefold cycle can be undertaken in sequences that vary in the time taken to complete the three processes and the number of times the practice is repeated.

Vyāsa provides an explanation that is slightly different from the usual understanding of *pūraka, kumbhaka,* and *recaka,* as he states that *bāhya* means that the breathing process is inhibited after breath has been exhaled, and *ābhyanatara* means that it is inhibited after breath has been inhaled. *Stambha* is the form of restraint in which both inhalation and exhalation are inhibited. He then explains that place means the area covered by the breath inside or outside of the body, whilst time and number refer to the duration of each threefold cycle and the number of times the cycle is repeated during the period of practice. He gives no further explanation of what is meant by *dīrgha* and *sūkṣma,* extended and subtle, presumably because he regards the meaning as obvious. Śaṅkara offers an explanation of what is meant by *deśa,* place, in this context, stating that it refers to the spread of the breath inside the body once it has been taken in through the nostrils. He explains *dīrgha* and *sūkṣma* in relation to the length of time one is able to extend the duration of the process of inhalation and exhalation. It is long in the sense of the time that one is able to carry out a single inhalation and exhalation, and it is *sūkṣma* in the sense that the breathing becomes very shallow during the practice of *prāṇāyāma*.

Vācaspati Miśra expands somewhat on Vyāsa's explanation by suggesting the exact dimensions of the space covered by the breath internally and externally, and the different durations of time for which *prāṇāyāma* may be practised. He also makes the point that proficiency in *prāṇāyāma,* and the level of restraint the adept is able to achieve, are developed only gradually over a period of time, and as a result of resolute practice frequently undertaken. As a committed practitioner of Yoga, Vijñāna

Bhikṣu comments at some length on this *sūtra*, providing a detailed discussion of the techniques of *prāṇāyāma* and presenting quotations from various Purāṇas relating to this element of yogic practice. Unfortunately, this discussion goes some way beyond the scope of the present study.

2.51 *bāhyābhyantara-viṣayākṣepī caturthaḥ*

> A fourth type of *prāṇāyāma* goes beyond the range of the external and internal movements.

The most obvious point about this *sūtra* is that it is referring to a fourth form of *prāṇāyāma*. However, the nature of this fourth element is far from clear as all we are told is that it goes beyond, *ākṣepī*, the range, the *viṣaya*, of internal and external breaths, the *bāhya* and the *ābhyantara*. It is hard to say exactly what this means in relation to the practice of *prāṇāyāma* and hence this is one of those occasions when the point is well made that the commentary is essential for the meaning of the *sūtras* to be properly conveyed.

So what do the commentators, and Vyāsa in particular, have to say? Vyāsa first makes the point that this fourth stage is possible only after the previous three have been mastered. He then defines it as follows: 'the fourth *prāṇāyāma* is a suspension of movement of breath after transcending both the earlier spheres' (Trans. Rukmani). What he seems to be saying is that, in this fourth stage, there is no longer either inhalation or exhalation. The suspension of the breath in this stage is a wholesale cessation of the breathing process. We will be aware that persons who dive for pearl-bearing oysters can hold their breath for several minutes, and what it seems is being said here is that the *yogin* who becomes an expert in the execution of *prāṇāyāma* develops a similar or even greater ability. We also hear of hibernating animals that suspend their breathing and heartbeats, and we might infer that *prāṇāyāma* enables the adept to withdraw from external perception to a considerable degree in a manner that allows for the inward perception leading to *viveka-khyāti*, discriminative knowledge, which is the real goal of Yoga.

Śaṅkara summarises Vyāsa's commentary. Vācaspati Miśra, however, makes the point that this fourth stage is not a new and different form of *prāṇāyāma* but rather the natural outcome of mastering the previous three stages. He also makes the point that the difference between the fourth and third stages is that the third is closely connected with the inhalation and exhalation, whilst the fourth goes beyond all three. Once again, Vijñāna Bhikṣu is expansive in his comments, referring to the later medieval yoga text *Vasiṣṭha Saṁhitā* to explain that this fourth stage is what is known as *kevala-kumbhaka*, complete suspension of the breath. He also gives more precise instructions as to the performance of *prāṇāyāma* as a daily exercise that allows the practitioner to progress towards this stage of *kevala-kumbhaka*.

2.52 *tataḥ kṣīyate prakāśāvaraṇam*

In this way, the covering of illumination is diminished.

The meaning of this *sūtra* is fairly straightforward. The first word, *tataḥ*, means 'from this' or 'as a result of this', and the verb *kṣīyate* means 'it wastes away' or 'it diminishes'. Then we have the subject, which is the covering, the *āvaraṇa*, of illumination, of *prakāśa*. Here again, we are presented with the familiar idea of the light of knowledge being present within each one of us. Amongst the major strands of Indian thought, we often encounter the idea that the spiritual quest entails the search for knowledge, realisation, awakening, or enlightenment, which in turn brings liberation from rebirth. The teachers of Vedānta assert that such knowledge is to be gained by study and realisation of the truths revealed in the

Bhagavad-gītā, the Upaniṣads, and the *Brahma Sūtras*, but an alternative line of thought insists that there is no need to look outside of oneself for knowledge, except perhaps for preliminary pointers that guide us in the right direction. Here the idea is that the highest knowledge already exists within ourselves and the process by which knowledge is realised is thus one of removing the coverings that prevent this inner knowledge from shining forth, as indicated here by the word *prakāśa*. These coverings are usually referred to as greed, malice, anger, and other similar qualities, which arise from *avidyā*, the lack of true knowledge. Here we are told that the advanced practice of *prāṇāyāma* is one of the means by which the coverings are removed and a state of knowingness attained as the light shines from within.

Vyāsa takes the view that the coverings referred to are in fact the karmic effects of previous actions, and that the knowledge they cover is the *viveka-jñāna* by which one perceives the absolute distinction between *puruṣa* and *prakṛti*. Śaṅkara is brief here, but he does go a little further than Vyāsa by explaining that karma is a source of ignorance, and it is this ignorance that is the covering referred to in the *sūtra*. Vācaspati Miśra confirms Vyāsa's view that the word *prakāśa* refers to the light of *viveka-jñāna*, but also draws our attention to the meaning of the *kṣīyate*, which is to dwindle or become less. Hence this does not mean that the coverings are destroyed, just thinned somewhat, and the need to undertake acts of *tapas*, austerity, is not removed through the execution of *prāṇāyāma*. Vijñāna Bhikṣu picks up on Vyāsa's view that karma is the covering of knowledge being referred to, and explains that we should understand that karma is the same as *adharma*, the absence *dharma*. Hence the coverings are in fact thoughts, words, and deeds that are wicked and harmful to others.

2.53 *dhāraṇāsu ca yogyatā manasaḥ*

And the mind becomes ready for various forms of *dhāraṇā*.

Here we are given a clearer insight into the transformative effect of advanced *prāṇāyāma,* as it carries the mental faculties towards a state in which *dhāraṇā,* focused concentration on a single object, can be performed. In fact, the next in the list of the eight limbs is *pratyāhāra,* withdrawal of the senses from external objects, but as this corresponds closely with *dhāraṇā,* there is a smooth enough transition from one topic to another. The point that is being made here would seem to be that *prāṇāyāma* has the effect of stilling the constant fluctuations of the mind and thereby allows the *yogin* to withdraw the mind from external perception so that it can be focused on internal concentration. Hence although *prāṇāyāma* is a physical form of practice, it can be clearly seen how it forms a part of the Yoga of the mind that Patañjali is teaching throughout his *Yoga Sūtras.* Vyāsa has nothing to add at this point, merely referring us back to an earlier *sūtra* (1.34) in which a similar point was made. Śaṅkara and Vācaspati Miśra follow Vyāsa in refraining from further comment, whilst Vijñāna Bhikṣu merely adds that the earlier *sūtra* referred only to the first three phases of *prāṇāyāma* and not to the fourth.

Sūtras 2.54–2.55: The Practice of Pratyāhāra

The final two *sūtras* of the *Sādhana-pāda* give a very brief account of what is meant by *pratyāhāra,* and of the results gained from its successful application. *Pratyāhāra* is the withdrawal of the senses from external perception, drawing them back into the mind, and the result of this is that one then gains control over the movements of the senses. At this point, we have now covered five of the eight *yogāṅgas*, which still leaves three to be considered, and it is this line of discussion that forms the first part of the third chapter, the *Vibhūti-pāda*.

> 2.54 *sva-viṣayāsaṁprayoge cittasya sva-rūpānukāra ivendriyāṇāṁ pratyāhāraḥ*
>
> *Pratyāhāra* is where the senses end their contact with their respective objects, and thus assume, as it were, the same nature as the mind.

This *sūtra* gives us a concise definition of what is meant by *pratyāhāra*, the fifth of the eight limbs of Yoga. The definition is twofold, the first of which is *sva-viṣaya-asaṁprayoge*. Each of the five senses has a particular object on which it focuses: sound, flavour, form and colour, aroma, and touch sensations. These are the *viṣaya*, the objects that are the focus of each of the senses, and the word *a-saṁprayoga* means the end to the contact between each sense and its respective object. Then, secondly, we have the phrase, *cittasya sva-rūpa-anukāra iva indriyāṇām*, which means that when the senses end their contact with their objects they appear to be non-different in form from the *citta*, the mind. We find this idea of the senses ceasing to have an independent existence and being taken back into the mind in a number of the Yoga treatises in the *Mahābhārata*, the idea being that these five *indriyas* are extended like tentacles out from the mind in order to bring perceptions into it for mental identification. *Pratyāhāra* is where those tentacles are taken back into the mind stuff, so that they are no longer distinguishable from it. The *Bhagavad-gītā* (2.58) compares this to a tortoise withdrawing its limbs back into its shell, as in that state it is as if the tortoise and its limbs are one and the same, just as the mind and the senses are one and the same when *prayāhāra* is successfully accomplished.

Vyāsa makes the point that when the senses are withdrawn back into the mind, the restraint of the movements of the mind is the same as exerting control over the senses. Śaṅkara confirms this latter point, but adds that withdrawal of the senses takes place as a part of the process of meditation and results from the *yogin*'s understanding of the limitations of sensory perception. Vācaspati Miśra points out that anger and attachment arise as a result of the contact between the senses and their objects. He further explains that the restrained senses come to share a common identity with the mind because, at that point, both are active only internally without any external activity. Vijñāna Bhikṣu states that this control of the senses is essential in the practice of Yoga, for without this mastery, one's meditation will be disturbed by the constant movement of the senses as they seek out their objects. Unless the senses are withdrawn into the mind by *pratyāhāra*, the *citta-vṛtti-nirodha*, the restriction of the movements of the mind referred to Patañjali in his second *sūtra*, cannot be accomplished.

2.55 *tataḥ paramā vaśyatendriyāṇām*

It is in this way that one gains absolute control over the senses.

This final *sūtra* of the second chapter now gives us the result gained through the successful practice of the *pratyāhāra* outlined in the previous *sūtra*. That result is *paramā vaśyatā indriyāṇām*. Here *paramā* means 'supreme', 'the highest', or 'absolute'; *vaśyatā* means 'control' or 'mastery'; *indriyāṇām* means 'of the senses', and so the meaning of the *sūtra* is readily discernible. It is interesting to note the manner in which the teachings here on regulation of the senses correspond to those encountered in the final eighteen verses of the second chapter of the *Bhagavad-gītā*, which are similarly concerned with the regulation of the senses. In the *Gītā*, however, the discussion moves beyond a strictly yogic context, at least in the conventional sense, and considers how this *paramā vaśyatā indriyāṇām* shapes the manner in which we live in the world day by day. Not only must the senses be controlled as an element of Yoga practice, but we must also recognise that it is the uncontrolled senses that are the root cause of selfish desire, avarice, anger, malice, and oppression. The *Yoga Sūtras* does not attempt to expand the idea beyond its own strict parameters of discussion, but it is interesting to note the wider implications suggested by the *Bhagavad-gītā*.

Vyāsa does in fact acknowledge the wider implications of gaining mastery over the senses, and gives a list of four or possibly five ways in which this might be understood. He concludes, however, that the *paramā*, the absolute, control of the senses is that referred to by a sage named Jaigīṣavya; it is not simply avoidance of pleasure or passionate hankerings, but is the internal restriction of all activity of mind and senses. When this is achieved, all the other worldly consequences that might be suggested naturally follow from that supreme achievement.

Śaṅkara here does little more than summarising Vyāsa's points, but Vācaspati Miśra pursues those ideas in further detail, pointing out that the avoidance of passion and the desirable sensations enjoyed through the senses represent an inferior or secondary form of mastery over the senses, standing in contrast to the *paramā vaśyatā* referred to by the *sūtra*. He reviews each of these in turn before confirming that it is the control advocated by Jaigīṣavya that is supreme or absolute. This is because it is not merely the restraint of sensory activity, but the wholesale suspension of the outward movement of the senses, so that there is no possibility of indulgence, and because it applies to all the senses simultaneously. Vijñāna Bhikṣu also provides a more detailed discussion of Vyāsa's list of the ways in which the senses can be restricted from their objects. Each one of these is superior to the preceding one until we arrive at the absolute control, which is achieved when the senses relinquish their independent existence and become nothing more than the mind.

Conclusion

The first half of the *Sādhana-pāda* dealt with *kriyā-yoga,* the afflictions that hinder the practice of Yoga, karma as a cause of suffering, and how liberation from this condition can be achieved. Then in *sūtra* 2.29, Patañjali expanded on this pathway to liberation by listing the eight limbs of Yoga around which his teachings on Yoga practice are based. This was followed by a fairly extensive discussion of the first two these eight, *yama* and *niyama,* describing the five principles of which each is comprised and the results that can be derived from a rigid adherence to these principles. Patañjali then moved on to provide shorter explanations of the next three limbs, *āsana, prāṇāyāma,* and *pratyāhāra,* showing how they form a part of the wider practice of Yoga that brings with it the ultimate realisation of our spiritual nature. And, at this point, we reach the end of the *Sādhana-pāda,* despite the fact that only five of the eight limbs have been discussed. The remaining three are the subject of the opening part of the next chapter, the *Vibhūti-pāda,* before it moves on to consider the mystical and magical powers acquired by the *yogins* as a result of their practice.

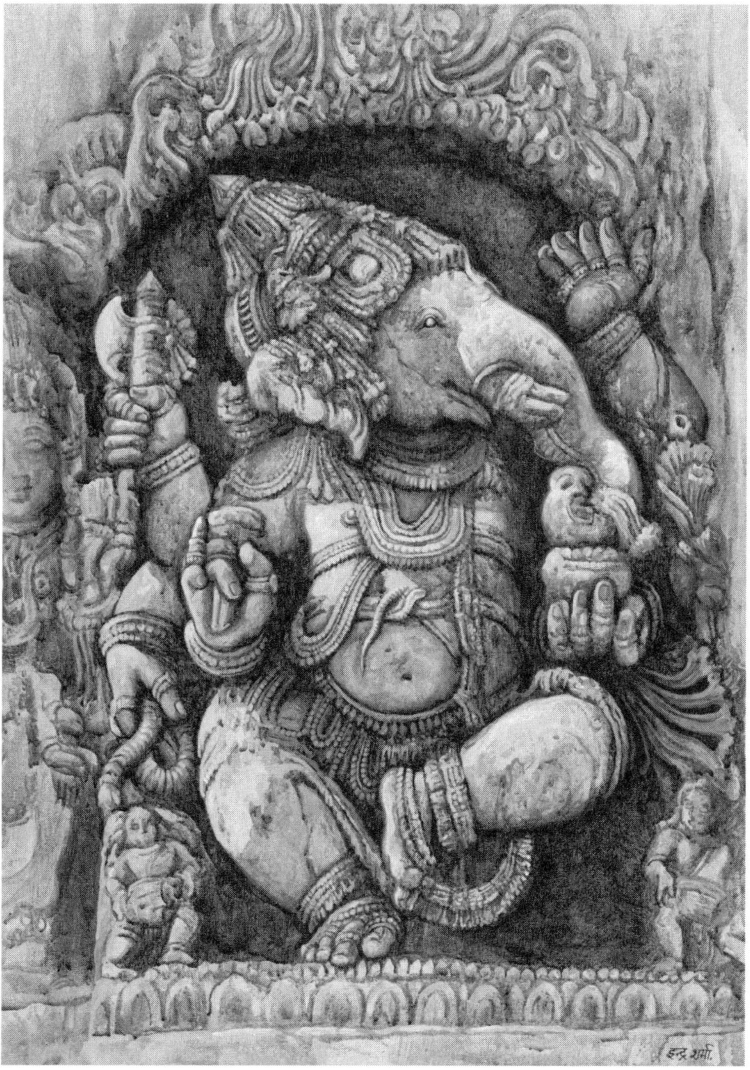

By saṁyama on the power of an elephant and other animals, one acquires their strength.—3.24

III
THE *VIBHŪTI-PĀDA*

As the name suggests, the main focus of this third chapter of the *Yoga Sūtras* is on *vibhūti*, a word that means 'might', 'glory', 'power', or 'wonderful ability'. In the context of Yoga discourse, *vibhūti* refers to the superhuman and supernatural abilities acquired by the successful *yogins* that enable them to experience a form of existence beyond the limitations generally imposed by the conventional laws of nature. These powers are delineated in succession from *sūtra* 3.16 through to *sūtra* 3.49, but before and after these *sūtras*, the chapter deals with other subjects that some might regard as being more significant, not least because the ideas here may be more acceptable to the modern mind.

We will recall that the *Sādhana-pāda* presented us with a list of what it called *yogāṅga*, the eight limbs of yoga, and then gave further information about the manner in which the first five of these are to be practised. So now the *Vibhūti-pāda* starts out with a discussion of the remaining three, *dhāraṇā*, *dhyāna*, and *samādhi*. These are briefly defined in the opening three *sūtras* of the chapter, but from this point onwards, are combined together into a single form of practice that is named as *saṁyama*. From *sūtra* 3.17, the transition is made to a presentation of the various *vibhūtis* acquired by the practitioner, the link being provided by the statement that it is *saṁyama* on a particular object or idea that brings a *vibhūti* that is broadly related to it.

The final six *sūtras*, 3.50 to 3.55, then move the discussion on a stage further by asserting that *saṁyama* is not only efficacious in granting the *yogin* supernatural powers related to existence in this world, but also provides the means by which discriminative knowledge is realised. In fact, the desire for such powers, as well as the powers themselves, is to be set aside, as one focuses exclusively on the highest goal of Yoga, for, as we have heard previously, it is this discriminative knowledge that reveals the absolute distinction between *puruṣa* and its material embodiments, and thereby allows *puruṣa* to gain liberation from this world and from the cycle of rebirth. This consideration of the means by which *saṁyama* leads to *kaivalya* carries the *Yoga Sūtras* forward into its fourth and final chapter, the *Kaivalya-pāda*. Although the *sūtras* that describe the supernatural powers and the means of obtaining them do not require extensive discussion, there is still a wide range of significant ideas to be encountered within the *Vibhūti-pāda* which carry the discussion forward towards its ultimate conclusion.

Sūtras 3.1–3.3: Dhāraṇā, Dhyāna, and Samādhi

In these opening three *sūtras* of the *Vibhūti-pāda*, we are given a very brief instruction on how the final three of the eight limbs of Yoga are to be understood. Very little information is actually given here, but what we can detect is that they represent a progressive development of the power of single-minded concentration, which begins with *dhāraṇā*, develops into *dhyāna*, and then concludes with the complete absorption of the mental faculties in the state known as *samādhi*. The reason for this brevity becomes clear from the subsequent *sūtras*, for Patañjali wants to combine these three together under the heading of *saṁyama*, and to then give a fuller account of that threefold combination.

3.1 *deśa-bandhaś cittasya dhāraṇā*

Dhāraṇā is the fixing of the mind on a single point.

This first *sūtra* of the chapter gives us a three-word definition of what Patañjali means by the term *dhāraṇā*, the sixth of the eight limbs listed in the *Sādhana-pāda*. It is the *deśa-bandha* of the *citta*, and the meaning of these words is quite clear. The term *citta* was given to us right at the start of the *Yoga Sūtras* where Yoga was defined as *citta-vṛtti-nirodha*, restraining the movements of the mind, and the *sūtra* here corresponds almost exactly with that opening statement, as *deśa* means a place or point and *bandha* means binding or keeping. Hence *dhāraṇā* is to be understood as a practice by which one keeps the mind fixed on a single point and prevents it from wandering off in the direction of different patterns of thought as is its usual wont; and anyone who has attempted such a practice will confirm that this is far easier said than done.

Vyāsa comments only briefly by suggesting single points or places on which the practitioner might fix the *citta* in concentration: the *nābhi-cakra* or navel-*cakra*, the *hṛdaya-puṇḍarīka* or lotus in the heart, the *mūrdhni-jyotis* or light in the head, the *nāsikāgra* or tip of the nose, and the *jihvāgra*, the tip of the tongue. Whether the first of these is a reference to the *cakra* system mentioned in later Yoga texts is doubtful, as the navel is itself quite frequently referred to as a wheel or circle without reference to that system. Precisely what is meant by the light in the head is unclear, although Śaṅkara gives an indication that his understanding of *nābhi-cakra* and *mūrdhni-jyotis* relates these to the system of subtle energy channels known as *nāḍīs*.

Vācaspati Miśra focuses his comments on Vyāsa's further observation that the single point to which the *citta* is to be bound may be something external rather than the points in the body in his list. Expanding on this, Vācaspati Miśra cites a passage from the *Viṣṇu Purāṇa* (6.7.75–85), which states that pure *dhāraṇā* is fixed concentration of the mind on the bodily form of Viṣṇu, with its well-established iconography as the four-armed Deity bearing a club, lotus, conch shell, and *cakra*. Vijñāna Bhikṣu provides supplementary quotations from the *Garuḍa Purāṇa* and the *Kūrma Purāṇa*, which provide instruction on various points and places on which the mind may be concentrated for the practice of *dhāraṇā*.

3.2 *tatra pratyayaika-tānatā dhyānam*

Dhyāna is where the focus of the mind remains constantly on that single object.

Here the clear line of continuity between *dhāraṇā* and *dhyāna* is expressed by the opening word *tatra*, which means 'there' or 'on that', and must be a reference to the single object of concentration that is the focus of *dhāraṇā*. *Dhyāna* is then defined as *pratyaya-eka-tānatā*, where *pratyaya* means the idea or thought and *eka-tānatā* means a single flow, to give the idea of a continuous flow of concentration that never wavers or deviates from the object that was the focus of *dhāraṇā*. So one might say that *dhyāna* is a continuous, undeviating flow of *dhāraṇā*. Vyāsa is again very brief in his comments on this *sūtra*, merely stating that *dhyāna* means that the meditation is untouched by the intrusion of any other form of thought or idea. Śaṅkara expands on this slightly by stating that in the practice of *dhāraṇā*, other ideas related to the object of concentration may arise, but where *dhyāna* is practised, there are no such intrusions, just an unbroken line of concentration. Vācaspati Miśra merely supplies a further quote from the *Viṣṇu Purāṇa* that complements the meaning of the *sūtra*; Vijñāna Bhikṣu takes a similar approach by supplying a verse from the *Garuḍa Purāṇa*, which provides an explanation of the development of *dhāraṇā* into *dhyāna*.

3.3 *tad evārtha-mātra-nirbhāsaṁ svarūpa-śūnyam iva samādhiḥ*

Samādhi is the same (*dhyāna*) where the object alone illuminates the consciousness, and which appears devoid of its form.

Here again we can see the clear connection between the final three *yogāṅga*, for just as *dhyāna* is a fully developed form of *dhāraṇā*, so *samādhi* is to be understood as *dhyāna* in its fully developed form, the ultimate conclusion of *dhāraṇā* and *dhyāna*. *Dhyāna* was shown to be a state of *dhāraṇā* in which the flow of thoughts relates only to the object of concentration and now we are told that *samādhi* is where the meditation becomes such that its form is *śūnya*, empty or absent. At this point, there is a single unwavering state that illuminates the mind, *artha-mātra-nirbhāsa*, a phrase that would appear to indicate that in the state of *samādhi* the flow of meditation ends and the object alone fills the mind without any specific thought being focused on that object.

Vyāsa provides us with a further explanation by stating that *samādhi* is that state in which the mind, the meditation, and the object of meditation are no longer distinct. In other words, the flow of thoughts focused on the object in the practice of *dhyāna* is now still and the object alone remains, completely filling the mind in a state of total absorption. Śaṅkara illustrates this point through the example of a crystal placed close to a coloured object. In that situation, the crystal becomes filled entirely with the colouration of the object, and in the same way, the mind becomes identical with the object of meditation. Vācaspati Miśra gives a similar understanding, stating that *samādhi* is reached when the distinction between contemplation and the object of contemplation no longer exists. Vijñāna Bhikṣu emphasises the point that *samādhi* is an advanced stage of *dhyāna,* the difference between them being that *dhyāna* involves a distinction between the knower, the object of knowledge, and the process of knowing, whilst in *samādhi,* all such distinctions vanish.

Sūtras 3.4–3.8: Saṁyama, the Essence of Yoga Practice

In these five *sūtras,* Patañjali draws together *dhāraṇā, dhyāna,* and *samādhi* under the single heading of *saṁyama,* which he refers to here as being almost the culmination of the Yoga path. One might feel that this discussion is anomalous in *Vibhūti-pāda,* but the point is that *saṁyama* in its varying forms is presented throughout the chapter as the means by which the practitioner becomes endowed with *vibhūtis.* So although there may appear to be an abrupt change of subject, there is a clear internal logic to the line of discussion followed here.

3.4 *trayam ekatra saṁyamaḥ*

When these three are applied to a single object, this is *saṁyama.*

This fourth *sūtra* is simple enough to comprehend, as it gives us the straightforward statement that when the three, *dhāraṇā, dhyāna,* and *samādhi,* are practised conjointly with a focus on a single object, then that is to be understood as *saṁyama.* Vyāsa merely reiterates this point, whilst Śaṅkara looks ahead to the main line of discussion in the *Vibhūti-pāda,* noting the central role of *saṁyama* in the progression of its *sūtras.* Vācaspati Miśra expresses the view that the use of the single term *saṁyama* in place of the other three is 'for brevity's sake' rather than having any greater significance, a view shared by Vijñāna Bhikṣu, who adds, 'The commentary is easy' in relation to this *sūtra*.

3.5 *taj-jayāt prajñālokaḥ*

When mastery in *saṁyama* is achieved, one's understanding is illuminated.

Here then is the first result of gaining proficiency or, more literally, conquest in the performance of *saṁyama*, which is given as *prajñā-ālokaḥ*. We have encountered the word *prajñā* a few times previously, and it means 'knowledge', 'wisdom', or 'understanding'; the word *āloka* here gives us the sense of 'spreading light' or 'illumination'. In other words, the first result of *saṁyama* is a form of enlightenment that enables us to perceive the world and our own lives in an undistorted manner, free of the passions and attachments that give us a vision of the world corrupted by selfish preoccupations.

Vyāsa gives a rather more elevated view of what is meant by *prajñā-āloka*, suggesting that in fact this refers to a special type of understanding, the *samādhi-prajñā*, which increases in proportion to *saṁyama* getting more stable. Even at this early point in the chapter, Śaṅkara feels able to direct the discussion towards the *vibhūtis* considered later on. He compares the idea of illumination in the word *āloka* to the shining of a lamp onto an object, so that the *yogin* gains powers of perception far beyond those of ordinary people. Vācaspati Miśra here notes that 'the commentary is easy', but emphasises the point that all these wonderful achievements gained through Yoga are the result of dedicated practice and a high level of commitment. Vijñāna Bhikṣu takes a similar line to Śaṅkara in suggesting that *āloka* means the illumination of objects that are subtle and beyond the range of normal perception.

3.6 *tasya bhūmiṣu viniyogaḥ*

This process is mastered through progressive stages.

The subject of this *sūtra* is *tasya viniyogaḥ,* the application or mastery of *saṁyama,* here referred to by the word *tasya,* meaning 'of that'. What we are told about success in the application of *saṁyama* is that it is *bhūmiṣu,* which here means 'in different levels or stages'. The clear meaning is thus that the mastery of *saṁyama* takes place step by step and that success in this practice is gradual, as one moves from one level of proficiency on to a higher level. Here one is reminded of a similar statement of the *Bhagavad-gītā* (6.25), which uses the phrase *śanaiḥ śanaiḥ,* meaning gradually or slowly. The point is that the results of Yoga practice are wonderful indeed, but one should not expect to achieve such results after practising these techniques for just a short amount of time.

Vyāsa makes the point that in making progress in *saṁyama,* it is impossible to move on to a higher level without first having gained proficiency in the previous stage. He also makes the interesting observation that this does not apply to those who have attained the state of *samādhi* through *īśvara-prasāda,* the grace of *īśvara,* because they have reached that point not through their own efforts but as a gift from a being other than themselves, *īśvara* himself. Śaṅkara suggests that the different levels referred to in the *sūtra* represent a progression from *saṁyama* on physical objects to *saṁyama* on objects of a more subtle nature, presumably mental constructs rather than actual objects. He also makes the point that the types of *saṁyama* that bring magical powers, such as telepathy, represent a lower level of *saṁyama,* and that these are set aside as one moves on to the higher level that brings realisation of the *ātman.* Curiously, or perhaps not so, Śaṅkara chooses to ignore Vyāsa's comments concerning *īśvara-prasāda.*

Vācaspati Miśra here returns to his earlier suggestion regarding *dhāraṇā* on the form of Viṣṇu and suggests that the different levels of *saṁyama* relate to the different parts of the form of Viṣṇu, as described in the *Viṣṇu Purāṇa*. He also states that the grace of *īśvara* carries one to the highest level of *saṁyama*, and it is for this reason that Vyāsa says that the progressive path does not apply to those who are recipients of divine grace. Vijñāna Bhikṣu compares progression in the practice of Yoga to the developing abilities of an archer who can only hit small targets after first gaining competence in hitting larger ones. He also confirms that the power of *īśvara* carries the recipients of grace to the highest stage of *saṁyama*, without their having to first pass through the lower stages.

3.7 *trayam antar-aṅgaṁ pūrvebhyaḥ*

These three are the very essence of Yoga,
transcending the other limbs.

Here the word *traya* obviously refers to the triad of *dhāraṇā*, *dhyāna*, and *samādhi*, and *pūrvebhyaḥ* means beyond the previous ones, which would be the first five limbs of Yoga. The meaning of the *sūtra* thus hinges on what is meant by *antar-aṅga*, literally 'within the body', or 'internal'. One very obvious meaning would be that whereas the first five limbs are external to the body, those that jointly comprise *saṁyama* are internal, being executed on a purely mental level. However, *antar-aṅga* also has the meaning of 'essential' and hence the suggestion here could well be that *yama*, *niyama*, *āsana*, *prāṇāyāma*, and *pratyāhāra* are preparatory processes that facilitate the essential practice of Yoga, which is the three elements of *saṁyama*.

Vyāsa gives little further guidance here except for noting that the triad of *dhyāna*, *dhāraṇā*, and *samādhi* are called *antar-aṅga* only in relation to the *saṁprajñāta samādhi*. Śaṅkara explains the *sūtra* to mean that even if the first five are not fully mastered, one should still attempt to practise *saṁyama*, implying that *saṁyama* is in one sense the true form of Yoga. Vācaspati Miśra suggests that the distinction between the earlier five and the later three is that it is only the combination of the three in *saṁyama* that can bring the adept to the state of *nirbīja samādhi*, the highest level of all, as is mentioned in the following *sūtra*. Vijñāna Bhikṣu takes the opportunity to consider the value of religious acts and the pursuit of higher knowledge in the quest for liberation. He equates the first five limbs of Yoga with spiritual action and the final three with the process of gaining realised knowledge, concluding that it is the knowledge gained through these three elements of *saṁyama* that yields the ultimate spiritual goal.

3.8 *tad api bahir-aṅgaṁ nir-bījasya*

> Though they in turn are external to the *samādhi* that is without seed.

Here we are informed that despite the fact that *saṁyama* was identified as *antar-aṅga*, internal or essential, in the previous *sūtra*, this is only in relation to *sa-bīja* or *saṁprajñāta-samādhi*, as was pointed out in Vyāsa's commentary to the previous *sūtra*. In relation to the supreme state of *samādhi*, which is *nir-bīja* or *asaṁprajñāta*, then the three limbs that collectively constitute *saṁyama* are to be regarded as *bahir-aṅga*, external or not of the essence. The point is that the *samādhi* that has been spoken of as the eighth limb is *saṁprajñāta* because there is still an object on which the mind is focused. In the highest stage, the *samādhi* takes the form of complete clarity of mind without there being any object on which it focuses.

Vyāsa provides only a very short explanation here, stating that *nir-bīja samādhi* can only appear when the three elements of *saṁyama* are no longer present. Śaṅkara, however, goes a little further than Vyāsa. He states that the first five limbs are not essential for the successful practice of Yoga; they are aids to success, but unlike the other three are not fundamental to the perfection of Yoga. Moreover, there are some individuals who attain the highest state of spiritual realisation without even undergoing the three components of *saṁyama*; this is because they have already reached a high state of spiritual awakening in a previous life, and here he refers his readers back to *sūtras* 1.18 and 1.19 of the *Samādhi-pāda*. Neither Vācaspati Miśra nor Vijñāna Bhikṣu has anything further to add beyond a recapitulation of what Vyāsa has said.

Sūtras 3.9–3.13: The Transformations Brought about by Saṁyama

The subject of this next group of *sūtras* is *pariṇāma*, which means a transformation, and the specific focus is on the transformations of the mind brought about by the practice of *saṁyama*. Postural Yoga brings about positive transformations of the body, and perhaps the mind as well, but Patañjali has been consistently emphasising the Yoga of the mind, and so it is to be expected that the form of practice he has taught would change the workings and very nature of the mind, and now this reconstruction of the mental faculties is outlined and explained.

3.9 *vyutthāna-nirodha-saṁskārayor abhibhava-prādurbhāvau nirodha-kṣaṇa-cittānvayo nirodha-pariṇāmaḥ*

The change brought about by restricting the movements of the mind consists of the overpowering of the latent impressions as they arise, and the appearance of the latent impressions of restraint. This condition of the mind arises at the moment when its movement is restricted.

As is often the case, the subject of this *sūtra* is to be found in the final word or phrase, in this case *nirodha-pariṇāma*, the transformation wrought by restraint. The word *nirodha*, of course, takes us back to Patañjali's opening definition of Yoga, and, in the present context, we can observe that such restraint is implicit in the description of *saṁyama*, for the total absorption of the mind on a single object, or indeed in *nirbīja samādhi*, must inevitably entail the restraint of all other movements of the mind. The *sūtra* as a whole gives us three pieces of information about *nirodha-pariṇāma*.

The first of these is *vyutthāna-saṁskāra ... abhibhava* and here again the word *saṁskāra* refers to the impressions on the mind left by each thought, perception, or idea, as it arises within the mind. The *vyutthāna-saṁskāras* are the arising or outgoing *saṁskāras* that are a feature of our conventional mental activities, and *abhibhava* means that these are overpowered or nullified. Hence *saṁyama* transforms the mind in such a way that the usual manner in which thought processes create *saṁskāras* is brought to an end. This is significant because it is these *saṁskāras* that generate future karma, and thereby perpetuate the cycle of rebirth. The second transformation caused by restraint is *nirodha-saṁskāra ... prādurbhāva* and here the phrase *nirodha-saṁskāra* indicates a different type of *saṁskāra* that is left by the practice of restraint, whilst *prādurbhāva* means generating or bringing into being. So the point is that the usual type of *saṁskāras* that generate karma and rebirth are inhibited, whilst a new type of *saṁskāra* based on restraint arises in the mind. These are the two primary transformations of the mind brought about by the practice of restraint inherent in *saṁyama*.

The third point made in the *sūtra* regarding the transformations caused by restraint is *nirodha-kṣaṇa-citta-anvaya*. Here *nirodha-kṣaṇa* means 'at the very moment that restraint occurs', and *citta-anvaya* means 'connected to the *citta*', giving us the meaning that the two types of transformation mentioned attach themselves to the mind at the very instant that they occur. In other words, the successful execution of *saṁyama* and the associated pattern of restraint yields its results from the very moment it occurs and not at some future point or in some future life.

Vyāsa makes the point that both types of *saṁskāra* attach themselves to the mind, but the practice of *saṁyama* causes a diminution of the outward or *vyutthāna-saṁskāras*, and the appearance of *saṁskāras* of restraint. Śaṅkara adds that these are not two independent processes, as it is the development of the *nirodha-saṁskāras* that inhibits and drives out the *vyutthāna-saṁskāras*. Vācaspati Miśra carries the discussion a stage further by explaining that the *nirodha-saṁskāras* not only prevent the *vyutthāna-saṁskāras* from appearing, but also act to erode those that are already present in the *citta*, thereby bringing freedom from karma to the adept in Yoga. Vijñāna Bhikṣu insists that what is being discussed here is *nirbīja* or *asaṁprajñāta-samādhi*, for *sabīja samādhi* still focuses on a particular object. Hence *sabīja samādhi* still produces *vyutthāna-saṁskāras* and it is only *nirbīja samādhi* that gives rise to the *saṁskāras* of restraint, the *nirodha-saṁskāras*.

3.10 *tasya praśānta-vāhitā saṁskārāt*

A flow of tranquillity arises in the mind from this new form of *saṁskāra*.

Here the word *saṁskārāt*, meaning from or as a result of the latent impression, must refer to the *nirodha-saṁskāra* that arises due to the practice of mental restraint inherent in *saṁyama*. The *sūtra* then gives one of the results arising from the appearance of that *nirodha-saṁskāra* with the words *tasya praśānta-vāhitā*, where *tasya*, meaning 'of that', refers to the *citta* and *praśānta-vāhitā* is a flow of tranquillity, giving us the meaning that the arising of *nirodha-saṁskāras* brings with it a flow of tranquillity into the *citta*. The idea would seem to be that our normal state of mind is one of constant transformation as we move from one thought or idea to another, but the *saṁskāra* of restraint makes the flow of the mind steady, constant, tranquil, and calm.

Vyāsa here makes the point that this flow of tranquillity is not necessarily a constant state, for the *nirodha-saṁskāras* may be weakened by the reappearance of various *vyutthāna-saṁskāras*, which have the effect of ending that tranquil flow. Śaṅkara adds that the perpetuation of this state of mental tranquillity is directly related to the degree of firmness by which the *nirodha-saṁskāras* are established by yogic practice. The tranquil flow will persist for as long as the *saṁskāra* of restraint can be maintained. Vācaspati Miśra merely asserts that what is being referred to here is the consequence of developing the *saṁskāra* of restraint. Vijñāna Bhikṣu again says, 'The commentary is easy', and that the idea of a flow of tranquillity clearly reveals the desirability of developing a succession of *nirodha-saṁskāras*.

> 3.11 *sarvārthataikāgratayoḥ kṣayodayau cittasya samādhi-pariṇāmaḥ*
>
> When the focus of the mind on all the objects of the world declines, and the state of single-mindedness arises, this is the transformation of consciousness towards *samādhi*.

The subject of this *sūtra* is again stated in the final phrase, *samādhi-pariṇāma*, which means the transformation that brings about the state of *samādhi*. The nature of this transformation is defined as being two-fold, both of which are related to the *citta*. The first of these is *sarva-arthatā ... kṣaya,* where *sarva-arthatā* means 'the state of having anything as its object', which refers to the normal state of the *citta* in which it shifts its focus from one object to another, and *kṣaya* means a dwindling or wasting away of that state of the mind. Hence it is stated that there must be a gradual diminution of the thoughts and ideas within the mind that relate to the affairs of this world. The second element of the transformation is *ekāgratā ... udaya,* where *ekāgratā* means 'one-pointedness' and *udaya* means the 'growth', 'expansion', or 'rising up', giving us the meaning of the expansion of the ability to direct the *citta* towards a single point, and to maintain it there fixedly. This is the transformation that takes place within the *citta,* bringing about the state of *samādhi.*

Vyāsa states that the spreading of the mind into a variety of thought processes and being fixed on a single point are both features of the *citta,* and with the rising up of one, the other declines to a corresponding degree. When the one-pointed state gains complete domination of the *citta,* that is *samādhi.* Śaṅkara points out that *kṣaya* means a dwindling but not a complete destruction, so there remains the possibility that the mind may once again start to seek engagement in a variety of external ways. The *pariṇāma* referred to in this *sūtra* is the transformation of the *citta* that carries it into the state of *samādhi.* Vācaspati Miśra has little to add here beyond Vyāsa's observations. Vijñāna Bhikṣu emphasises the point that the *pariṇāma,* the transformation, being mentioned here is a gradual one that takes place progressively as one's practice develops. He also points out that the word *kṣaya,* meaning diminishing, shows that the eradication is not yet complete and this is what distinguishes the transformation mentioned here from that which is the subject of the following *sūtra.*

3.12 *tataḥ punaḥ śāntoditau tulya-pratyayau cittasyaikāgratā-pariṇāmaḥ*

Furthermore, the transformation of the mind towards one-pointedness occurs when an idea takes the same form whether at peace or arising.

The subject of this *sūtra* is *ekāgratā-pariṇāma,* the transformation that brings about one-pointedness. As Vijñāna Bhikṣu noted in his comment on the previous *sūtra,* there could be some difficulty in distinguishing this transformation of the mind from the *samādhi* transformation discussed in the *sūtra* 3.11. Here the word *tataḥ,* meaning 'then' or 'from that', could provide us with the answer, as it suggests that this *ekāgratā-pariṇāma* follows on as a natural consequence of *samādhi-pariṇāma.* And we will then recall Vijñāna Bhikṣu's explanation that this next transformation is more complete, or more absolute, than that related to *samādhi.* What then does this transformation related to one-pointedness entail? The answer is given with the words *śānta-uditau tulya-pratyayau,* where *śānta* and *udita* mean 'at peace' and 'uprising', and *tulya-pratyaya* means equal conceptions, and these conceptions are of the *citta.* Exactly what this means is not immediately apparent from the *sūtra* itself. Vyāsa explains that an earlier *pratyaya* of the concentrated mind ceases and subsequently a similar *pratyaya* arises. Where there is single-pointed concentration on the part of the *yogin,* both of these manifestations of the idea will remain the same. In other words, there is no movement of the concentrated mind regardless of whether the object of concentration is fixed or reappearing. The focus remains constant on that single point, as represented by the word *ekāgratā.*

Śaṅkara explains the *sūtra* and Vyāsa's commentary in relation to the process by which thoughts enter the mind. As this occurs, a thought is made tranquil by the act of concentration and then, as the next idea enters, it is brought to the same state by the practitioner, as indicated by the phrase *tulya-pratyaya*. Vācaspati Miśra adds further clarity by explaining that as each new idea arises, it is transformed into the same tranquil state as the previous idea and in this way all thoughts are transformed into a single state, one after another. Vijñāna Bhikṣu confirms that the word *tataḥ* indicates that this *ekāgratā-pariṇāma* follows on as a result of the *samādhi-pariṇāma* referred to in the previous *sūtra*, and explains that the *ekāgratā* means that all the diverse thoughts that enter the mind are made into a single, unified flow rather than the complex diversity of movements of the mind in its conventional state.

> 3.13 *etena bhūtendriyeṣu dharma-lakṣaṇāvasthāpariṇāmā vyākhyātāḥ*
>
> In this way, I have now explained the transformations of the fundamental nature, the temporality, and the condition of the material elements and the senses.

At this point in his presentation, Patañjali takes the opportunity to broaden out his discussion of the transformatory results gained through Yoga practice, and to refer briefly to a major theme of Sāṁkhya/Yoga philosophy. This is the theory of *pariṇāma*, transformation, and in particular, what is known as the *satkārya-vāda*, which states that all effects are pre-existing in their cause. The idea is that nothing comes into being out of nothing; this applies in particular to the Sāṁkhya understanding of how the world originates in the evolution of the single substance of primal *prakṛti* into the form of the twenty-four basic elements. On the basis of the *satkārya-vāda*, it is asserted that each of these twenty-four elements exists in a latent state within the primal *prakṛti*, and hence they emerge through the transformation, the *pariṇāma*, of *prakṛti* rather than coming into existence from a state of non-existence.

Here Patañjali states *etena ... pariṇāmā vyākhyātāḥ*, where *etena* means 'by this' or 'in this way', with reference to the previous group of *sūtras*, and *pariṇāmā vyākhyātāḥ* means 'different forms of *pariṇāma* have been explained'. What he is saying is that the previous discussion of the transformation of the mind can be expanded so as to be applied to other categories of transformation, specifically those of the *bhūta* and the *indriya*, the five fundamental elements of matter (earth, water, fire, air, and space) and the five senses (taste, scent, sight, touch, and hearing). Moreover, this doctrine of transformation, the *pariṇāma-vāda*, relates to three specific categories, *dharma*, *lakṣaṇa*, and *avasthā*.

The word *dharma* is usually understood as 'right conduct' or 'proper way of living' but it has a number of other meanings as well, and in this case, it can be translated as 'an attribute' and means the fundamental character of any specific object, that which defines something as what it is, so that heat and light might be taken as the *dharma* of the sun or of fire. And as an interesting aside, when this idea is applied to humanity, we can notice that *dharma* in the sense of compassion and acts of kindness is the defining quality that makes a human being fully human. This is the true meaning of 'human nature'.

The word *lakṣaṇa* usually means the 'qualities or characteristics of an object', but here Vyāsa states that it means its position in relation to time, in the past, present, or future, and he takes the opportunity to embark on a lengthy discussion of the process of transformation in relation to these three phases of time. Then *avasthā* means 'the particular status or condition of an object at a given time', as, for example, gold can exist as a solid lump of metal or as a beautifully crafted item of jewellery. And again we can see how this relates to the concept of *pariṇāma* and also the *satkārya-vāda*, for the item of jewellery is not a creation out of something else, but existed in a latent state within the lump of gold from which it was formed.

As must surely be apparent, this line of philosophical debate takes us some distance beyond the exposition of Yoga that is the central theme of the *Yoga Sūtras*. Vyāsa takes this opportunity to present one of his longer passages of commentary in which he outlines the philosophical ideas discussed above in line with the Sāṁkhya/Yoga doctrines of *pariṇāma-vāda* and *satkārya-vāda*. Each of the commentators follows Vyāsa's lead by providing extensive discourses on these lines and, at the same time, attempting to show the shortcomings of alternative schools of thought, notably Buddhism and Nyāya/Vaiśeṣika, which do not accept the *satkārya-vāda*. Unfortunately, the scope of the present work does not allow us to pursue these lines of argumentation in any further detail, as they carry us some distance away from the text of the *Yoga Sūtras* itself.

Sūtras 3.14–3.16: Knowledge of Past and Future Achieved through Saṁyama

These three *sūtras* mark the transition from the earlier line of discussion to the main theme of the chapter, which is the miraculous powers achieved by the successful practitioner of Yoga. *Sūtras* 3.14 and 3.15 continue the discussion of the essential nature of a substance, the *dharmin*, or that which possesses a *dharma*, an attribute. Despite the transformations an object undergoes through the three phases of time, the fundamental substance, the *dharmin*, remains unchanged. Now when the intense concentration of *saṁyama* is focused on the three factors of *dharma*, *lakṣaṇa*, and *avasthā*, referred to in *sūtra* 3.13, the *yogin* acquires knowledge of the past and of the future, and this is the first of the miraculous powers that may be acquired by the expert practitioner of Yoga presented in this chapter.

3.14 *śāntoditāvyapadeśya-dharmānupātī dharmī*

The *dharmin* is that which remains constant as the *dharmas* pass through the stages of cessation, arising, and beyond designation.

The meaning of this *sūtra* is rather difficult to comprehend, and here the explanations of the commentators are particularly valuable. The subject here is the *dharmin*, which means 'that which has a *dharma*' or perhaps all *dharmas*, and here we must take *dharma* to mean an attribute which makes an underlying substance into a specific object. The essential meaning again comes from the Sāṁkhya understanding of the nature and origins of this world. The ultimate *dharmin* is the original substance, primal *prakṛti*, out of which the elements of matter evolve through the process of *pariṇāma*, the transformation by which the single substance of primal *prakṛti* becomes the different elements of the variegated world.

The first phrase of the *sūtra* contains the words *śānta*, *udita*, and *avyapadeśya*, meaning ceased, arisen, and beyond designation. Vyāsa explains that these terms refer to the condition of an attribute, a *dharma*: in the past, which has now gone and hence is *śānta* or ceased; *udita*, in the present which has arisen; and in the future, which is unknown and hence *avyapadeśya*, beyond designation. Each substance in this world, each *dharmin*, undergoes the transformations arising from these three phases of time, assuming various attributes or forms, *dharmas*, but the *dharmin* retains its constant original identity. Therefore, Patañjali states that the *dharmin* is *anupātin*, meaning that it remains the constant substance of the changing attributes, *dharmas*.

Vyāsa again takes the opportunity to embark on a lengthy philosophical discussion of the process of transformation, which includes the phrase *sarvaṁ sarvātmakam*, which is a way of saying 'everything has the same nature as everything else'. Lest this be taken as confirmation of the idea of the unity of *ātman* and Brahman, it must be pointed out that what Vyāsa means here is that every one of the diverse objects of which this world is comprised is of the same substance of *prakṛti*, despite the superficial differences of appearance. The other commentators again follow Vyāsa by including lengthy philosophical discussions of the relationship between the *dharmin*, the primal substance, and the *dharmas* that become attributes of the *dharmin*. And once again these discussions would carry us well beyond the scope of the present study.

3.15 *kramānyatvaṁ pariṇāmānyatve hetuḥ*

It is differences in the nature of progression that cause differences in the nature of the transformation achieved.

Now Patañjali concludes this opening section of the *Vibhūti-pāda* by making a final point regarding the process of transformation, which is fundamental to understanding how it is that miraculous powers are acquired. These *vibhūtis* represent forms of transformation that go far beyond anything that is usually encountered, and the reason that these are possible for the *yogin* relates to the differences in the process of transformation. We have been informed that all features of this world are no more than transformations of the single substance of primal *prakṛti*. In this *sūtra*, it is stated that we observe diversity rather than the unity of *prakṛti* alone because of the differing ways in which *prakṛti* becomes transformed, so that it appears as the different objects visible around us.

Such transformations take place according to a particular succession, such as ageing or the creation of a pot from clay, and this is referred to here as *krama-anyatvam*, the change in the sequence of progression, and this is the cause, the *hetu*, of *pariṇāma-anyatvam*, which is the change in the nature of the transformation. The practitioner of Yoga brings about a transformation of the mind from diverse forms of concentration to the single-pointedness of *saṁyama*. This transformation of the *citta* or *buddhi* has far-reaching consequences. In Sāṁkhya thought, *buddhi* is a feature of the mental faculties of each living being, but it is also the first evolute, or transformation, from primal *prakṛti*. Hence when *buddhi* is transformed from concentration in diverse ways to concentration on a single point, this can affect *prakṛti* as a whole because *buddhi* is both individual and universal according to Sāṁkhya doctrine.

This is a complex line of discussion, but it is important because it reveals why it is that Patañjali includes these *sūtras* on the transformation of the mind, the *buddhi*, through one-pointed concentration as a preface to his chapter on the *vibhūtis* developed by the *yogin*. For those who are particularly interested in the link between Sāṁkhya ideas and the acquiring of miraculous powers, Edwin Bryant's discussion of this and *sūtra* 3.16 is highly recommended. Here again Vyāsa and the other commentators provide lengthy commentaries, which carry us into the realm of the complexities of Indian philosophy, particularly with regard to the Sāṁkhya teachings on the process of transformation through which the world as we know it comes into existence. And again we must forego any indulgence in that particular line of discussion.

3.16 *pariṇāma-traya-saṁyamād atītānāgata-jñānam*

> Through *saṁyama* on the three transformations, one acquires knowledge of the past and future.

Here then we have the first direct statement regarding a *vibhūti*, which, in this case, is the ability to acquire knowledge of things that have faded into the past, beyond our normal perception, and things that are yet to be. So the *vibhūti* here includes the ability to foretell the future through the application of the mind to *saṁyama*, one-pointed concentration. The object of that *saṁyama* is here described as *pariṇāma-traya*, the threefold transformation, and this might refer either to the three phases of time, past, present, and future, or the *dharma*, *lakṣaṇa*, and *avasthā*, the attribute, the temporality, and the condition of an object, as referred to in *sūtra* 3.13. Given the nature of the *vibhūti* acquired by this means, one might naturally conclude that it is the three phases of time that are the object of *saṁyama*, but Vyāsa holds to the view that it is in fact the latter three that are the focus of concentration in this case. The point would be that this *saṁyama* on the full threefold nature of the object, as it is in the present, will bring to the fore knowledge of the nature of its past and future, which are latent in that present form.

Vyāsa in fact comments only briefly here, reminding us of the three elements of *saṁyama* as *dhāraṇā*, *dhyāna*, and *samādhi*, and repeating the claim made in the *sūtra* itself. Śaṅkara adds to this point by stating that *saṁyama* on an object goes far beyond the normal sensory perception of that object, and hence brings full knowledge of its nature and identity, past and future included. Vācaspati Miśra makes the point that full knowledge of an object includes its past and future, and this wider knowledge comes from the heightened level of concentration that is inherent in *saṁyama*. Vijñāna Bhikṣu further elaborates on the point by stating that *saṁyama* on the transformations undergone by an object brings knowledge of its past transformations into its present form, and also knowledge of the transformations it will undergo in the future due to the progression of time.

SŪTRAS 3.17–3.32: THE ACQUISITION OF HIGHER POWERS

This next group of *sūtras* follows the pattern established by *sūtra* 3.16 by revealing the various miraculous powers that come to the advanced practitioner through the application of *saṁyama* to different ideas and objects. On some occasions, the commentators take the opportunity to consider the specific points in greater detail, but for the most part, they are content to let *sūtras* speak for themselves, as the basic idea remains more or less the same throughout.

Patañjali's discussion of magic and supernatural powers inevitably raises doubts in the rational mind about the authenticity of his teachings. Many people today are instinctively dubious about claims of miracles, and indeed one of the attractions of Yoga is that it is a form of spirituality that does not depend on faith in the supernatural, but on verifiable experience. So what then are we to make of these passages of the *Yoga Sūtras*? For the most part, the treatises on Yoga in the *Bhagavad-gītā* and the *Mahābhārata* make no mention of these *vibhūtis*. An exception to this rule is to be found in Chapters 228 and 289 of the *Mahābhārata*'s *Śānti-parvan*, and we should be aware that various narratives within the *Mahābhārata* refer to *yogins* possessing such powers, notably the story of Śuka's yogic path to liberation in chapters 309-320 of the *Śānti-parvan*. Moreover, in modern India, the idea of saints and holy men being capable of supernatural feats is widely accepted, and at times even expected. Still, however, the question remains as to whether the claims made in this passage somehow undermine the validity of the *Yoga Sūtras* as a whole. After all, if Patañjali is deemed to be making impossible claims for Yoga here, why should we think that he is doing anything different in other sections of his work?

There is no obvious solution to this question, and different individuals will reach different conclusions. Some may feel that to exclude the possibility of supernatural occurrences is overly dogmatic, while others may hold the view that even if the claims made here are exaggerations, or no more than theoretical assumptions based on Sāṁkhya doctrine and cultural perspectives, this does not invalidate other teachings on Yoga that can be substantially verified based on personal experience. I do not have any clear-cut solutions to offer on this point, but I do think the question is one we need to raise and consider in developing a full understanding of the *Yoga Sūtras*.

On some of these *sūtras*, the commentators provide quite extensive discussion, not so much of the *vibhūti* itself, but of the object on which the *saṁyama* is to be focused. As these tend to move the discussion some distance away from the text of the *Yoga Sūtras* itself, we will try to proceed through this passage without delving too deeply into the additional ideas they set forth.

3.17 *śabdārtha-pratyayānām itaretarādhyāsāt saṅkaras tat-pravibhāga-saṁyamāt sarva-bhūta-ruta-jñānam*

> Because of the superimposition of one onto the other, the word, its meaning, and the concept it represents become confused, but by the application of *saṁyama* to the distinctions between these, one acquires knowledge of the speech of all beings.

Here again there is ample opportunity to engage in philosophical discussion of the relationship between a word and the idea or object it represents, a consideration that is of particular importance in Vedānta, which bases its conclusions on the proper interpretation of the meaning of Vedic texts. Vyāsa takes the lead in this with a detailed exposition on this subject, which is followed and expanded upon by the other commentators. For our purposes, we can confine ourselves to noticing that fixing the mind in unwavering concentration on the connection between word and meaning enables the *yogin* to understand the speech of all beings, a phenomenon that is frequently encountered in narratives contained within the *Mahābhārata* and Purāṇas.

> 3.18 *saṁskāra-sākṣāt-karaṇāt pūrva-jāti-jñānam*
>
> Through direct perception of the latent impressions on the mind, one gains knowledge of one's previous births.

We have previously discussed the idea of *saṁskāras*, which are impressions left on the mind by all previous thoughts, ideas, and experiences, even those of past lives. These are generally latent in the sense that we cannot directly remember our past lives, nor indeed many of the experiences we have undergone in the present life, but nonetheless all of these have left a mark on the mind that, at some point in the future, will effect the enactment of karmic results. *Saṁyama* is not directly mentioned here but the word *karaṇa* means causing or making, whilst *sākṣāt* means direct as opposed to latent. The point here is that by intense internal concentration, the latent impressions are brought to the surface so that one gains *pūrva-jāti-jñāna*, knowledge of one's previous births. Here one might be reminded of Marcel Proust eating a madeleine cake dipped in lime tea, the experience of which brought countless lost memories flooding into his conscious mind. Vyāsa here recounts at some length the story of a sage named Jaigīṣavya who gained knowledge of his past lives in a similar way, and one will probably be aware of the accounts of the enlightenment of the Buddha, a part of which was knowledge of all his previous births.

3.19 *pratyayasya para-citta-jñānam*

And by direct perception of their overt ideas, one acquires knowledge of other people's minds.

In this short *sūtra*, there is a presumption of continuity from the previous *sūtra*, which gave the idea of *sākṣāt-karaṇa*, making something direct or overt, which in turn was a direct result of *saṁyama*. So here we can see that the object of *saṁyama* is *pratyaya*, a word that means 'an idea', 'concept', or 'conviction within the mind', and the result gained by this is *jñāna*, knowledge, of *para-citta*, the mind or *citta* or another person; in other words, the ability to read minds. Vyāsa adds very little here, but Vijñāna Bhikṣu explains that the *saṁyama* that brings this ability is to be focused on one's own ideas rather than those of the other. By intense concentration on an idea within one's own mind, one gains the ability to perceive ideas in the minds of others. Here again, we may recall the Sāṁkhya basis of this *sūtra*, which indicates that the individual *buddhi* is a transformation of the absolute *buddhi*, which would include the *buddhi* of another.

3.20 *na ca tat sālambanaṁ tasyāviṣayībhūtatvāt*

But this knowledge does not apply to the nature of the object the other is thinking of, as this is not the object of the practitioner's perception.

Here Patañjali qualifies the assertion of the previous *sūtra* by stating that the knowledge acquired in the mind of another is not knowledge of the exact object the other person has conceptualised. The knowledge is of the other person's mental state and not of the object itself. Vyāsa and the other commentators go even further than this by suggesting that what the *yogin* actually gains knowledge of is the *raktaṁ pratyayam*, the emotional response of the other to a particular idea or object rather than an understanding of the idea or object itself that has given rise to the emotional response.

3.21 *kāya-rūpa-saṁyamāt tad-grāhya-śakti-stambhe cakṣuḥ-prakāśāsaṁprayoge 'ntardhānam*

Through *saṁyama* on the form of the body when its ability to be perceived is suspended and there is no contact between the eye and its illumination, one acquires the power to become invisible.

Here the miraculous power being referred to is the ability to become invisible, and this again is achieved by *saṁyama*, in this case on the *kāya-rūpa*, the form of the body. This involves a suspension of the perceivable nature of the bodily form, its *grāhya-śakti*, and a dissociation of the eye from the illumination that enables it to see, the *cakṣuḥ-prakāśa*. Vyāsa explains that it is the separation of the eye from its power of illumination that brings about the suspension of the visibility of the body, and that this separation is a direct consequence of *saṁyama* on the form of the body. Vijñāna Bhikṣu further explains that having achieved perfection in this *saṁyama*, the *yogin* can become invisible by his will alone, and that the disjunction of the eye from the illumination takes place in the eye of the person who is looking at the *yogin*.

3.22 *sopakramaṁ nirupakramaṁ ca karma tat-saṁyamād aparānta-jñānam ariṣṭebhyo vā*

Karma may or may not have yet produced a result. By *saṁyama* on both types of karma, one acquires knowledge of the time of death. Such knowledge can also be derived from omens.

This *sūtra* first divides karma into two types, which can be understood in two ways: either as dormant karma that has yet to produce a result and karma that is currently being experienced; or else as rapidly fructifying karma and karma that emerges very slowly. Vyāsa clearly takes the second view and compares the process to the drying of one cloth spread in the sun and another squeezed into a ball. Both will eventually become dry, but the rate at which this occurs will be quite different. The main point here is that by applying *saṁyama* to these two types of karma, one acquires *aparānta-jñāna*, knowledge of the time of one's death, because the duration of life is determined by fructifying karma, and deep concentration on that karma will bring knowledge of the full nature of one's karma, including the time of death. The point is also made that knowledge of the time of one's death can also be gained from an understanding of portents and omens. There are a number of passages in the Purāṇas that refer to such portents and what they mean, and the commentators, including Vyāsa, take the opportunity to expound further on these.

3.23 *maitry-ādiṣu balāni*

By *saṁyama* on goodwill and other such qualities, one acquires specific powers.

The word *maitrī* means 'friendliness' and 'goodwill', whilst we could translate *ādi* as 'etc.', or 'of the same type'. As a result of *saṁyama* on such qualities, one acquires what are referred to as *balāni*, a word that means 'strengths' or 'powers'. It is not clear from the *sūtra* exactly what this means, but Vyāsa explains that *maitrī-ādi* means *maitrī, karuṇā,* and *muditā,* 'goodwill', 'compassion', and 'delight'. These were mentioned in *sūtra* 1.33. The powers that are acquired by expressions of these states of mind and *saṁyama* upon them are the power of goodwill, *maitrī-bala,* the power of compassion, *karuṇā-bala,* and the power of delight, *muditā-bala*. Vācaspati Miśra further explains these powers, stating that the power of friendship brings happiness to everyone he encounters, the power of compassion delivers distressed people from their suffering, and the power of delight imparts a sense of detachment to others, so that they are also delighted.

3.24 *baleṣu hasti-balādīni*

By *saṁyama* on the power of an elephant and other animals, one acquires their strength.

The *sūtra* here merely refers to *saṁyama* 'on powers', *baleṣu,* but one must take it that the statement of *hasti-bala-ādīni,* the power of the elephant etc., means that *saṁyama* on the power of one mighty beast brings the power of that particular creature. In line with this view, Vyāsa adds that through *saṁyama* on the power of Garuḍa, the bird who is the carrier of Viṣṇu, one acquires the power of Garuḍa. He then expands further by saying that it is not just the power of animals that is being referred to here, but even the power of the wind that can be acquired by *saṁyama* on that power.

3.25 *pravṛtty-āloka-nyāsāt sūkṣma-vyavahita-viprakṛṣṭa-jñānam*

By utilising the illumination of one's mental activity, one acquires knowledge of things that are subtle, concealed, and far distant.

Here the *vibhūti* to be acquired is knowledge of things that are *sūkṣma,* subtle, *vyavahita,* concealed, and *viprakṛṣṭa,* far distant, but the means of acquiring that power is not referred to as *saṁyama* but as *pravṛtty-āloka-nyāsa.* Here *nyāsa* means 'application' or 'utilisation', *āloka* means 'illumination', and *pravṛtti* means 'activities', which Vyāsa takes to mean 'the activities of the mind'. When these are applied to objects that are normally beyond our range of vision because they are too subtle, hidden by obstruction, or too far away, the *yogin* can still gain perception of them. The meaning would seem to be that even though an object is beyond our normal range of vision, it still becomes perceptible to the higher vision of the *yogins* who focus their enhanced mental faculties on that object. Vijñāna Bhikṣu explains that *saṁyama* is not referred to in this case because the advanced practitioner is able to gain knowledge of concealed objects just by turning his attention to them, without the need of a more intense form of practice.

3.26 *bhuvana-jñānaṁ sūrye saṁyamāt*

Knowledge of different worlds is acquired through *saṁyama* on the sun.

A recurring theme within the eighteen major Purāṇas is a description of the different regions of the universe and the living beings who inhabit them. Vyāsa here provides a fairly extensive presentation of this Purāṇic cosmology, but the essential point made by the *sūtra* itself is a fairly simple one. By applying the practice of *saṁyama* to the sun, *sūrya*, one acquires *bhuvana-jñāna*, knowledge of these different worlds. Śaṅkara makes no additions to Vyāsa's cosmological discourse, but both Vācaspati Miśra and more especially Vijñāna Bhikṣu pursue that discussion in some detail, the latter providing citations from various Purāṇas related to Vyāsa's commentary.

3.27 *candre tārā-vyūha-jñānam*

Saṁyama on the moon brings knowledge of the position of the stars.

The *sūtra* here gives a simple enough instruction, although the word *saṁyama* is implied rather than stated. When *saṁyama* is applied to the moon, the *vibhūti* acquired by the practitioner is *tārā-vyūha-jñāna,* where *tārā* means 'the stars' and *vyūha* means 'their respective positions'. This *sūtra* is clearly connected to *sūtra* 3.26, as both reveal yogic practices that bring knowledge of the physical universe. Neither Vyāsa nor the other commentators see the need for any further explanation.

3.28 *dhruve tad-gati-jñānam*

Saṁyama on Dhruva, the polestar, brings knowledge of the movements of the stars.

Here again the word *saṁyama* is implied rather than stated, and in this case the *vibhūti* is acquired through intense concentration on the polestar, which is known as Dhruva in Indian cosmology. The *vibhūti* gained thereby is *tad-gati-jñāna,* where the word *tat* means 'of them' and refers to the stars previously mentioned, whilst *gati* means 'movements' or 'tracks'. Hence the meaning of the *sūtra* as a whole is relatively simple, a view shared by all the commentators including Vyāsa.

3.29 *nābhi-cakre kāya-vyūha-jñānam*

Saṁyama on the circle of the navel brings knowledge of the workings of the body.

In this *sūtra,* the object of *saṁyama* is said to be the *nābhi-cakra,* the circle of the navel, and one might conclude that this is a reference to the idea of there being seven *cakras,* or subtle energy points, within the body, as mentioned in the *Haṭha-yoga-pradīpikā* and other later texts that incorporate tantric concepts. This, however, is most unlikely, as we cannot detect any tantric influence on the *Yoga Sūtras,* and the use of the word *cakra* most likely refers only to the circular shape of the navel. The *vibhūti* acquired by this application of *saṁyama* is knowledge of the *kāya-vyūha,* the arrangement of the body, a phrase which Vyāsa explains in Āyurvedic categories as the three humours (*doṣas*), namely, wind (*vāta*), bile (*pitta*), and phlegm (*śleṣman*; also known as *kapha*), and the seven constituents of the body, *dhātus* – skin, blood, flesh, sinew, bone, marrow, and semen. The internal workings of the body and the functioning of its various organs are beyond our range of perception, but here it is said that intense concentration on the navel allows the *yogin* to acquire a clear understanding of the organs and substances of which the body is comprised.

3.30 *kaṇṭha-kūpe kṣut-pipāsā-nivṛttiḥ*

Through *saṁyama* on the pit of the throat, hunger and thirst cease to have any effect.

Again this is a fairly straightforward statement regarding the *vibhūti* acquired through *saṁyama* on the region of the body just below the throat. Again one might be tempted to see here a reference to the *cakra* system, but Vyāsa in particular makes it quite clear that he regards the *sūtra* as indicating *saṁyama* on a specific part of the physical body. And in this case, that practice allows the *yogin* to be free from the effects of hunger and thirst. The commentators see little need for any further elaboration, though Vijñāna Bhikṣu suggests that the precise technique is one that has to be learned from a *guru*.

3.31 *kūrma-nāḍyāṁ sthairyam*

Through *saṁyama* on the tortoise channel, one acquires steadiness.

It is not immediately apparent what is meant here, either with regard to the *vibhūti* or the object of *saṁyama* that leads to its acquisition. Vyāsa suggests that the *kūrma-nāḍī*, literally the tortoise channel, is located in the chest and is so named because it is in the shape of a tortoise. He further explains that the *sthairya*, the steadiness, referred to here is akin to that of a snake or iguana, and one must presume that this means the ability of those creatures to remain without movement for considerable periods of time. He does not connect the term *nāḍī* to the tantric idea of the channels of subtle energy running throughout the body, and, in the absence of any other viable interpretation, I see no reason not to accept Vyāsa's explanations. Vijñāna Bhikṣu, however, does seem to want to identify a tantric element here, suggesting that the word *kuṇḍalita* should be added to the example of a snake, thereby bringing in some suggestion of the idea of the *kuṇḍalinī* energy that is often represented as a coiled serpent lying dormant at the base of the spine. In considering this interpretation, we should of course be aware that Vijñāna Bhikṣu was active at a much later time than the other commentators.

3.32 *mūrdha-jyotiṣi siddha-darśanam*

> Through *saṁyama* on the light within the head,
> one becomes able to see higher beings.

Again both the *vibhūti* itself and the object of *saṁyama* are not immediately comprehensible, as questions naturally arise regarding the nature of the *mūrdha-jyotis*, the light in the head, and the identity of the *siddhas*, the higher or perfected beings who become visible. Vyāsa offers only a very brief explanation by stating that there is an aperture in the skull that is filled with light; the *siddhas* are mystical beings who exist in the space between the earth and the realm of the gods. Vijñāna Bhikṣu adds that the light in the skull is not from an external source, but is *sva-prakāśaka*, self-illuminating, a form of inner light. Vācaspati Miśra suggests that the word *mūrdhan*, the head, should here be understood to indicate the *suṣumnā-nāḍī*, though it is not clear on what basis he makes that assertion.

Sūtras 3.33–3.37: Attaining Spiritual Powers

I have chosen to isolate this group of *sūtras* from Patañjali's wider discussion of *vibhūtis* because the emphasis here appears to be rather different. The distinction is by no means clear cut, but I do think we can detect here something of a move away from the miraculous abilities that relate to our existence in this world towards the stages of spiritual enlightenment that have been the focus of Patañjali's teachings in previous chapters. It may be that the distinction I am perceiving here is not the intention of the text itself, but, nonetheless, I think it is a point worth considering and, for this reason alone, it is worthwhile looking at these *sūtras* as a passage somewhat apart from the main thrust of this section of the chapter.

3.33 *prātibhād vā sarvam*

Otherwise, all things can be acquired through intuitive knowledge.

The use of the word *vā* here, meaning otherwise, reminds us of a similar use of it made by Patañjali when he introduced *īśvara-praṇidhāna*, devotion to the Deity, as an alternative means of achieving *samādhi*. The word *sarva*, meaning all, suggests that all the *vibhūtis* previously outlined, or even omniscience, can also be attained by what is referred to as *prātibha*. This of course raises the question of what is meant by the word *prātibha*, intuitive knowledge, suggesting that the fruits of *saṁyama* can also be attained by a flash of intuition, the lightning flash or wink of the eye mentioned by the *Kena Upaniṣad* (4.4). Vyāsa suggests that *prātibha* is the knowledge that is a precursor of the development of full knowledge of the distinction between *prakṛti* and *puruṣa*, like the dawn light appearing before the sun, a view that further suggests that here we are moving into the domain of purely spiritual discourse. Śaṅkara follows this view by stating that *prātibha* is the intuitive knowledge that comes from *saṁyama* on the *ātman*, or through devotion to *īśvara*. Vācaspati Miśra is quite brief here, but Vijñāna Bhikṣu makes the point that *prātibha* means 'knowledge that comes from within' rather than the instruction of the *guru*, and notes Vyāsa's description of *prātibha* as *tāraka*, that which carries us across, as indicating the highest spiritual goals.

3.34 *hṛdaye citta-saṁvit*

> Through *saṁyama* on the heart, one acquires understanding of the thought processes.

Here, however, we seem to be seeing a return to the previous line of discussion, as the *vibhūti* acquired through *saṁyama* on the heart, *hṛdaya*, is revealed. This *vibhūti* is *citta-saṁvit*, where *citta* means the mind or thinking process, and *saṁvit* means knowledge, understanding, or perception. Vyāsa merely indicates that the heart is the seat of mental activity and that this *vibhūti* amounts to a constant awareness of the movements of the *citta*, but Vijñāna Bhikṣu is quite clear in stating that the yogic perfections now being considered are of a higher nature to those previously delineated, which he refers to as *kṣudra-siddhis*, minor achievements. The significance of *citta-saṁvit* is that it is a preliminary stage in developing knowledge of the distinction between *citta* and *puruṣa*.

3.35 *sattva-puruṣayor atyantāsaṅkīrṇayoḥ pratyayāviśeṣo bhogaḥ parārthatvāt svārtha-saṁyamāt puruṣa-jñānam*

> Because worldly experience is based on the misidentification of *sattva* with *puruṣa*, which are entirely distinct, it is for the purpose of another. Through *saṁyama* on one's own purpose, one acquires knowledge of *puruṣa*.

Clearly this *sūtra* carries us back to the earlier discussion of the absolute distinction between *puruṣa* and *prakṛti*, a form of dualism that is a fundamental precept of Sāṁkhya and Yoga. In this case, the word *sattva* is used in place of *prakṛti* as one half of the duality, a usage that is sometimes seen in Sāṁkhya and Yoga treatises in the *Mahābhārata*. Making reference to the three *guṇas*, Vyāsa uses the compound *buddhi-sattva* to indicate that, in this case, *sattva* is to be taken as the mental faculties and their particular illumination. The *sūtra* itself first includes the assertion that worldly experience is based on the misidentification of *puruṣa* with *sattva*, so that one seeks to gratify that which is not the true self. *Saṁyama* is then applied to *sva-artha*, that which is beneficial to the true self, and this then brings *puruṣa-jñāna*, knowledge of *puruṣa*, which one would naturally presume is the *viveka-jñāna*, the knowledge of distinction, that has been a central focus of the earlier chapters. Hence, once again, we can observe that there seems to have been a shift of emphasis here away from miraculous powers related to existence in this world towards the spiritual enlightenment that brings liberation.

Vyāsa offers a refinement of this idea by explaining that the *puruṣa* that is known by this *saṁyama* is not *puruṣa* itself, but the reflection of *puruṣa* present within the *buddhi-sattva*. According to Vyāsa, the state of *parārthatva*, which means 'being for the sake of another', characterises *sattva* which exists for the sake of *puruṣa*, whereas in his commentary to 2.20, Vyāsa explained that the adjective *svārtha*, being for its own sake, characterises *puruṣa*. The other commentators then follow Vyāsa's lead by further considering the relationship between *puruṣa* and *buddhi*, which is one of intimate co-existence but ultimate distinction in line with the precepts of Sāṁkhya doctrine.

3.36 *tataḥ prātibha-śrāvaṇa-vedanādarśāsvāda-vārtā jāyante*

> When this is achieved, intuitive knowledge and higher powers of hearing, touch, seeing, tasting, and smelling arise.

Now we have what appears to be a return to the idea of powers that operate in this world rather than those which bring transcendence of the world, although perhaps the inclusion of *prātibha*, intuition, suggests that the separation between them that I have suggested is based on an artificial dichotomy. What I mean by that is that the manner in which Patañjali has constructed his discourse seems to suggest that the acquisition of miraculous powers in this world and the realisation of higher, spiritual knowledge are two parts of the same process. Here the word *tataḥ*, meaning 'as a result of that', indicates that the *puruṣa-jñāna* mentioned in the previous *sūtra* brings with it heightened abilities in relation to all five of the senses. So a viable conclusion might be that whilst a distinction between supernatural abilities and spiritual enlightenment is certainly to be recognised, this distinction is less than absolute.

Vyāsa informs us that the higher sensory abilities are to be understood as those which are *divya*, divine or related to the gods, so that one's powers of perception are elevated to the level of those of the gods. Vācaspati Miśra makes a significant contribution here by suggesting that the enhanced abilities of sight, hearing etc. are preliminary stages prior to the awakening of intuitive knowledge, *prātibha*, which in itself has been referred to as the dawn of full enlightenment. He thus indicates that the development of miraculous powers related to this world is a preliminary stage of yogic progression prior to the final goal of the realised knowledge of the spiritual identity of *puruṣa*.

3.37 *te samādhāv upasargā vyutthāne siddhayaḥ*

These are obstacles in the state of *samādhi*, but they are *siddhis* when the mind is active.

This *sūtra* is sometimes cited to show that Patañjali held the view that the *siddhis* or *vibhūtis* he has revealed in this chapter are lesser stages of yogic development, which are in fact obstacles blocking the attainment of the ultimate goal of Yoga, which is spiritual enlightenment through *samādhi*. Again, however, I do not think that this is quite the case, for what is being said here is that these powers are *siddhis*, perfect achievements, when the mind is active, and only become obstacles if they intrude into the focused mind of the *yogin* during the state of *samādhi*. So there is certainly some reservation being shown about the development of miraculous abilities, but Patañjali does not go so far as to say that these must therefore be entirely rejected. It is more a warning of the potential dangers they pose as the *yogin* enters the state of *samādhi*.

In his short commentary, Vyāsa makes exactly that point, but Śaṅkara goes a little further by stating that the *vibhūtis* 'are antagonistic to vision of *puruṣa*' (Trans. Leggett). Vācaspati Miśra expands on Śaṅkara's observation by explaining that if a *yogin* achieves these higher powers, he may then consider himself to have achieved the goal of Yoga and thereby become deviated from achieving the highest result attained through Yoga, which is liberation from rebirth. Vijñāna Bhikṣu is of the same opinion, expressing the view that the *yogin* should show *upekṣā*, indifference or even contempt, towards the *vibhūtis*, and continue his pursuit of the higher goal of *puruṣa-darśana*, perception of *puruṣa*.

Sūtras 3.38–3.42: Five Further Powers

Despite the reservations expressed in the previous *sūtra*, Patañjali now returns to his previous line of discussion by revealing further *vibhūtis* that are acquired by the practitioner. Given the view of the *vibhūtis* expressed in *sūtra* 3.37, one might naturally wonder why the text should now simply reveal further miraculous powers. What seems the most likely explanation is that Patañjali sees his statement in *sūtra* 3.37 not as a wholesale rejection of the attainment of *vibhūtis*, as suggested by Vijñāna Bhikṣu's use of the word *upekṣā*, but simply a warning of the potential dangers they pose if they arise during a *yogin*'s absorption in a state of *samādhi*.

> 3.38 *bandha-kāraṇa-śaithilyāt pracāra-saṁvedanāc ca cittasya para-śarīrāveśaḥ*
>
> By loosening the causes of bondage, and by perceiving the movements of the mind, one's mind can enter another person's body.

The *vibhūti* being referred to here is quite easily identified. It is the ability to transfer one's mind, *citta*, to another body and take control of that body. The means by which this is achieved is said to be twofold: first of all, *bandha-kāraṇa-śaithilya*, loosening the causes of bondage, and, secondly, *pracāra-saṁvedana*, gaining awareness of the movements, which, according to Vyāsa, are the movements of one's own mind, *sva-citta*. These are somewhat different from the usual means of gaining *vibhūtis*, which is *saṁyama* on a particular object or idea, and what is meant here is not readily apparent; hence we must turn to the commentators for guidance.

Vyāsa explains that the cause of bondage referred to is the residue of karma present in the mind in the form of *saṁskāras*, latent impressions. This keeps the *citta* bound within the body of a person, but when that karma is eroded by the attainment of *samādhi*, then the mind is set free. This brings the *yogin* full knowledge of his mental processes and also allows him to transfer his own *citta* into the bodies of others. And here one is reminded of a story told in the biographies of Śaṅkarācārya when he was challenged to a debate on the erotic arts by the wife of one of his philosophical opponents. Śaṅkara then entered the body of a dying king, and gained knowledge of eroticism through his association with the queens. He was then able to return to his own body and triumph in a debate on that subject area. One may certainly have doubts as to the absolute veracity of this account. Here our Śaṅkara does little more than summarise Vyāsa's comments, and Vācaspati Miśra adopts the same approach. Vijñāna Bhikṣu, however, suggests that the powers referred to in the remaining *sūtras* of this chapter are predominantly based on *kriyā*, the activities the *yogin* is able to perform, rather than the application of intense mental concentration.

3.39 *udāna-jayāj jala-paṅka-kaṇṭakādiṣv asaṅga utkrāntiś ca*

> By controlling the *udāna* air, one can raise oneself upwards and remain untouched by water, mud, thorns, and other obstacles.

Here we will recall Vijñāna Bhikṣu's comment regarding this group of *vibhūtis* being related to *kriyā*, action, for the *vibhūti* revealed here is the power of levitation, and the means by which it is acquired appears related to *prāṇāyāma* rather than *saṁyama*. The *udāna* air is the upward breath that, according to Vyāsa, reaches up to the region of the head. Here we are told that mastery or conquest, *jaya*, of the *udāna* brings *utkrānti*, which could mean the ability to levitate so that one is untouched, *asaṅga*, by water, mud, and thorns, *jala*, *paṅka*, and *kaṇṭaka*. *Utkrānti* is also a common yogic term which refers to a form of voluntary dying by exiting one's body upwards. Vyāsa has little to say on the details, but remarks that *utkrānti* takes place at *prāyaṇa-kāle*, at the time of death. In this case, the ability to remain untouched by such obstacles as water and mud should probably be understood as a separate *siddhi*, which he unfortunately does not describe in more detail. Vyāsa also takes this opportunity to explain the nature of all five of the bodily airs, but adds little else to the statement of the *sūtra* itself, and Śaṅkara expands only slightly on Vyāsa's comments. Vijñāna Bhikṣu adds an extensive discussion of the nature and functions of the bodily airs.

3.40 *samāna-jayāj jvalanam*

By controlling the *samāna* air, there is illumination.

This *sūtra* follows on from the previous one by referring to mastery over the *samāna* air, the air in the lower part of the torso, which, according to Vyāsa, distributes nourishment to all parts of the body. This is again understood by the commentators to mean *saṁyama* on the *samāna* air, whilst the *jvalana*, the illumination that is the result of *samāna-jaya*, is an effulgence that emanates from the body of the *yogin*. This idea of elevated spiritual practitioners displaying a bodily effulgence is one that is frequently referred to in Purāṇic descriptions of such saints and sages. The commentators are all very brief on this *sūtra*, but Vijñāna Bhikṣu reminds us of the story of Satī, the wife of Śiva, who burned her own body to ashes by meditating on the fire within the body.

3.41 *śrotrākāśayoḥ saṁbandha-saṁyamād divyaṁ śrotram*

Through *saṁyama* on the connection between hearing and space, one acquires celestial powers of hearing.

This *sūtra* speaks of the *vibhūti* by which one acquires *divyaṁ śrotram*, celestial hearing, which Vijñāna Bhikṣu explains as the hearing of subtle sounds that are not overtly manifest and are thus beyond the normal range of auditory perception. Here again the method of acquiring this *vibhūti* is a form of *saṁyama*, in this case, on the interconnection between hearing and the element of space. In understanding this idea, we are drawn again into the domain of Sāṁkhya analysis, in which the element known as *ākāśa*, space or sky, is linked to sound and to the sense of hearing, *śrotra*. The intense concentration of *saṁyama* directed towards this inherent linkage is the means by which this heightened sense of hearing is obtained. Vyāsa takes this opportunity to discuss the connection between *śabda*, *śrotra*, and *ākāśa*, sound, hearing, and space, and the other commentators follow this lead, with Vācaspati Miśra and Vijñāna Bhikṣu writing at some length on the subject.

3.42 *kāyākāśayoḥ saṁbandha-saṁyamāl laghu-tūla-samāpatteś cākāśa-gamanam*

> Through *saṁyama* on the connection between the body and space, and absorbing oneself in the lightness of cotton, one gains the power to travel through the sky.

The *vibhūti* referred to by this *sūtra* is easily identified as *ākāśa-gamana*, travelling through space or the sky, and the means by which this miraculous ability is achieved is said to be twofold. Firstly, there is *saṁyama* on the connection between the body and space, *kāya* and *ākāśa*, and in the *Mahābhārata* we do find passages in which the presence of the great elements of space, air, water, fire, and earth within the body are discussed, as in Chapter 239 of the *Śānti-parvan*, where it is stated that within the body, space is represented by sound, hearing, and bodily cavities (v9). Secondly, there should be *samāpatti* on the lightness of cotton. The difference between *samāpatti* and *saṁyama* is not that marked, but *samāpatti* implies absorption of the mind to the point of virtual identity, and this in turn suggests that the mind becomes so absorbed in the idea of the lightness of cotton that this attribute is acquired by the *yogins* themselves, thereby granting thc *vibhūti* of levitation. And it is somewhat interesting to note that the Transcendental Meditation group uses this *sūtra* as a part of their Yogic Flying programme, though one cannot be sure as to the degree of success.

Vyāsa suggests that the connection between the body and space is such that the body cannot exist without space within which to exist. He also states that this *vibhūti* is achieved gradually so that first one can walk on water, then on a spider's web, and eventually on the rays of the sun. The other commentators just summarise Vyāsa's observations, although Vijñāna Bhikṣu indicates that the two elements of this process are alternatives rather than both being required.

If we pause now for a moment to follow the logical progression of the *Vibhūti-pāda,* we can note that it started by continuing the discussion of the eight limbs of Yoga by providing succinct definitions of *dhāraṇā, dhyāna,* and *samādhi* before explaining that these three can be understood conjointly under the heading of *saṁyama*. It is then explained that the effective practice of *saṁyama* gives rise to a transformation of the mental faculties of the adept, as it creates *saṁskāras* of restraint, which restrict and nullify the *saṁskāras* generated by conventional mental activities. After a brief consideration of the reality and permanence of objects, Patañjali then moves on to outline the manner in which the transformations of the conscious mind brought about by *saṁyama* can bestow a range of miraculous powers upon the *yogin*. At the same time, it is noted that the power of *saṁyama* can also be applied to the awakening of the spiritually enlightening knowledge that brings freedom from karma and liberation from rebirth. It is this understanding of the spiritual potency of *saṁyama* that dominates the remaining *sūtras* of the *Vibhūti-pāda,* and it is to this line of discussion that we will now turn our attention.

Sūtras 3.43–3.46: Achieving the Perfection of the Bodily Form

The next four *sūtras* may be taken as leading up to the statement about the body of the perfect *yogin* in *sūtra* 3.46, although they can equally well be taken independently. First there is a statement about the *mahā-videhā*, the great detachment from the body, then there is the *vibhūti* of gaining mastery over the five primary elements, then reference to the miraculous powers related to the body, and finally a statement regarding the nature of the perfect bodily form. And again the question would arise as to how closely the ideas presented here are related to the understanding of the ultimate goal of Yoga, which is the knowledge of the distinction between *puruṣa* and *prakṛti* that brings liberation from rebirth.

> 3.43 *bahir akalpitā vṛttir mahā-videhā tataḥ prakāśāvaraṇa-kṣayaḥ*
>
> The great detachment from the body, the *mahā-videhā*, occurs when the movements of the mind are external, but are not artificial. When this is achieved, the covering of illumination dwindles.

There are two parts to this *sūtra*. The first part gives some indication of what is meant by the term *mahā-videhā*, literally 'the great separation from the body', and the second part, introduced by the word *tataḥ*, meaning 'from that', gives the result derived from *mahā-videhā*, which is *prakāśa-āvaraṇa-kṣaya*, destruction or diminution of the coverings of the light. Vyāsa claims that *mahā-videhā* is the name of a particular concentration, *dhāraṇā*. The *sūtra* explains that *mahā-videhā* is a form of *vṛtti*, a movement of the mind, which is *bahir*, external, but not artificial, *akalpitā*. The mind frequently moves beyond the body as, for example, when we think about some distant place we have visited, but this external movement is *kalpitā* because the mind does not actually become located in that distant place, it is just an internal recollection. For such a movement of the mind to become *a-kalpitā*, real and not imagined, the mind must actually be transferred to that other external location so that it can observe exactly what is taking place there at the present time.

The cultivation of this supernatural ability erodes the coverings that obscure the light, and, on this point, all the commentators agree that the light in question is the light of *sattva*, the highest of the three *guṇas* and the gateway to enlightenment. The *sattva-guṇa* represents light, clarity, wisdom, compassion, and gentility, but it becomes covered over by the other two *guṇas* of *rajas*, passionate longing, and *tamas*, the darkness of ignorance. What is therefore being said in this *sūtra* is that the miraculous ability of the mind to move out of the body brings with it a diminution of the covering influence of *rajas* and *tamas*, so that the light of *sattva* becomes predominant within the mind. Hence we can see again from this *sūtra* how Patañjali draws together and combines the attainment of *vibhūtis* with spiritual enlightenment, and indeed moral upliftment. Vyāsa adds here that it is this *mahā-videhā* that allows *yogins* to enter the bodies of others, and Vācaspati Miśra qualifies this by pointing out that entering the body of another is not the only form of *mahā-videhā*. Vijñāna Bhikṣu here emphasises the point that the coverings referred to are the *guṇas* of *rajas* and *tamas* in their various manifestations, which prevent the light of *sattva* from illuminating the mind.

3.44 *sthūla-svarūpa-sūkṣmānvayārthavattva-saṁyamād bhūta-jayaḥ*

Through *saṁyama* on their gross form, their essential nature, their subtle form, their relative presence, and their functions, one acquires mastery over the material elements.

Here another *vibhūti* and the means of attaining it through *saṁyama* is described. The *vibhūti* in question is *bhūta-jaya*, mastery over, or conquest of, the five great elements of *prakṛti*, space, air, water, fire, and earth, which one presumes means mastery over these basic elements as they exist both in the *yogin*'s own physical body and in the wider world. What then of the *saṁyama* that brings this *vibhūti*? This is said be on five aspects that define the great elements: *sthūla*, the gross form, *svarūpa*, their fundamental identity, *sūkṣma*, their subtle form, *anvaya*, their relative presence, and *arthavattva*, their functions. In explaining the meaning of these five, Vyāsa resorts again to Sāṁkhya ideas on the nature of the elements which form a part of manifest *prakṛti*. It is not appropriate here to delve into the lengthy explanations provided by Vyāsa and his successors, so I will try to give a brief explanation of what is meant by these five terms just to add some clarity to the meaning of the *sūtra* itself.

First of all, *sthūla*, the gross form, is explained as meaning the overt form of the element as it is directly perceived, along with the qualities such as aroma or sound associated with each of them in Sāṁkhya teachings. *Svarūpa*, inherent nature, is said to mean the specific quality that defines each element, such as the quality of liquidity inherent in water. *Sūkṣma*, subtle, is a little more difficult to define, but this relates to the idea that the overt manifestation of the elements appears due to a transformation of a subtle form, or *tan-mātra*. The subtle form is the prior stage of the gross manifestation. Precisely what is meant by *anvaya* is not clear here, as this term usually means a sequence, connection, or progression, but the commentators take it as referring to the three *guṇas*, the essential qualities that are pervasive throughout *prakṛti* in all its forms, and, in the absence of any other clear explanation, we might as well accept that view. The term *arthavattva* means the role or function, and Vyāsa explains this in relation to *prakṛti* as a whole, which has the dual function of, on the one hand, providing living beings with experience and, on the other, providing a means for living beings to gain liberation from this world. One further point of interest here is that in his commentary, Vyāsa refers to the views of Patañjali, mentioning the author of the *Yoga Sūtras* by name. This could be taken as evidence against the view that Patañjali and Vyāsa were one and same person, although it is not absolutely conclusive.

3.45 *tato 'ṇimādi-prādur-bhāvaḥ kāya-saṁpat tad-dharmānabhighātaś ca*

> At this point, powers such as making the body minute also appear; the body achieves a perfect state, and the limitations imposed by its inherent nature are overcome.

The word *tataḥ*, meaning 'from that', at the start of this *sūtra* indicates that it is speaking of the consequences of the mastery gained over the five elements referred to in *sūtra* 3.44. First of all, there is *aṇimā-ādi-prādur-bhāva*, meaning the appearance of *aṇimā* and others. This is a reference to a group of eight *siddhis* or *vibhūtis*, miraculous powers, that are frequently mentioned in early Indian texts. They are as follows:

1. *aṇimā*, the ability to become minutely small
2. *mahimā*, the ability to become large in size
3. *laghimā*, the ability to become light and float through the air
4. *garimā*, the ability to become heavy and immovable
5. *prāpti*, the ability to acquire objects from distant places

6. *prākāmya*, the ability to do whatever one desires without restriction
7. *vaśitva*, the ability to bring others under one's control
8. *īśitṛtva*, the ability to achieve mastery over the world.

Clearly the notion of these eight *siddhis* is closely related to the idea of the *vibhūtis*, as presented in this chapter. The second and third results of *bhūta-jaya* mentioned here are *kāya-saṁpat*, perfection of the body, and *tad-dharma-anabhighāta*. In this latter phrase, *tad-dharma* means 'the normal condition or inherent nature of the body', whilst *anabhighāta* means 'the absence of limitations or restrictions'. The idea would seem to be that bodily activities are limited due to the nature of the body, the *dharma* of the body, but when the elements are mastered, one can transcend all such restrictions. This would appear to be very much in line with the idea of the *siddhis* outlined above. Vyāsa, however, implies that the pronoun *tad* in the compound *tad-dharma-anabhighāta* refers back to the elements (*bhūtas*) mentioned in the previous *sūtra*, and explains overcoming the characterstics of the elements as, for example, the *yogin* not being burnt by the heat of fire.Vyāsa also lists these eight *siddhis*, but adds that the *yogin* will not use these to alter the fundamental nature of the world, recognising that this is the sole prerogative of *īśvara*. Śaṅkara builds on this final point by stating that the *yogin* even acquires the power to make fire cold, but refrains from doing so in deference to the creative acts of *īśvara*. Vācaspati Miśra expands a little on the explanation of the eight *siddhis*, but does not venture far beyond Vyāsa's comments, whilst Vijñāna Bhikṣu cites the *Vedānta Sūtras* (4.17), which asserts that a liberated being possesses all powers except the ability to create the world.

3.46 *rūpa-lāvaṇya-bala-vajra-saṁhananatvāni kāya-saṁpat*

The perfect state of the body includes beauty, grace, strength, and the hardness of diamond.

This *sūtra* merely provides an explanation of one of the phrases used in *sūtra* 3.45, *kāya-saṁpat,* meaning perfection of the bodily form, and the list given of the qualities of that bodily form requires little by way of further explanation. Here Vyāsa merely repeats the statement of the *sūtra,* and the other commentators follow his lead in seeing no need for further elucidation.

Sūtras 3.47–3.49: The Perfection of Spiritual Awakening

These next *sūtras* mark a move back from the discussion of powers that pertain to this world towards a renewal of the focus on spiritual awakening. Both of these are regarded as *siddhis,* perfections, but clearly the ideas here are more closely related to the spiritual quest for absolute liberation. It is said that this is achieved, first, through mastery of the senses, which otherwise absorb the mind in thoughts of this world; then through gaining mastery over *prakṛti* as a whole which is the locus of our bondage; and finally through gaining knowledge of the distinction between our true spiritual identity, which is *puruṣa,* and our physical and mental embodiment.

3.47 *grahaṇa-svarūpāsmitānvayārthavattva-saṁyamād indriya-jayaḥ*

Through *saṁyama* on their perception of objects, their inherent nature, the sense of ego, their relative presence, and their functions, one achieves mastery over the senses.

In this case, the *vibhūti* presented by Patañjali is not so much a supernatural power as a stage in the adept's progression towards yogic perfection. We will recall his initial definition of Yoga as *citta-vṛtti-nirodha,* restricting the movements of the mind, and the mastery over the senses, *indriya-jaya,* referred to here is an essential element in the path of progress towards that outcome, as it is the senses and the perceptual stimuli they constantly present that are a major feature of the usual activities of the mind. The *Bhagavad-gītā* frequently speaks of the necessity of controlling the senses, using phrases such as *nigṛhītāni ... indriyānīndriyārthebhyaḥ* (2.68), holding back the senses from their objects such as sounds, tastes, sights, and aromas. What is interesting about the *Gītā*'s discussion, however, is that mastery over the senses is not strictly confined to the practice of Yoga techniques, but is applied equally to the way in which one lives one's life. Mastery of the senses is essential for restricting the movements of the mind, but mastery of the senses also means the gradual diminishing of avarice, self-centred thinking, and indifference to the plight of others. This, I think, is one of the great contributions to Indian thought made by the *Gītā,* showing that Yoga is not just a form of personal spiritual practice, but that Yoga shapes the way we live our lives and interact with the world and those who share it with us.

The achievement of mastery over the senses is achieved by *saṁyama* on five features of the senses, three of which are the same as those referred to in *sūtra* 3.44 in relation to gaining mastery over the five elements. The five mentioned here as objects of the *saṁyama* that brings mastery over the senses are as follows:

1. *grahaṇa,* literally 'grasping', this is the process of perceiving objects in the outside world;
2. *svarūpa,* the inherent nature of each of the senses, which means the general nature of the sense that is common to each being that possesses that sense,

as opposed to the differing ways in which that sense is manifest in different beings, even those of the same species;

3. *asmitā*, the sense of ego or the concept of 'I'. Vyāsa explains that this relates to the particular manner in which senses exist in an individual being as opposed to their general characteristics that is their *svarūpa*;
4. *anvaya*, again Vyāsa takes this term as indicating the relative disposition of the three *guṇas* within a person's senses;
5. *arthavattva*, the functions of the senses; each of the five has a particular object such sound or flavour that it perceives, and this is its specific function on behalf of *puruṣa*.

Śaṅkara is quite brief here, summarising Vyāsa's explanations, but both Vācaspati Miśra and Vijñāna Bhikṣu provide more detailed discussions of the precise manner in which knowledge of the objects of this world is acquired by the senses and then conveyed to the mind, which acts on behalf of *puruṣa*.

3.48 *tato mano-javitvaṁ vikaraṇa-bhāvaḥ pradhāna-jayaś ca*

When the senses are mastered, one gains the speed of the mind, one's existence does not rely on the senses, and one gains mastery over primal matter (*pradhāna*).

Starting with the word *tataḥ*, meaning 'from that', this *sūtra* gives us the results that come as a consequence of achieving mastery over the senses, as discussed in the previous *sūtra*. These are said to be threefold, *mano-javita*, speed of mind, *vikaraṇa-bhāva*, existing without reliance on the senses, and *pradhāna-jaya*, control over *pradhāna*, which is *prakṛti* in its primal, unitary state before it evolves into the variegated forms we see in the world around us. Speed of mind could mean the ability to move one's thought processes at a rapid rate, but Vyāsa explains that it means the ability to move one's body at the speed of the mind, the idea being that one only has to fix one's mind on a location in order to become present there. In the phrase *vikaraṇa-bhāva*, the word *bhāva* means a state of being or existence, whilst in this context *vikaraṇa* almost certainly means not relying on the senses. Hence the idea is that whilst in our present state of being we rely on our senses to gather information about the world around us, the adept in Yoga gains the ability to know things without requiring sensory perception. The word *pradhāna* means the primary object or the essential feature, and in Sāṁkhya treatises it is used to refer to *prakṛti* in its primal state, from out of which all the diverse elements of the evolved world come into being. So where Patañjali here includes *pradhāna-jaya* as one of the powers gained from mastery over the senses, what this means is that the *yogin* then gains mastery over all aspects of the manifest world.

Vyāsa and Śaṅkara comment very briefly on this *sutra*. Vācaspati Miśra, expanding on Vyāsa's commentary on the second of the three perfections mentioned in the *sutra*, explains that one who is endowed with the perfection of not having to rely on the senses is able to gain knowledge of events that occurred in the past and in the present, as well as events now taking place in Kashmir or some other distant location.

3.49 *sattva-puruṣānyatā-khyāti-mātrasya*
sarva-bhāvādhiṣṭhātṛtvaṁ sarva-jñātṛtvaṁ ca

When there is a full understanding of just the distinction between *puruṣa* and its mental embodiment, one acquires mastery over all that exists, and knowledge of all things as well.

Quite clearly this *sūtra* takes us back to the earlier discussion of gaining realised knowledge of the absolute distinction between *puruṣa,* the spiritual self, and *sattva,* a term which is deemed by the commentators to mean *buddhi,* the intellect that forms the mental embodiment. This knowledge was earlier referred to as *viveka-khyāti,* realisation of the distinction, and here the term *viveka* is expanded into *sattva-puruṣa-anyatā,* realisation of the ultimate distinction (*anyatā*) of *sattva* and *puruṣa.* It is this idea that lies at the heart of Sāṁkhya teachings, which insist that liberation from rebirth comes only when we fully realise that our true identity is neither the body nor the mind, but is *puruṣa,* the changeless, spiritual being that gives life to the mental and physical embodiments. Hence we must take it that the results of this realisation of the duality of matter and spirit are equivalent to *mokṣa,* or *kaivalya,* liberation from rebirth. This is expressed here in two ways, firstly, *sarva-bhāva-adhiṣṭhātṛtva,* which means 'having control over all states of existence', and, secondly, *sarva-jñātṛtva,* the state of knowing all things. In other words, omnipotence and omniscience, and this we can understand as the state of liberation from all the constraints imposed upon *puruṣa* by its continued existence within the domain of matter.

Vyāsa claims that this *sūtra* describes a special *siddhi,* perfection, called *viśokā,* 'free of sorrow' and that the *yogin* who attains it is free from the bonds of the *kleśas* and dwells being omniscient and powerful. As explained in the next *sūtra,* this state of being is just one step removed from *kaivalya,* final liberation. Śaṅkara adds very little to Vyāsa's commentary, but Vācaspati Miśra makes the point that the *vibhūtis* previously delineated are subordinate to the spiritual realisation mentioned in the present *sūtra.* Vijñāna Bhikṣu further adds that we should understand that the awakened knowledge of the distinction between *buddhi* and *puruṣa,* mind and spirit, is gained through *saṁyama* on that distinction, as the most advanced feature of the yogic endeavour.

Sūtras 3.50–3.55: Renouncing the Powers and Achieving Kaivalya

The final section of this second chapter builds on what was said in *sūtra* 3.49 regarding the knowledge that discriminates between matter and spirit, and thereby looks forward to the *Kaivalya-pāda*, the final chapter of the *Yoga Sūtras* that focuses on the spiritual conclusion of Yoga practice, liberation from rebirth.

3.50 *tad-vairāgyād api doṣa-bīja-kṣaye kaivalyam*

> And when, as a result of renouncing even such powers as these, the seed of contamination dwindles, one attains *kaivalya*.

The subject of this *sūtra* is once again the final word, *kaivalya*, which means the separation of *puruṣa* from *prakṛti* so that *puruṣa* gains liberation from suffering and rebirth. The first phrase here is *tad-vairāgyād api*, meaning 'as a result of renouncing even that', and here one can take *vairāgya*, renunciation, to refer either to the whole concept of *vibhūtis* acting in the material sphere, or else, more specifically, to the omniscience and omnipotence referred to in *sūtra* 3.49. In either case, the meaning is the same: however great one's achievements might be within the material domain, they must be set aside if one is to wholly transcend that domain and achieve *kaivalya*. The other point made here is *doṣa-bīja-kṣaye*, meaning that when the seed of faults or contamination dwindles away, then *kaivalya* will arise. The idea would seem to be that Yoga practice removes all the *doṣas*, the faults, obstacles, or contaminations existing within the mind, but the seed from which all such expressions of materialism arose may still exist in a latent state. The primary seed of material existence is the ignorance of one's true identity that lurks within the deepest recesses of the mind, and this also must disappear if *kaivalya* is to be attained.

Vyāsa does not clearly gloss the word *tad* from the *sūtra*, and ancient and modern interpreters have understood his commentary in different ways. The phrase *tad-vairāgyād api*, 'by renouncing even that', is understood by Śaṅkara to refer to the powers of omniscience and omnipotence referred to in the previous *sūtra*. This understanding informs the translation of the *sūtra* given above. Rukmani understands that Vyāsa refers to renouncing *sattva*, placing this word in the brackets of her English translation of Vyāsa's commentary. According to Vijñāna Bhikṣu, what is renounced is the two *siddhis* of omniscience and omnipotence as well as the knowledge of the distinction between *puruṣa* and *sattva* mentioned in the previous *sūtra*. One might naturally presume that it is this knowledge that brings *kaivalya*, but, according to this interpretation, Vyāsa makes the point that this type of knowing still takes place on the level of mental activity and that *kaivalya* actually means the absolute transcendence of all thought processes, even those that are most enlightening. Vācaspati Miśra adds that the knowledge by which *kaivalya* is finally attained is intuitive rather than being based on any form of thought process, which would be categorised as a movement of the mind. Vijñāna Bhikṣu adds that one must first develop the discriminative knowledge, the *viveka-khyāti*, before one abandons even that mental process prior to attaining the state of absolute *kaivalya*.

3.51 *sthāny-upanimantraṇe saṅga-smayākaraṇaṁ punar aniṣṭa-prasaṅgāt*

If one receives invitations from higher beings, one should not take pleasure in such contacts, for they may again arouse unwanted consequences.

This *sūtra* again warns against the allurements that may beset the successful practitioner, in this case, contact with the higher beings of this world who may offer the enticing prospect of celestial delights. If such divine entities approach the *yogin*, after the manner that is frequently described in the Purāṇas, he should remain aloof, literally not smiling, for such contacts may lead to the reappearance of unwanted consequences. The real point here again is that *kaivalya* means complete dissociation from the domain of matter so that even the most heady delights of this world become a matter of indifference to the *yogin*.

Here Vyāsa refers to progressive stages in the development of yogic abilities and states that the gods and other higher beings become envious of the *yogin*'s spiritual attributes, and hence try to allure him with the prospect of celestial pleasures. Many such stories can be found in the Purāṇas. The *yogin*, however, understands that falling victim to temptation will condemn him to a repetition of the constant cycle of suffering and rebirth, and so rejects these invitations. Śaṅkara does not add to Vyāsa's comments, but Vācaspati Miśra confirms that such temptations are presented only to those in the earlier stages of progression and not to those approaching yogic perfection. Vijñāna Bhikṣu draws our attention to the word *smaya* in the *sūtra*, which literally means smiling, and says that this indicates that the adept may feel a sense of pride in his achievements when approached by higher beings. Such pride is also to be avoided, as it is a further form of material attachment that keeps one bound to this world.

3.52 *kṣaṇa-tat-kramayoḥ saṁyamād viveka-jaṁ jñānam*

Through *saṁyama* on instants of time and their sequence, one acquires the knowledge born of discrimination.

Here we return to the pattern of discourse whereby a particular *vibhūti* is acquired by *saṁyama* on a designated object. There is a difference here, however, as the *vibhūti* in question is one that is closely related to yogic enlightenment and liberation. This *vibhūti* is the knowledge that arises from the ability to perceive the distinction between matter and spirit, *prakṛti* and *puruṣa*. To achieve this knowledge, *saṁyama* is to be focused as an intense form of concentration on the existence of time, the moments of which time is comprised, *kṣaṇa*, and the sequence of the passage of such moments, *tat-krama*.

Turning to the commentators for further explanation of why this form of *saṁyama* yields this particular result, we find that Vyāsa focuses mainly on the idea of time. He states that moments of time can never accumulate, for one moment only comes to exist after the disappearance of the preceding moment, and he concludes, therefore, that time has no reality beyond the processes of the *buddhi*, the intellectual faculty. It is a mental construct. It is *saṁyama* on the reality of time that brings the knowledge, the *jñāna*, that arises from the realisation of distinction between *puruṣa* and *prakṛti*. Following Vyāsa's lead, our other commentators assert that because the reality of this world is based on the progression of time, when realisation of time is achieved through *saṁyama*, this will bestow upon the *yogin* realisation of the true nature of all things.

3.53 *jāti-lakṣaṇa-deśair anyatānavacchedāt tulyayos tataḥ pratipattiḥ*

> Then one gains the ability to properly perceive two identical entities that cannot be distinguished by their birth, characteristics, or place.

The word *tataḥ* in this *sūtra*, meaning 'from that', again reveals that what is being described here is a consequence of the subject of the previous *sūtra*, namely the knowledge born from discrimination. And what is attained from that knowledge is *pratipatti*, proper knowledge or perception in relation to identical objects that cannot otherwise be distinguished in terms of origin, characteristics, or position in space. The idea would seem to be that the identity of all objects in this world is defined by the time in which they are present and their physical identity. The previous *sūtra* referred to the movement of time and, in this *sūtra*, it is position and physical identity that are considered. Conventional perception allows us to detect a distinction between objects by differences of origin, characteristic marks, and the place where they are located, but even where such differences do not exist and two objects are otherwise indistinguishable, the higher perception of the *yogin* allows him to gain knowledge of the distinction. The conclusion here would thus be that the successful application of *saṁyama* brings to the practitioner full knowledge of all aspects of the world, as defined in relation to both time and space. Still, I think, the underlying focus remains on the absolute realisation that brings liberation, but for this to be achieved, the true nature of the world must be understood by means of the *viveka-ja jñāna*, the discriminative wisdom referred to in the previous *sūtra*.

Vyāsa explains that the physical nature of an object constantly undergoes change as the atoms of which it is comprised fluctuate moment by moment. This pattern of constant transformation is beyond our normal range of perception, but the perfect *yogin* becomes aware of every aspect of the world through the *saṁyama* that brings discriminative knowledge. Vācaspati Miśra builds further on Vyāsa's analysis and makes the point that whereas there is always a degree of doubt in conventional knowledge of objects, the higher perception of the *yogin* is perfect and free from any possibility of fault or limitation. Vijñāna Bhikṣu provides further philosophical discussion of the nature of time and space, and the interaction between them, taking the opportunity to challenge the Vaiśeṣika idea of the way in which objects in this world are composed of atoms.

3.54 *tārakaṁ sarva-viṣayaṁ sarvathā-viṣayam akramaṁ ceti viveka-jaṁ jñānam*

The knowledge born of discrimination allows one to cross beyond the world, it includes all objects and all times, and is not confined to any form of sequential reasoning.

In this *sūtra,* Patañjali gives us a clearer insight into what he means by *viveka-ja jñāna,* the knowledge born of discrimination that has been the main subject of the previous two *sūtras,* and here again, we get a clear indication that if this is one of the *vibhūtis* of this chapter, it is of a much higher nature than most of those previously described. The word *iti,* here combined with *ca* to make *ceti,* indicates that the words and phrases given previously are to be taken as defining *viveka-jaṁ jñānam.* The first of these is *tāraka,* a noun formed from the verb 'to cross', which means 'the carrier or the transporter across'; this must mean that this knowledge carries one across from this world of bondage to the spiritual domain. Then we have the compound *sarva-viṣaya,* which means 'all objects', and indicates that the *viveka-ja jñāna* embodies and encapsulates knowledge of all things. Next is *sarvathā-viṣaya,* which means that this universal knowledge is not confined to the present, but includes knowledge of the past and future as well. Then finally we have *akrama,* which means 'without sequence', and probably indicates that this knowledge is not arrived at by a process of step-by-step reasoning, but comes as a flash of intuition from within, rather than from without through the application of the senses.

Vyāsa confirms that this form of knowledge is an intuitive sense of knowing that comes from within, and takes the word *tāraka* as making that exact point, thereby giving a different meaning to that term. Śaṅkara builds on that by saying that this is knowledge that cannot be received from the instruction of a *guru*, or from the words of sacred text. Vijñāna Bhikṣu, however, is quite emphatic in his view that the word *tāraka* is meant to indicate the liberating potency of this knowledge. He writes of *viveka-ja jñāna*: 'By the direct perception of defects and through the superior detachment it becomes the saviour (*tāraka*) from the round of births and deaths – this is the meaning' (Trans. Rukmani).

3.55 *sattva-puruṣayoḥ śuddhi-sāmye kaivalyam iti*

When there is equality in the purity of *sattva* and *puruṣa*, this is *kaivalya*.

This final *sūtra* of the *Vibhūti-pāda* is of great interest because it further defines what is meant by *kaivalya*. What I find particularly interesting here is the idea that *kaivalya* is not based on the understanding of absolute distinction between *puruṣa* and *prakṛti*, for the word *sattva* is said by the commentators to mean *buddhi*, the intellectual faculty, in its purest state, free from the influence of the lower qualities of *rajas* and *tamas*. What seems to be suggested here is that this purified *sattva* comes to possess the same transcendent purity as the spiritual *puruṣa*. Hence the phrase *śuddhi-sāmye*, meaning of equal purity, but what does this mean?

It could indicate that when free of impurity *buddhi* attains the same spiritual nature as *puruṣa*, but Vyāsa explains that *kaivalya* is attained when all the impurities of the mind are cleansed away; in that state, the mind, or *buddhi*, is as free from impurity as is *puruṣa*, our spiritual identity that is always absolutely pure. So we are not to understand that *buddhi* becomes 'spiritualised', but just that it attains the same freedom from impurity as is always the attribute of the spiritual entity that is *puruṣa*. Śaṅkara adds that the purity referred to means the removal of the influence of *rajas* and *tamas*, and the eradication of the *saṁskāras* that may give rise to any future results of karma. It is as a result of this complete eradication of all the blemishes in the mind that *kaivalya* is attained.

Vācaspati Miśra further clarifies the ideas presented in this chapter by stating that *kaivalya* does not depend on first attaining the other miraculous powers previously discussed. Whether or not such powers have been achieved, *kaivalya* will be attained when the mind is made free of all blemishes. Vijñāna Bhikṣu adds that although the word *sāmya* is used here, meaning sameness or equality, that should not be misunderstood as meaning absolute equality or identity between the mental faculties and *puruṣa*, for *prakṛti* and *puruṣa* are absolutely distinct. The sameness is only in relation to the state of purity achieved.

Conclusion

The *Vibhūti-pāda* opened with a consideration of the final three of the eight limbs of Yoga, *dhāraṇā, dhyāna,* and *samādhi,* which were grouped together under the single heading of *saṁyama*. When the practice of *saṁyama* is fully mastered, the mind becomes transformed so that it no longer generates the *saṁskāras* that create future karma and rebirth, but instead manifests *saṁskāras* of restraint, *nirodha-saṁskāras,* which severely limit the effect of the *saṁskāras* produced by the conventional movements of the mind. Furthermore, the ability to apply intense *saṁyama* to given ideas and objects brings supernatural abilities that give the adept a position in this world far beyond anything that is possible for those who do not gain success in Yoga practice. Wondrous as they are, these miraculous *vibhūtis* are not the supreme goal of *saṁyama,* for this intense concentration culminating in *samādhi* brings with it intuitive knowing of the distinction between *prakṛti* and *puruṣa* and of one's true spiritual nature. In this way, the *Vibhūti-pāda* comes to its conclusion by turning the focus of the discourse onto *kaivalya,* the state of absolute liberation that carries the practitioner of Yoga far beyond the range of the miraculous powers that have been presented here. It is *kaivalya* that forms the main subject of the fourth and final chapter, which is appropriately named the *Kaivalya-pāda,* and it is on to this subject that we now follow Patañjali's line of instruction.

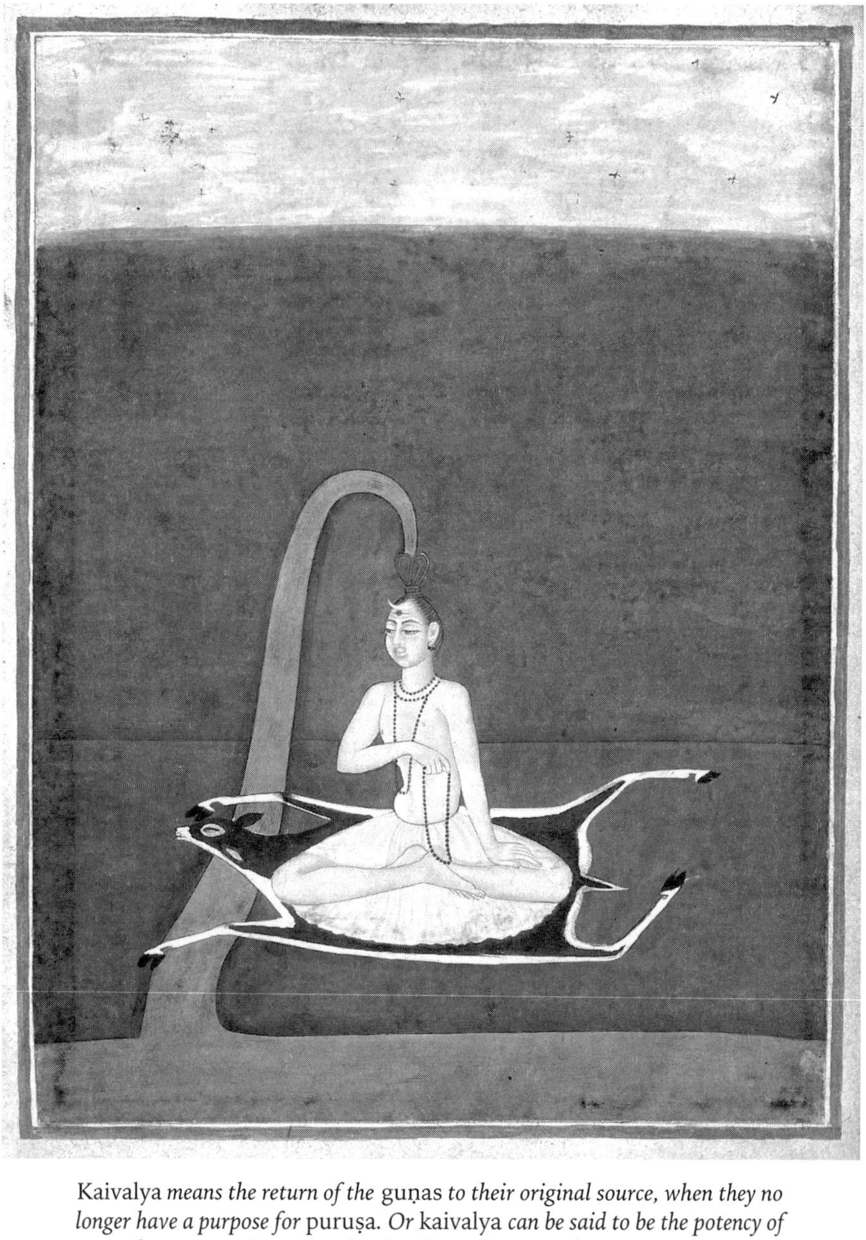

Kaivalya *means the return of the* guṇas *to their original source, when they no longer have a purpose for* puruṣa. *Or* kaivalya *can be said to be the potency of the true consciousness when it achieves its natural position.—4.34*

IV
THE *KAIVALYA-PĀDA*

The fourth and final chapter of the *Yoga Sūtras*, the *Kaivalya-pāda*, is the shortest of the four, but it is here that the preceding lines of discussion find their conclusion in the explanation of how it is that the yogic practices previously considered culminate in the adept's achievement of liberation from death and rebirth. This state of liberation is typically referred to as *mokṣa* or *mukti*, meaning 'release', but in Sāṁkhya and Yoga treatises *kaivalya* is more commonly used because its literal meaning of aloneness emphasises the idea of *puruṣa*'s separation from its relationship with *prakṛti*. When that position of bondage within the domain of *prakṛti* is ended, *puruṣa* then stands alone, free of all miseries and, according to the *Bhagavad-gītā* (6.21), experiencing a sense of joy that has no limit. We might be somewhat discouraged by this assertion, thinking that we can never reach such heights of spiritual awakening, but it is made clear that the experience of that joy comes little by little to each practitioner so that even a small amount of success in Yoga practice can bring some limited experience of that beatific state.

The chapter itself does not directly address the subject of *kaivalya* until *sūtra* 4.24, starting off instead with a consideration of the nature of the bondage from which the *yogin* is seeking release. Hence the initial focus of this discussion is on karma and rebirth, and the manner in which karma produces future results. It is explained again that action and the transformations of the mind that give rise to action produce *saṁskāras*, subtle impressions on the mind, which are themselves the causes of rebirth, as these latent impressions become manifest in our lives. There is also an assertion of the reality of this world as it is experienced, a view that contradicts the later *vivarta-vāda*, or doctrine of illusory transformation, of Advaita Vedānta and the *śūnya-vāda*, or doctrine of emptiness, of Buddhist teachings. Much of this chapter can be read as polemics agains Buddhist philosophy in particular.

From *sūtra* 4.18, Patañjali turns his attention to the relationship between *citta* and *puruṣa*, the mind and the spiritual entity. *Puruṣa* is absolutely distinct from the mind, but imbues the mind with sentience due to its proximity. And then in the final section of the chapter, the conclusion of this prior discussion is reached, as it is explained how the restraint of the mind, and its imbibing true knowledge of the distinction between *puruṣa* and *citta*, brings *puruṣa* to a state of enlightenment and liberation. As stated in the final *sūtra* of the *Vibhūti-pāda*, *kaivalya* is achieved when the mind is freed from all impurities, for at that point its movements, its *vṛttis*, no longer serve as a barrier to liberation. This, undoubtedly, is the point to which Patañjali has been moving throughout his exposition on Yoga, for Yoga in its highest form is a spiritual practice that is designed to yield spiritual results in the form of enlightenment and freedom from rebirth.

Sūtras 4.1–4.5: The Progression of Rebirth

The subject of these first five *sūtras* is the manner in which karma unfolds and thereby leads to the cycle of repeated births and deaths. Although the subject of the *Kaivalya-pāda* as a whole is liberation, it is necessary to first consider the nature of the problem from which one is seeking liberation, and that problem is karma and rebirth. The explanation given here rests on the understanding of karma set forth in the Sāṁkhya and

Yoga traditions, which also forms the basis of the *Bhagavad-gītā*'s detailed explanations of karma, non-karma, and *karma-yoga*. The idea is not that karma is a system of judgement, with punishment and reward enacted by some higher deity, but rather a process of self-transformation brought about by the thoughts and ideas that pass through mind. These thought processes give rise to physical actions, but it is not the action that creates karma but rather the subtle impression, the *saṁskāra*, left on the mind by idea that generated the action. So it is not so much the physical action of giving charity that produces future karma, but rather the benign state of mind that stimulated that action, which leaves a subtle impression on the mind; and it is that *saṁskāra* that subsequently produces a result in the form of positive karma. It thus becomes apparent how it is that control of the mind directs the progression of karma, and it is this specific point that these first five *sūtras* are concerned with.

4.1 *janmauṣadhi-mantra-tapaḥ-samādhi-jāḥ siddhayaḥ*

The higher powers arise from birth, herbs, *mantras*, austerity, and achieving *samādhi*.

This opening *sūtra* of the chapter is very much a continuation of the *Vibhūti-pāda*, with Patañjali adding a footnote to that previous line of discussion. We have heard of the *siddhis*, the superhuman powers that can be acquired through *saṁyama* culminating in *samādhi*, and here it is being added that these are acquired by other means as well, and may even be inherent in an individual from birth, particularly where birth is amongst the higher beings of this world. It is interesting therefore to note the extent to which, despite its complex philosophical lines of discourse, the *Yoga Sūtras* remains very much rooted in the enchanted world of the Purāṇas, *Mahābhārata*, and *Rāmāyaṇa*. Vyāsa here elaborates somewhat by outlining the specific *siddhis* that can be attained by each of the means listed in the *sūtra*, and the other commentators follow Vyāsa's lead by citing examples from Purāṇic texts, whilst Śaṅkara makes specific mention of the particular herbs believed to possess this potency.

> 4.2 *jāty-antara-pariṇāmaḥ prakṛty-āpūrāt*
>
> The transformation into another birth is caused by the flooding over of nature.

This second *sūtra* is comprised of two phrases, the first of which is easily understood, the second rather less so. The compound *jāty-antara-pariṇāmaḥ* means transformation into a different birth or bodily form, and this is followed by *prakṛty-āpūrāt*, where the *āt* ending gives the sense of 'because of', or 'due to'. So what is *prakṛty-āpūra*? We will readily identify the word *prakṛti* as the term used to designate the material substance out of which this world is formed, but it can also have the meaning of a person's individual nature, and it is in this latter sense that I think it is being used here. In the *Bhagavad-gītā*, Kṛṣṇa frequently uses the word *prakṛti* to refer to matter, but in verse 59 of Chapter 18, he says to Arjuna, *prakṛtis tvāṁ viyokṣyasi*, your nature will compel you to act in a certain way. We can then note that *āpūra* means a flooding over or a filling in, so what is being said here is that throughout one's life the thoughts and ideas that shape the mind thereby create a particular *prakṛti*, or personal nature, and the transformation into the next birth occurs when that *prakṛti* floods over to a new body and thereby creates the new identity. We are in that sense our own creators because the way in which we develop our mind and identity determines the nature of our next incarnation. The way we cultivate our mind fills it up with positive or negative traits, which eventually flood over to shape our future identity. This and the following *sūtra* can be understood as describing the process of rebirth, or they can be linked with *sūtra* 4.4 which talks about the *yogin*'s power of creating new minds. The latter interpretation is explored by Gokhale.[1]

Vyāsa adds that it is *dharma* and other factors that are the causes of this process, and we should note that this is exactly in line with what has been said above, for *dharma* is a state of mind as much as it is a set of righteous actions. Vācaspati Miśra gives the example of a great tree growing from a seed to illustrate how a causal factor such as *dharma* can produce a distinct future result. Vijñāna Bhikṣu, however, offers us a slightly different understanding, suggesting that here *prakṛti* does in fact refer to the material elements that form a body and that this body is 'filled up' by the type of personality formed in a previous life. The central meaning is not changed fundamentally by this reading of the text.

4.3 *nimittam aprayojakaṁ prakṛtīnāṁ varaṇa-bhedas tu tataḥ kṣetrikavat*

There is, however, no external cause that directly brings about these different natures. It is just like when a farmer breaks the field boundaries, allowing the water to take its natural course.

Here Vyāsa is particularly useful in explaining the precise meaning of the *sūtra* and he does so by describing the actions taken by a farmer in cultivating crops. What could be expected to be the external cause of transformation is *dharma* and other qualities (including, of course, *adharma*, the opposite), but this does not directly create the new state of being, it just removes the barriers to attaining that other state. In cultivating crops, a farmer does not always directly water them, but he removes the boundary around a field or plot of land so that water from a

1 Gokhale, *The Yogasūtra of Patañjali*.

higher station flows naturally into it. And he does not directly apply moisture from the ground to the roots of his crop, but he removes the weeds that form a barrier to his own plants' absorption of water. In the same way, *dharma* does not directly create the transformation of existence, but it removes barriers, such as wickedness, so as to allow a natural flow into that new state of being. It is really about purification of the mind by the removal of barriers such as greed, self-centredness, and a lack of compassion, so that there is then a natural movement towards a higher state of being.

Picking up on Vyāsa's comments, Śaṅkara reminds us that tendencies towards wickedness, *adharma,* will have the effect of breaching the barriers of *dharma* so that there is a transformation into an iniquitous state of being. Vācaspati Miśra recognises the theistic implications of this *sūtra* and states that when a tendency towards *dharma* arises, it is *īśvara* who removes the barriers. Hence the role of *īśvara* does not impinge upon individual free will, but *īśvara* does act as the facilitator of the expression of that free will in the form of tendencies towards *dharma* and *adharma*. In relation to that point, we might look to 18.61 of the *Bhagavad-gītā,* which would seem to confirm what Vācaspati Miśra is saying here. Vijñāna Bhikṣu takes the opportunity to present a complex discussion of the relationship between cause and effect with regard to material objects, states of mind, and the role of *īśvara,* but this discussion goes some way beyond our present scope.

4.4 *nirmāṇa-cittāny asmitā-mātrāt*

Created minds are formed solely from the sense of 'I'-ness.

The literal meaning of this *sūtra* is not that difficult to identify. *Nirmāṇa-cittāni* means created *cittas,* or mentalities, and *asmitā-mātra* means 'only the sense of I', with the *āt* ending giving it the meaning of 'because of' or 'due to'. So the created *cittas* are solely the result of *asmitā*, the sense of 'I am'. Easy enough then, but what does it actually mean? All the commentators take this *sūtra* as referring back to the *siddhis* gained by *yogins*, one of which is the ability to expand the mind so as to take on multiple forms and personalities. The *yogin* uses his *asmitā* as a means of generating these multiple personalities, and the commentators then look at the question of whether these newly manifested forms have their own mental nature or whether they are simply the same person in a different form. The conclusion they reach is that these secondary forms possess their own independent mental faculties, as well as their own physical form, and Vijñāna Bhikṣu cites the example of the Rāma *avatāra* who did not appear to possess the same omniscience as Viṣṇu, of whom he was an expanded form. According to Vjñāna Bhikṣu, all living beings and all mental faculties are expansions of the mind of *īśvara*, but each of us has his or her own independent mentality.

4.5 *pravṛtti-bhede prayojakaṁ cittam ekam anekeṣām*

In the varying types of action performed by many different entities, it is the single element known as *citta* that is the causal factor.

Here Vyāsa follows the line established in relation to the previous *sūtra* by explaining that it is the single *citta* of the *yogin* that controls the different actions in the different bodies manifested through his own *siddhi*-potency. Thus although each of the new forms generated has its own distinct mental faculties, all of them still fall under the purview and guidance of the one *citta* of the *yogin*. If one were to separate the *sūtra* from Vyāsa's commentary, one might also recognise the view that although many different types of action are performed by different limbs and organs of action, in all cases, the cause of the action is *citta*. In this reading of the *sūtra*, we can again identify the understanding that all action is merely a reflection of a state of mind, and it is in that sense that karma is to be understood as primarily a mental rather than a physical process. The commentators all follow Vyāsa's lead here, with Śaṅkara stating that 'the other projected minds ... are all obedient to the controller mind' (Trans. Leggett), while Vācaspati Miśra makes a comparison with *īśvara* and the multiplicity of living beings. All living beings are projected from *īśvara*, and, whilst being wholly distinct from him, remain under his strict control. Vijñāna Bhikṣu again refers to the *avatāras* of Viṣṇu who are all projected out from the Deity, and are controlled and again withdrawn through the will of Viṣṇu.

Sūtras 4.6–4.8: The Influence of Yoga on Karma

In these next three *sūtras*, Patañjali returns to the subject of karma, discussing different forms of karma and how the practitioner of Yoga can be free from all karma, and thereby gain liberation from this world that is sustained by karma. Here we read that karma is of three types, a confirmation of a statement found in the *Bhagavad-gītā* (18.12), which asserts that the fruits of action are *aniṣṭa, iṣṭa*, and *miśra*, undesirable, desirable, and mixed. Here Patañjali confirms the *Gītā*'s view along with Kṛṣṇa's insistence that one should aspire towards *a-karma*, transcendence of all three manifestations of karmic results. The early chapters of the *Gītā* teach that this state of *a-karma* can be attained through *karma-yoga*, the performance of action as a duty for the good of the world without any trace of selfish desire, but in these *sūtras*, Patañjali reveals that *a-karma* is also achieved through meditation.

4.6 *tatra dhyāna-jam anāśayam*

But the mental state shaped by *dhyāna* leaves no impression.

The first word here, *tatra,* means 'there' or 'in this regard', and this is followed by the phrase *dhyāna-ja,* which means 'arising from meditation'. Then *an-āśaya* in its typical usage in yogic discourse means 'devoid of any stock or impression', the idea being that the movements of the mind create *saṁskāras,* which in turn develop into future karmic results, but the practice of meditation leaves no such *saṁskāra* and is hence *a-karma.* Here Vyāsa takes the word *tatra* to refer to the *nirmāṇacitta,* the created mind, that was the subject of the previous two *sūtras.* He claims that there are five types of *nirmāṇacitta* that correspond to the five means by which *siddhis* are developed as outlined in *sūtra* 4.1 of this chapter. Where a mind is created using *siddhis* that are obtained through birth, herbs, *mantras,* or acts of austerity, *saṁskāras* will be left on that mind, but where a *nirmāṇacitta* is created using *dhyāna,* this mind will be free from *saṁskāras.* This observation is perfectly reasonable, but we should also be aware of the wider significance of this *sūtra* in relation to generation of future karma and achieving the state of *a-karma,* which the *Bhagavad-gīta* states is achievable through *karma-yoga,* desireless action. The *sūtra* here is making the point that *dhyāna-yoga* is also a means by which that *a-karma* state may be attained.

As is to be expected, the other commentators all follow Vyāsa's lead in relating the *sūtra* to the five means by which *siddhis* are gained. Śaṅkara has little to add, but Vācaspati Miśra emphasises the point that because *dhyāna* leaves no *saṁskāra,* and is thus free of karma, it is to be regarded as a pathway to liberation. Vijñāna Bhikṣu further explains that when *siddhis* are sought through higher birth, herbs, *mantras,* or austerity, there is a desire for such *siddhis* that is the motivation, and it is this desire that creates the *saṁskāra* that will perpetuate rebirth.

> 4.7 *karmāśuklākṛṣṇaṁ yoginas tri-vidham itareṣām*
>
> Action performed by *yogins* is neither white nor black, but action performed by others is of three types.

This *sūtra* confirms what has been said previously about karma and *a-karma*. The words *a-śukla* and *a-kṛṣṇa* indicate that the karma of the *yogin* is neither white nor black, positive or negative, meaning that the *yogin* enters the state of *a-karma* and thereby escapes from the cycle of action and reaction. For other types of person, for non-*yogins*, karma is of three types, which are defined by the *Gītā* (18.12) as undesirable, desirable, and mixed. Hence Patañjali is here indicating that in its ultimate phase Yoga practice carries the adept beyond the domain of karma, positive and negative. Vyāsa explains that the karma defined here as black, *kṛṣṇa*, is due to actions that harm others, whilst the white karma, the *śukla* that brings a desired result, is action that benefits others or belongs to those who engage in *tapas*, *svādhyāya* or *dhyāna*. Action that is neither white nor black is the karma of the *yogin* who has completely renounced the world to focus absolutely on spiritual pursuits. It is interesting to note here that Vyāsa makes a reference to *phala-saṁnyāsa*, the renunciation of the result of one's action, which is a central feature of the path of *karma-yoga* presented in the *Bhagavad-gītā*, whereby the *yogin* remains active in the world, performing actions for the welfare of others without any attachment or selfish desire, but renouncing the rewards of all actions in Kṛṣṇa (3.30). Vyāsa uses the concept of *phala-saṁnyāsa* to explain how the yogin escapes, specifically the results of good acts, the *śukla* or white karma. As for black karma, the *yogin* simply does not perform it.

Śaṅkara takes this opportunity to take up one of the principal themes of his writing as a whole (if indeed this commentary is the work of Ādi Śaṅkarācārya), namely rejection of the view that ritual action forms a part of the path to liberation. For Śaṅkara, realised knowledge is the only means of gaining liberation; rituals have specific aims behind them and hence they may fall under the heading of *śukla-karma*, but this is still karma, and hence ritual acts are a barrier to *mokṣa*, and should be given up in the final stage of spiritual awakening. It is to be noted that, on this issue, Śaṅkara's view is at odds with the teaching of the *Bhagavad-gītā* (18.5–18.6) in which Kṛṣṇa insists that such acts should never be abandoned, only the selfish desire that might be the motivation behind their performance. Vācaspati Miśra does, however, draw our attention to another of the *Gītā*'s ideas on karma by pointing out that where the action is performed as an offering to *īśvara*, the karma is neither white nor black. Here one presumes that he has in mind verses such as 9.27, 18.46, and 3.30 of the *Bhagavad-gītā*. Vijñāna Bhikṣu is well aware of the conflicting views about the performance of action as a part of the yogic path, and cites a verse from the *Bhagavad-gītā* (5.11) which states *yoginaḥ karma kurvanti*, meaning '*yogins* perform action', to support his view that action should be performed as a part of the process of purification. He also points out that *yama* and *niyama*, the first two of Patañjali's eight limbs, are primarily concerned with modes of action.

4.8 *tatas tad-vipākānuguṇānām evābhivyaktir vāsanānām*

Latent impressions manifest as a result of these three types of action, and these ripen only in the form of the results that correspond to them.

At first glance, this looks to be quite a difficult *sūtra* to grasp, but according to Vyāsa's explanation, the idea being expressed here is relatively straightforward. The subject of the *sūtra* is *abhivyaktir vāsanānām*, the appearance or manifestation of *vāsanās*. The word *vāsanā* sometimes appears to be used interchangeably with *saṁskāra*, the difference being that *vāsanā* means the collection or group of different latent impressions that arise from a pattern of actions, and the thought processes that generate actions. The word *tataḥ*, meaning 'from that', refers to the three types of karma mentioned in the previous *sūtra*, and so the meaning of this *sūtra* as a whole is that the *vāsanās* created in the mind are directly correlated with the three types of action that generate them, and then in turn, the *vāsanās* are directly correlated with the *karma-phala*, the fruits of action that we experience day by day, lifetime after lifetime. The point here is to establish a direct line of continuity between action and its motivating states of mind, the *vāsanās* formed by that action, and the results arising from the *vāsanās* in this or a future life. Vyāsa explains that only some *vāsanās* become manifest at any given moment. For example, when somebody experiences divine karma and becomes a deity, only the *vāsanās* related to the divine existence will become manifest, but not those that pertain to human, animal or demonic existence.

Śaṅkara uses his commentary to emphasise this binding relationship between action performed, *vāsanās* generated in the mind by that action, and then the karmic results that are born of the *vāsanās*, the collection of *saṁskāras* arising from a pattern of action. Vācaspati Miśra closely follows the line of explanation presented above, and Vijñāna Bhikṣu simply re-emphasises the exact correlation between action performed, the *vāsanā* thereby generated, and the karmic experience encountered in the future when the *vāsanā* ceases to be latent and produces a manifest result.

Sūtras 4.9–4.13: Saṁskāras and the Results of Action

In this next group of *sūtras*, Patañjali continues his consideration of the process by which karma fructifies into specific results that correlate exactly with the *saṁskāras* formed by the performance of action. Essentially, what he is doing here is seeking to precisely establish the nature of the problem for which the Yoga system is designed to provide a solution. Understanding that problem is an essential prerequisite for the presentation of *kaivalya* that appears in the final part of this chapter. This discussion inevitably draws in a consideration of the origins of the progression of rebirth and of the nature of time, subjects that are also referred to in this next phase of the discourse.

4.9 *jāti-deśa-kāla-vyavahitānām apy ānantaryaṁ smṛti-saṁskārayor eka-rūpatvāt*

> Although there may be separation in terms of birth, place, and time, because the *saṁskāras* have a form identical to memory, they still remain in direct contact.

The words *smṛti-saṁskārayor eka-rūpatvāt* indicate that what is being said here is 'because of the identitiy of memory and *saṁskāra*'. And the consequence of that identity of memory and *saṁskāra* is the absence of dissociation, *ānantaryam*, despite their being separated in terms of birth, place, and time. All the commentators, however, understand that the *ānantarya* refers to the causal continuity of *saṁskāras*, although this leaves the role of memory unclear. What is being considered here is the manner in which the experience of one life has an influence over a future life by dint of the fact that *saṁskāras* of the mind, of the subtle body, move with the *puruṣa* from one body to another. Even in old age, we will have memories of our childhood despite the transformations we have undergone over the ensuing years and, as with memory, the *saṁskāras* we generate move with us even beyond this life to another bodily form in another time and another place.

Vyāsa adds to this idea by referring to the possibility of rebirth in the form of a cat. Although any previous birth as a cat may have been hundreds of lifetimes previously, and in an entirely different setting, still the *saṁskāras* that shape a cat identity remain, and so the mental faculties once more take the form appropriate for life as a cat. To this, Śaṅkara adds the observation that 'there is no nearness or remoteness of *saṁskāra*-groups, because they are equally stored in the mind' (Trans. Leggett). Vācaspati Miśra responds to an imagined objector who argues that when rebirth occurs in any form, the *saṁskāras* that are prominent should be those from the birth immediately preceding it. To this, Vācaspati Miśra responds by stating again that there is no temporal or locational precedence in relation to the mass of *saṁskāras* stored in the mind and retained over countless lifetimes. Vijñāna Bhikṣu adds that the *saṁskāras* that come to the fore in shaping the mental faculties for any given birth correspond exactly to the fructifying karma that is giving rise to birth in that particular form.

4.10 *tāsām anāditvaṁ cāśiṣo nityatvāt*

And because of the eternal nature of desire,
these *saṁskāras* have no beginning point.

One might naturally ask when this progression of action, *saṁskāra*, and rebirth began. Was there some point prior to this sequential progression when there were no *saṁskāras* at all? To this inquiry, Patañjali answers, *tāsām anāditvam*, there is no beginning point in relation to 'these' which according to Vyāsa refers to *vāsanās* that can be taken as a synonym of the *saṁskāras* mentioned in the previous *sūtra*. Patañjali then explains that this is because of *āśiṣo nityatva*, the eternal nature of desire as an inherent feature of the mind. The point is that *saṁskāras* are created as a result of desire, *āśis*, and desire is inherent in the mind as well as its being generated by external factors derived from sensory perception. Vyāsa further explains that the primary desire is the desire to exist, which is seen in all living beings; this might be understood as primal desire, whilst the many desires that arise in the mind along with perceptions are secondary. He then repeats a point that he has made earlier by stating that the fact that fear of death is present in all beings is evidence that they have experienced death before. Those experiences of death have left *saṁskāras* which awaken fear of death even in a young child who knows nothing of its own mortality. Śaṅkara follows Vyāsa in a consideration of theories as to how it is that the subtle body that transmigrates with *puruṣa* takes on a form appropriate to the physical body, and both Vācaspati Miśra and Vijñāna Bhikṣu are similarly preoccupied with that line of debate, which takes us some steps away from the primary meaning of the *sūtra* itself.

4.11 *hetu-phalāśrayālambanaiḥ saṁgṛhītatvād eṣām abhāve tad-abhāvaḥ*

> Because *saṁskāras* are dependent upon the cause, the result, the foundation, and the support, if these cease to exist, then the *saṁskāras* will also cease to exist.

Here Patañjali moves on to make an implicit explanation of how Yoga practice can arrest the constant progression of action and reaction via the generation of *saṁskāras*. These are said to be dependent upon four factors: their cause, their result, their foundation or basis, and their support, *hetu*, *phala*, *āśraya*, and *ālambana* respectively. When these four factors cease to be present, when there is *abhāva*, non-existence, of these, then the *saṁskāras* also cease to exist. This, of course, is about the means by which liberation, *kaivalya*, is achieved, for existence in this world is sustained by the progression of individual karma and this progression of karma is itself sustained by the repeated manifestation of *saṁskāras* arising from prior action and the states of mind that give rise to action. Hence if the means can be found by which the development of *saṁskāras* can be checked, then karma will end and liberation attained; and, in order to achieve this goal, one must look towards the suspension of the four causal factors through which *saṁskāras* are generated.

Adding a valuable further elucidation, Vyāsa explains that the cause, the *hetu*, is *avidyā*, the primal ignorance that causes *puruṣa* to mistakenly consider itself as *buddhi* and thereby partake of the experiences of life in this world, from which it is entirely distinct. The results, the *phala*, are the karmic consequences, good, bad, and mixed, which arise from adherence to or deviation from *dharma*. The foundation, the *āśraya*, is the mind, for the *saṁskāras* rest upon the mind, and the support, the *ālambana*, is any perceived object that affects the movements of the mind and thereby gives rise to the manifestation of an associated *saṁskāra*. We cannot, of course, surround ourselves with positive sounds and sights that create positive *saṁskāras*, but the aim of the Yoga system is to remove all *saṁskāras*, for it is only in this way that one can gain liberation from the constant progression of karma.

Śaṅkara expands slightly on Vyāsa's observations, noting that all unrighteous acts that are contrary to *dharma* arise from *avidyā*, regarding the body and mind as the self, and hence *avidyā* is the primal cause of karma. Vācaspati Miśra raises the question of whether the fact that *saṁskāṛas* are without any beginning means that it is not possible to bring their progression to a point of final conclusion. His view is that the absence of a beginning point does preclude the possibility of ending the cycle of karma, and that this is the meaning of this particular *sūtra*. Vijñāna Bhikṣu enters into a detailed analysis of Vyāsa's comments, noting that *avidyā* is essentially the lack of discriminating knowledge that would identify the distinction between *puruṣa* and its embodiment formed of *prakṛti*. He also reminds us that 'there is a mutual connection between deeds and *vāsanās* (i.e., *saṁskāras*)' (Trans. Rukmani), for actions create *saṁskāras*, and these *saṁskāras* then give rise to future reactions and further forms of action. Hence the sequence continues until the means be found by which the four factors that give rise to *saṁskāras* are arrested.

4.12 *atītānāgataṁ svarūpato 'sty adhva-bhedād dharmāṇām*

> The reality of past and future is established because of the temporal distinctions of the attributes.

Here Patañjali turns his attention to the question of time, which is, of course, central to his line of discussion related to the progression of karma through the generation of *saṁskāras*. One might argue that in the present, the past is gone and the future does not exist, but Patañjali denies this with the statement that both the *atīta*, the past, and the *anāgata*, the future, do have a *svarūpa*, a reality to their existence. The evidence he gives to confirm this statement is *adhva-bhedād dharmāṇām*, and here the word *dharma* is not used in the more usual sense of 'right action', but in the sense of an attribute which makes an underlying substance, *dharmin*, into a specific object, as seen in the *sūtras* 3.13-14. Then *adhva-bheda* means a difference or distinction (*bheda*) with reference to the three 'paths' (*advan*) of time – past, present, and future. Thus, following Vyāsa, while the same underlying substance (*dharmin*) can by its nature manifest certain attributes, they do not all manifest at once, some belonging to the past and some belonging to the future. Here again we can think about, for example, gold as a substance, *dharmin,* that takes on different *dharmas* as it manifests as different gold-made objects in the course of time.

Vyāsa emphasises the fact that the very idea of karmic progression rests on the understanding of there being three phases of time: past, present, and future. Confirming the Sāṁkhya view that nothing can come into being without being previously existent in a latent form, he also makes the point that past and future are themselves inherent in the present. Śaṅkara takes this opportunity to expound at some length on philosophical ideas regarding the nature of causation and the progression of time. Vācaspati Miśra similarly comments at some length on the idea of *satkārya-vāda,* which asserts that effects must pre-exist within their causal factor, applying this understanding to the progression of time and the fructification of karmic results. Vijñāna Bhikṣu also writes at length on this subject, and points out that it is the latent reality of past and future within the present that allows *yogins* to develop the supernatural power of perceiving past and future states.

4.13 *te vyakta-sūkṣmā guṇātmānaḥ*

These attributes are manifest or subtle, and are pervaded by the *guṇas.*

Here the opening word *te,* meaning 'they', refers to the attributes previously mentioned, and the *sūtra* tells us three things about them: they can be manifest, *vyakta,* or subtle, *sūkṣma,* and their very nature is pervaded by or consists of the *guṇas,* as they are *guṇa-ātmānaḥ*. Vyāsa confirms the assumption that *vyakta,* manifest, refers to the present attributes that we are directly perceiving through the senses, whilst the past and future are subtle in the sense that they exist only in a latent form. All attributes, *dharmas,* are *guṇātmānaḥ,* shaped by the *guṇas,* because this manifest world consists of the evolutions of primal *prakṛti*. In both its primal and evolved forms, *prakṛti* is pervaded by these three *guṇas* of *sattva, rajas,* and *tamas,* and hence all phenomena at all phases of time are similarly pervaded by them.

Vyāsa is very brief here, merely explaining the meaning of manifest and subtle in this context and asserting the pervasive nature of the *guṇas*. Śaṅkara considers the presence of the *guṇas* in this world in a little more detail, pointing out that the *guṇas* themselves are not subject to sense perception, but their presence is evident in the varying manifestations of the world around us. Vācaspati Miśra raises the question of how it can be that such a variegated world as we see moment by moment can have emerged from the single substance of primal *prakṛti,* and answers this potential objection by stating that the *guṇas* are present even when *prakṛti* is in its primal, undifferentiated form, and hence the potential for infinite variegatedness is latent within the fluctuations of the three *guṇas*. Vijñāna Bhikṣu here expounds at some length on the nature and influence of the *guṇas* in the evolution of the world from the single, primal substance of *prakṛti,* but makes the point that from this *sūtra* onwards, the object of discussion is *viveka-jñāna,* the discriminating knowledge that is *mokṣa-kāraṇa,* the cause of liberation.

The *sūtras* of the first phase of the *Kaivalya-pāda* began by providing an insight into the workings of karma, showing how it is that the states of mind that give rise to different forms of action leave marks on the mind, *saṁskāras,* which are the causal factors in generating future karmic reactions. For the *yogin,* however, the practice of meditation leaves no such *saṁskāra,* and hence the mind shaped by meditation is free of the causes of future karma; it is in this way that progress towards *kaivalya* through yogic techniques can be made. As we move forward from this point, we will see how this line of discussion is continued towards its ultimate conclusion: the understanding that Yoga practice limits the generation of *saṁkāras,* and thereby puts an end to the continuous progression of karmic action and reaction. This is *kaivalya,* which is the final stage of the Yoga system in its entirety, as it becomes apparent that all the previous themes and lines of discussion have been leading us to this single point of spiritual emancipation. It is only in the last group of *sūtras* (4.24–4.34) that *kaivalya* becomes the exclusive topic of consideration, but as we read carefully through the preceding passages of the chapter, we can observe that everything that has been said so far is building up to this final point.

Sūtras 4.14–4.17: Objects and the Perception of Objects

The subject of this group of *sūtras* is the reality or otherwise of the objects perceived in this world, and here we find a clear assertion of the *satya-vāda* that states that the world and the objects of this world are indeed entirely real. This rejection of idealist understandings of the present existence as being no more than a creation of the mind is directed primarily against the Buddhist idealism of Yogācāra, but many will be aware that it is on this subject that the Sāṁkhya philosophy underlying the *Yoga Sūtras* differs from the later Advaita Vedānta of Śaṅkarācārya. There can be no doubt that Patañjali adheres strictly to the Sāṁkhya view of the world as real, a true manifestation of *prakṛti.* Our commentator Śaṅkara does not challenge this assertion and joins in with Vyāsa in focusing on a rejection of the Buddhist view of momentariness, which argues that there are no real objects because everything is subject to a constant process of transformation. One must be aware that Patañjali and almost certainly Vyāsa lived prior to Śaṅkarācārya's formulation of an idealist expression of

Vedānta, the *vivarta-vāda*, and hence their words here will not be aimed in that direction.

4.14 *pariṇāmaikatvād vastu-tattvam*

Because it retains a single identity through various transformations, there is reality to an object.

There can be little doubt that this *sūtra* is an overt denial of the Buddhist view of the non-reality of objects. The Yogācāra or Vijñāna-vāda school of Buddhism in particular rejects the idea stated here of *vastu-tattva*, the reality of an object, on the grounds that everything changes moment by moment so that there can be no permanent reality. In particular, Vyāsa mentions the view that any object is just a mental construction like an object appearing in a dream, and Gokhale remarks that 'Vyāsa here is probably referring to Vasubandhu's argument in *Viṁśatikā* (verses 1 and 3) which compares cognitions with dream and regards objects as unreal.'[2] Here Patañjali argues for *vastu-tattva* and explicitly denies the Buddhist view with the statement *pariṇāma-ekatvāt*, there is an essential unity running through the moment-by-moment transformations. A particular object may have a minutely different form from that which it held in the previous moment, but the essential sameness of that object is not to be denied on the basis of imperceptible transformations. Hence that essential oneness establishes the principle of *vastu-tattva*, the reality of an object.

For Vyāsa, the main point made by this *sūtra* is to deny the view of the idealists who, like Berkeley in a more modern era, claim that reality itself is no more than a mental construct: outside of its conception within the mind, an object has no ontological reality, and its perceived reality persists only so

2 Gokhale, *The Yogasūtra of Patañjali*, 172.

long as it is held within the mind. Patañjali and Vyāsa reject this view by stating that whether or not an object is conceived of within the mind, the reality of its existence remains unadulterated. Vyāsa forcefully concludes: 'How can these people who reject the reality of the object which exists as it is by its own authority do so on the strength of fancied cognition without force of proof; while prattling about the very thing they deny, how can they inspire confidence in their own words?' (Trans. Rukmani) Śaṅkara here engages in a debate with the *vijñāna-vāda* of an imagined Buddhist opponent, supporting Patañjali and Vyāsa, but without revealing any hint of the *vivarta-vāda* of the Advaita Vedānta, which argues that the world is real because it is Brahman, but is unreal in terms of the variegated forms in which it is perceived, for all things are Brahman, and Brahman alone. Vācaspati Miśra and Vijñāna Bhikṣu both follow a similar line of debate, confronting and rejecting the Buddhist view, although Vijñāna Bhikṣu includes Śaṅkarācārya's Advaita Vedānta in the debate, asserting that this is to be rejected along with Buddhism.

4.15 *vastu-sāmye citta-bhedāt tayor vibhaktaḥ panthāḥ*

> An object has the same identity in all circumstances, but due to differences of mentality between two persons, the paths of perception diverge.

Following on from his previous statement, in this *sūtra*, Patañjali addresses the question of why it is that if an object has a single reality, it is perceived in different ways by different persons, and exists in their minds in differing forms. His response is a relatively simple one: the reality of the nature of the object does not change; it is the transformations and distinctions of mental processes that are the sole cause of such divergences. Hence his opening phrase is *vastu-sāmye*, meaning 'whilst the object remains the same'; the divergent paths, or experiences, *vibhaktaḥ panthāḥ*, are due to differences of *citta, citta-bhedāt*. Thus here again the idealist view that all objects exist only in the mind of the beholder is rejected, and the reality of objects is again asserted in line with the core precepts of Sāṁkhya teachings.

Vyāsa elaborates on this point by noting that different minds will have different perceptions on coming into contact with the same object. For one person, the object may bring joy, whilst for another person it will bring sorrow; the object itself is neither inherently sorrow-making nor inherently joy-bringing; it is the same in both cases, and the variation exists between the perceiving minds. Moreover, if an object were the creation of one mind, how could it be that the same object is experienced by a different mind? Hence the conclusion again must be *vastu-tattva*, the object is inherently real.

Śaṅkara continues his rejection of the Buddhist *vijñāna-vāda*; the Buddhist may argue that if an object were real, in the sense of constant, then it would evoke the same reaction in all perceivers, and the fact that reactions vary demonstrates that objects exist only as mental constructions. This argument is to be rejected because a variety of mentalities is well established, and it is this that gives a very obvious explanation of differing perceptions of the same object. Vācaspati Miśra illustrates this point by using the example of perception of the same woman. When her male lover sees her, he experiences a sense of joy over anticipated pleasure, but rival mistresses feel pain on seeing her, recognising her as an obstacle to their hopes. The object of perception is one and the same; it is the nature of the perception that varies. Vijñāna Bhikṣu explains that differing perceptions and differing experiences arising from the same constant object are due to differences of karma. Where karma is positive, a person derives pleasure from an object, but negative karma causes the same object to bring pain to another person.

Hence it can be seen that there are different perceivers and different perceptions, but the object itself is one and the same.

> 4.16 *na caika-citta-tantraṁ vastu tad-apramāṇakaṁ tadā kiṁ syāt*
>
> An object cannot be shaped by one mind alone. If that were the case, what would happen if it were not perceived by that mind?

Here again Patañjali continues his philosophical debate with those who hold to the idealist view that objects do not exist beyond their conception within the mind. This view is rejected here with the words *na ca eka-citta-tantram,* there cannot be any creation of objects by one mind alone. The reason why this is the case is a very obvious one: What would happen to that object when it was no longer present in the mind that created it? Would it then not exist? Vyāsa takes up Patañjali's argument with some gusto, pointing out that if the creating mind became distracted, the object would then cease to be and if that mind returned to it later on, it would be impossible because its existence would have vanished during the period of distraction. His conclusion is: 'Therefore, the object is independent of the mind and is common to all purposes' (Trans. Rukmani).

Śaṅkara goes further with this rejection of idealism, pointing out that if that view were accepted, then the world would be constantly coming into being and then disappearing as the minds of individuals moved from one object to another. He concludes: 'So *puruṣa* is the experiencer, mind is the instrument, and the object is its field; the categories of experiencer, instrument, and object are distinct' (Trans. Leggett). Vācaspati Miśra adds the point that consciousness of an object usually means consciousness of a specific part of that object, and so the implication would be that parts of an object come into being and disappear as the mind examines the various parts of that object. Vijñāna Bhikṣu takes a similar line, but identifies the philosophical opponents by name as the Vijñāna-vāda Buddhists, which is interesting as at the time when he lived, there were very few Buddhists left in India, so it is unlikely that he would ever have encountered them directly.

4.17 *tad-uparāgāpekṣitvāc cittasya vastu jñātājñātam*

An object is either known or unknown by the mind, depending on the extent to which it colours the mind's perception.

This is really the conclusion of the previous discussion and the denial of the idealist position. What is being said here is that objects do exist, sometimes being known and sometimes being unknown or unperceived, dependent on whether or not they influence the mind. The point is that the existence of the object does not vary or fluctuate; what does fluctuate is the extent to which it enters the mind, depending on perception, memory, and other fluctuating factors. The conclusion is once again emphatically *vastu-tattva*, objects have an inherent reality regardless of whether or not they enter the mind of an individual. Vyāsa comments only briefly here, confirming the assertion of the *sūtra* itself, whilst Śaṅkara sees fit to continue his dismissal of the ideas of those who support the theory that objects exist only as mental constructs. Śaṅkara's response to these *sūtras* has been interesting inasmuch as he has taken them, certainly correctly, as a rejection of the Vijñāna-vāda school of Buddhism, but has not taken them as in any way challenging the alternative form of idealism advocated by his own school of Advaita Vedānta.

Vācaspati Miśra comments at greater length, but essentially rehearses the previous argument that if objects had no inherent reality beyond mental conception, then they would be constantly fluctuating in line with the constant fluctuations of the mind. Vijñāna Bhikṣu here detects an indication of the distinction between the mind and *puruṣa,* the spiritual entity that is the true self beyond the mind. The knowledge of objects that becomes present in the mind comes and goes and is subject to fluctuation, but *puruṣa* possesses a different form of knowing, which is constant, all-pervasive, and changeless. The problem is of course that this state of absolute knowingness is covered by the veil of *avidyā*. It is this distinction between the mind and *puruṣa* that is the main topic considered in the next group of *sūtras*.

Sūtras 4.18–4.23: The Mind and Puruṣa

In this group of six *sūtras,* the question of the difference between *citta* and *puruṣa* is considered. When we contemplate our own selves, our thoughts, our ideas, and our identity, this is usually in relation to the *citta,* the mental faculties, and to a lesser extent, perhaps the physical body. It appears that *citta* is a fully conscious entity because it displays the signs of sentience and of life, but according to the Sāṁkhya understanding, sentience and life belong solely to *puruṣa,* the spiritual entity beyond the *citta,* and *citta* only displays the marks of consciousness by way of reflection because of its proximity to *puruṣa*. The *viveka-jñāna,* the discriminative knowledge, that has been referred to repeatedly as the goal of Yoga practice enables the practitioner to see the reality beyond the *citta,* and thereby come to understand the spiritual nature of *puruṣa* as the true self of all beings. It is this distinction between *citta* and *puruṣa* that is now considered in these next *sūtras,* and this in turn leads to the point of realised knowledge that is the key to *kaivalya*. Here again much of the discussion is directed towards refuting the arguments of Buddhist teachers who put forward a doctrine of momentariness in order to demonstrate that there is no existence of an *ātman* distinct from the mind. A central pillar of the doctrines set forth in the *Yoga Sūtras* is the idea of *puruṣa* as a spiritual entity, the true self that is distinct from mind and body. For Patañjali and our commentators, it is the realisation of the distinction between *puruṣa* and its embodiment that is the primary goal of Yoga, for this realisation brings liberation from rebirth.

4.18 *sadā jñātāś citta-vṛttayas tat-prabhoḥ puruṣasyāpariṇāmitvāt*

The movements of the mind are always known to *puruṣa*, the master of the mind. This is because *puruṣa* is never subject to transformation.

This *sūtra* states that the *citta-vṛttis*, the movements of the mind, are always known, *jñāta*, to the *puruṣa* because *puruṣa*, the master of *citta*, *tat-prabhu*, is by nature changeless, *apariṇāmin*. The idea here is of *puruṣa* being solely a witness rather than a participator in the mental fluctuations that flow constantly through the *citta*. These *vṛttis* bring about transformations of the mind, but *puruṣa* remains unchanged by them, *a-pariṇāmin*. The false identity with the *citta* adopted by *puruṣa* in its state of ignorance does not alter the changeless state of *puruṣa*, for it is always the witness and never truly the participator in mental processes. Hence, from its changeless position, it possesses knowledge of the movements of the mind, and falsely identifies with them, but is in fact untouched by them. The *Bhagavad-gītā* (5.10) gives the example of a drop of water on a lotus leaf, which touches the leaf but does not penetrate its waxy surface, leaving it unchanged by the contact.

Vyāsa makes only a brief addition to the *sūtra*, stating that the fact that *puruṣa* is always aware of the movements of the mind proves that it is unchanging, for its knowledge is constant. Śaṅkara comments at greater length, but arrives at the same conclusion, stating that the fact that the knowledge gained by the mind is flickering, whilst the knowledge inherent in *puruṣa* is unchanging, demonstrates the distinction that must be recognised between them. Vācaspati Miśra here highlights the logical progression that Patañjali is following in presenting his ideas. Previously, he has demonstrated that the mind and the objects perceived by the mind are entirely distinct, and here he is highlighting a further distinction, namely that between mind and *puruṣa*. Thus, the path of discriminative knowledge, *viveka-jñāna*, is being shown. Vijñāna Bhikṣu makes an important observation here by pointing out that if *puruṣa* were dependent on *citta* for its acquisition of knowledge, then the gaining of liberation from association with *citta* would in fact represent a diminution on the part of *puruṣa*, thus deprived of its means of knowing. This cannot be the case, and hence it is to be concluded that the knowingness of *puruṣa* is independent of the movements of the mind.

4.19 *na tat svābhāsaṁ dṛśyatvāt*

Because the mind is itself an object of perception,
it cannot be regarded as self-illuminating.

Here the view that the mind is self-illuminating is rejected, and this may well be a specific rejection of the teachings of Buddhism, which seek to deny the existence of the *ātman* by saying that consciousness is inherent in the mind without the need for any other entity to imbue it with consciousness. This view is countered here by the word *dṛśyatvāt*, which means, because of its nature as an object of perception'. One may recognise the *citta* as a faculty that makes perceptions, but, at the same time, it is possible for the *citta* itself to be perceived. Therefore, there must be some other entity that is the perceiver of the *citta*, and that again demonstrates the distinction to be understood between *puruṣa* and *citta*. In order to confirm Patañjali's assertion, Vyāsa then provides examples of what is meant here. He says: 'living beings ... say 'I am angry', 'I am afraid', 'I feel attached to that person', 'I am angry with that person'. This cannot be explained unless there is a knowledge of one's own *buddhi*' (Trans. Rukmani). Anger, fear, and attachment are modifications of *citta*, or *buddhi*, and because we can observe those modifications, the ultimate observer cannot be *citta* but must be something higher than *citta* and distinct from it. That is *puruṣa*.

Śaṅkara explores at greater length the possibility of a self-illuminating mind that is capable of perceiving itself, concluding that the arguments presented by Vyāsa show that this notion cannot be applied to the *citta*. He looks at the example of fire, which might be cited as an example of a self-illuminating object that requires nothing external to itself for its perception, pointing out that, although fire can be regarded as self-illuminating, there still must be an external perceiver if fire is to be perceived. Vācaspati Miśra takes the opportunity to enter into further debate with Buddhism, using Vyāsa's arguments to insist that the mind cannot be the ultimate perceiver when the mind itself is an object of perception. Vijñāna Bhikṣu follows that lead in adding to the criticism of Buddhist ideas. Like Vācaspati Miśra, he refers to Buddhists as *vaināśika*, believing in destruction because they deny the existence of the *ātman* that transmigrates after death. There is no doubt that the statement of the *sūtra*, and more especially Vyāsa's commentary, can be taken as arguments put forward to counter the Buddhist doctrine of *an-ātman*.

4.20 *eka-samaye cobhayānavadhāraṇam*

And it is unable to perceive both itself and its object at the same time.

This *sūtra* can be readily identified as forming a continuation of the previous line of argument. Is the mind a perceiver or an object of perception, or is it both, as the Buddhists will claim? Here Patañjali argues that it cannot have both roles simultaneously; it must either be an object of perception, as in the statement, 'I am angry', or else a perceiver, as in the statement, 'I see the jar'. Patañjali here states *ubhaya-anavadhāraṇam*, there cannot be both self-perception and perception of external objects at the same time, *eka-samaye*. Therefore, the unavoidable conclusion is that there must be another, external perceiver, distinct from *citta*. That is *puruṣa*.

Here Vyāsa simply repeats the statement of the *sūtra* itself, but names those who oppose this view as *kṣaṇika-vādins*, those who hold to the doctrine of momentariness – in other words, the Buddhists. Śaṅkara further explains that each single thought or perception fully occupies a single moment; therefore, it is impossible for the mind to perceive itself and an external object at the same time. Vācaspati Miśra continues this critique of Buddhist momentariness, insisting that the mind cannot perceive an object and at the same moment perceive its own perception. Hence there must be another perceiver, external to the mental processes. And addressing the argument of those who regard the mind as self-illuminating, with no need for an external source of illumination, Vijñāna Bhikṣu refutes the view that the mind may at one instant focus on an object and at the next instant focus on itself as the perceiver. Any such idea would wholly undermine the doctrine of momentariness, and hence the central thesis of these *kṣaṇika-vādins* would be negated.

4.21 *cittāntara-dṛśye buddhi-buddher atiprasaṅgaḥ smṛti-saṁkaraś ca*

If one *citta* were subject to the perception of another *citta*, then there would be infinite regress of one

> *buddhi* being perceived by another *buddhi*, and their memories would be mixed up.

Here again we have a continuation of the refutation of the Buddhist ideas of momentariness and *an-ātman*, which involve an insistence that there is no spiritual entity existing beyond the mental processes. As the entire doctrine of the Sāṁkya and Yoga systems rests on the idea of the existence of such a *puruṣa*, both Patañjali and Vyāsa see the need to refute the Buddhist position in order to assert the validity of everything that is said in the *Yoga Sūtras*. This is not just factional squabbling, for the debate here is fundamental to the teachings of the text as a whole. Here the idea that is being challenged is the potential suggestion that the observer of the mental activity of *citta* could be another manifestation of *citta* that occurs in the following instant. Patañjali's counter-argument is that if this were the case, there would be an infinite stream of *buddhis*, each one observing its predecessor. The central point here is to reject the Buddhist idea of the existence of an infinite line of manifestations of *citta* or *buddhi*, each separate from its predecessor, as is a central tenet of the doctrine of momentariness. This doctrine asserts that an object or a *citta* exists only in the moment, and is then succeeded by another *citta* caused by its predecessor, and Patañjali is here aiming to show the shortcomings of this idea.

Vyāsa continues Patañjali's refutation, again naming the opponents as *vaināśikas*, those who believe in destruction because no *ātman* continues after death. He explains that confusion of memory would be the inevitable outcome of there being an infinite number of separate manifestations of *buddhi*, for there would then be an infinite number of memories, each distinct from the other, rather than there being a single projection of memory, as is the general experience. He also challenges the Buddhist idea that there is rebirth and eternal existence in this world without an eternally existing entity in the form of *puruṣa*. The schools of Sāṁkhya and Yoga, he says, accept 'the existence of *puruṣa*, the master, who is the experiencer of the mind' (Trans. Rukmani). Following on from Vyāsa's refutation of *vaināśika* thought, Śaṅkara rejects the idea of momentariness by asking how it can be that if ever-new *cittas* emerge moment by moment, there is a transmission of memories. Surely, such continuation of memory contradicts the idea of momentariness, for the next moment's encounter with the same object will engender a separate memory and, as Patañjali says, confusion will reign.

Vācaspati Miśra similarly takes up the point regarding the transmission of thoughts and memories in relation to the idea that a new *citta* emerges in each new moment of time, whilst Vijñāna Bhikṣu includes a lengthy commentary at this point, taking the opportunity to scrutinise different schools of Buddhist thought, and expose, in his mind, the shortcomings of each. He moves on from this, however, to include Advaita Vedānta within the scope of his critiques, writing, 'By the same argument, the present day Vedāntins are also known as illogical' (Trans. Rukmani), and then presenting arguments to show that the idea of non-duality also crumbles under precise examination of its precepts.

4.22 *citer apratisaṁkramāyās tad-ākārāpattau sva-buddhi-saṁvedanam*

As consciousness is unwavering, *puruṣa* has knowledge of its own *buddhi* by pervading the *buddhi*.

This is a rather difficult *sūtra* to grasp, and indeed to translate, but what appears to be said here amounts to a response to a potential critique from the Buddhist teachers whose ideas Patañjali has just sought to refute. 'How is it', they might ask, 'that if consciousness in the form of the *puruṣa* you postulate is unchanging, it can gain possession of the knowledge acquired by *buddhi*? Surely the acquisition of knowledge by *puruṣa* from *buddhi* would mean that the transformations experienced by *buddhi* would similarly affect *puruṣa*'. In the response given by the *sūtra*, Patañjali confirms that consciousness, *citta*, is indeed unwavering because the knowledge is not transmitted in some way from *buddhi* to *puruṣa*, but is inherently present in *puruṣa*, because it is the conscious nature of *puruṣa* that gives *buddhi* the appearance of consciousness. It is for this reason that we typically regard our own mind as conscious and sentient, when in fact it possesses such attributes only in the form of a reflection from the consciousness of *puruṣa*. Clearly this was an important line of debate at the time of the composition of the *Yoga Sūtras*, when Buddhism still held a significant position throughout India. These might appear to be rather insignificant details to the modern reader, but we must be aware that the central line of Patañjali's teachings rests on the understanding of the true self, *puruṣa*, being a spiritual entity that is entirely distinct from its mental and physical embodiments. Hence this discussion of *puruṣa* as the true locus of consciousness is absolutely central to the text as a whole.

Vyāsa comments relatively briefly here, emphasising the point that *puruṣa* is not affected directly by the movements of the mind and that the mind appears to be endowed with consciousness only as a reflection of the consciousness of *puruṣa*. He also cites a verse which states that Brahman is not hidden in any of the remotest regions of creation, but is concealed beneath the movements of the mind. Śaṅkara clarifies the ideas presented here by explaining that when *buddhi* becomes aware of an object, it takes on the form of that object and is transformed thereby. This transformation pertains only to *buddhi*, however, for *puruṣa* is unchanged in all circumstances. Vācaspati Miśra illustrates the idea of the consciousness of *puruṣa* being reflected in *buddhi* with the example of the moon being reflected in pools of water. When the wind blows, these reflections flicker and change, but the moon itself is unchanged; so it is that the reflection of consciousness in *buddhi* moves and fluctuates whilst *puruṣa*, the true source of consciousness, remains unmoved. Once again, Vijñāna Bhikṣu comments at some length here, presenting a detailed analysis of the relationship between *puruṣa* and *buddhi*, and of how it is that the constant movements of the *buddhi* do not cause any transformation in *puruṣa*, despite the relationship existing between them.

4.23 *draṣṭṛ-dṛśyoparaktaṁ cittaṁ sarvārtham*

> When the *citta* is thus coloured by both the seer and the seen, it becomes capable of perceiving all objects.

What is being established in this *sūtra* is that there are three factors involved in the process of perception; the seer that is *puruṣa*, the means of perceiving that is *citta*, and the object that is perceived. Perception only takes place when *citta* is under the influence of both *puruṣa*, which gives it consciousness, and the object that affects *citta* when perception occurs. The important point of doctrine is to understand the respective roles of each of the three and the distinction between them, for this understanding is the basis of *viveka-jñāna*, the discriminating knowledge that brings liberation from rebirth. It is in this way that perception of all objects, *sarva-artha*, is possible for *citta*.

Vyāsa gives the reasons why this explanation is required. It is because there are others who do not understand the nature of the mind, or the relationship between *puruṣa* and its embodiment. Some hold the view that *citta* is itself possessed of consciousness, whilst there are others who assert that objects exist only in the form of mental perceptions; 'they are to be pitied', he says. Those who recognise that the three – *puruṣa*, *citta*, and the object of perception – are all distinct and fully real have the true understanding: '*puruṣa* has been realised by them' (Trans. Rukmani). Our other three commentators all grasp the opportunity provided by Vyāsa's words to enter into lengthy polemical debates with various potential opponents. These discussions are very interesting from the wider perspective of a study of Indian philosophy, but they are somewhat tangential to the principal line of thought that Patañjali is following here.

Sūtras 4.24–4.28: Approaching Kaivalya

Now that the proper understanding of the distinction between *puruṣa* and *citta* has been established at a theoretical level, Patañjali is able to carry his presentation forward towards the main topic of this chapter and indeed the *Yoga Sūtras* as a whole: *kaivalya,* liberation from rebirth. The proper understanding is that of the Sāṁkhya and Yoga systems, defined as *viveka-jñāna,* which is the recognition of the transcendent nature of the true self as distinct from mind and body. It is not enough, however, to merely accept this idea as a principle of philosophical analysis, it must be wholly absorbed and made a part of one's very existence, and it is for this purpose that the Yoga system exists. There are obstacles to overcome, for past *saṁskāras* continue to afflict the mind, but if these can be negated, then the full realisation of *viveka-jñāna* begins to awaken, and *kaivalya* is in sight.

4.24 *tad asaṁkhyeya-vāsanābhiś citram api parārthaṁ saṁhatya-kāritvāt*

> Although the *citta* becomes variegated due to the influence of the countless *vāsanās* it bears, it serves the purpose of another because it acts in a state of combination.

In this *sūtra*, the short word *api* means 'although' or 'in spite of' and this is applied to the fact that the *citta* mentioned in the previous *sūtra* is variegated or divided in various ways, *citra*, due to the presence of innumerable *vāsanās*, a term we have encountered before, which means a chain or combination of *saṁskāras*. Despite this stream of constant variations that it experiences, it is still to be understood that *citta* serves the purpose of something else that is distinct from itself, which is of course *puruṣa*. Hence Patañjali uses the compound *para-artham*, serving the purpose of another. And *citta* is able to act in this way because it exists in a state of combination. We might take the word *saṁhatya*, combination, to refer to the proximity of *citta* to *puruṣa*, which gives *citta* the semblance of consciousness, or it might refer to the combination of *citta* with the five senses that supply it with perceptions. The *sūtra* itself gives no clear indication as to which of these is the correct reading, but the commentators all understand the combination referred to as being that between the mind and the organs of perception, as *puruṣa* remains entirely distinct from all mental faculties, and is hence never in reality in combination with *citta*.

Vyāsa adds that the phrase *para-artham* means that *citta* serves the purpose of *puruṣa* in two ways, by providing experience of the external world and also by allowing for the cultivation of the higher knowledge, the *viveka-jñāna*, which allows *puruṣa* to achieve *kaivalya*. *Citta* has no purpose of its own to fulfil, but exists solely to serve *puruṣa* in terms of either worldly or spiritual pursuits. He also refers again to the contrary ideas of the Buddhists, the *vaināśikas*, who regard the mind as acting for itself in the absence of a higher spiritual self, and Śaṅkara is thereby prompted into a further refutation of the Buddhist doctrine of *an-ātman*, which denies the existence of *ātman* as a spiritual entity beyond the mind. Vācaspati Miśra similarly offers a robust defence of the idea of *puruṣa* as a transcendent entity that is served by the mind whilst remaining always distinct from it. Vijñāna Bhikṣu sees the phrase *saṁhatya-kāritva,* acting in association with others, as further evidence that *citta* acts only on behalf of *puruṣa,* citing an assertion of the *Sāṁkhya Sūtras* that states, 'Anything that functions in combination with others is for the sake of another' (Trans. Rukmani). And it is interesting to note here that Ādi Śaṅkarācārya writes on this same point at some length in the prose portion of his *Upadeśa Sāhasrī,* suggesting again that our commentator may indeed have been the original Śaṅkarācārya.

4.25 *viśeṣa-darśina ātma-bhāva-bhāvanā-vinivṛttiḥ*

When a person perceives the distinction, there is no further contemplation of the nature of his own existence.

This *sūtra* is about the *viśeṣa-darśin,* the person who sees the distinction between the *citta* and *puruṣa,* as referred to in the previous *sūtra,* in terms of the former existing only for the sake of the latter. What we are told about such a person is that there is cessation, *vinivṛtti,* of *ātma-bhāva-bhāvanā.* Precisely what this phrase means is unclear from the *sūtra* itself, and all subsequent commentators rely on Vyāsa's reading of the text to determine the meaning. The two words *ātma-bhāva* mean 'one's own existence', whilst *bhāvanā* can mean 'the cause' or 'origin', or else 'contemplation', 'consideration', or 'thought'. It is in this latter sense that Vyāsa understands the *sūtra,* and if we follow his lead, then we may take it as indicating a progression from theoretical reasoning to direct perception, which might in turn be taken as a progression from Sāṁkhya theory to the direct perception of *puruṣa* achieved through Yoga. If a *yogin* achieves the state of being able to directly perceive the existence of *puruṣa* at the very core of his being, then there is no further need of contemplating the theoretical reasoning of the Sāṁkhya system, for the truths they expound are now an object of direct realisation. This is very much in line with the teachings on Yoga in Chapter Six of the *Bhagavad-gītā* (6.20), which describe the *yogin* as *ātmānaṁ paśyann ātmani*, seeing the *ātman* within himself.

Vyāsa further explains that when ignorance of the distinction between *citta* and *puruṣa* is removed, *puruṣa* no long identifies itself with *citta* and no longer has such thoughts about himself as 'Who was I?' or 'How was I'?. Śaṅkara confirms this view, pointing out, 'when there is a desire to know something, and that thing is ascertained, the desire to know it ceases' (Trans. Leggett). Vācaspati Miśra here chooses to continue his refutations of Buddhism by asserting that such persons never even contemplate the distinction of *puruṣa* and *citta*, because they do not accept the existence of *puruṣa*. Therefore, there is no possibility of them ever reaching the end of such contemplation. Vijñāna Bhikṣu here confirms an indication in Vyāsa's commentary that the contemplation of one's own state of being is not confined to an understanding of what one is, but also relates to an understanding of previous lives and of future destiny. All such contemplation is irrelevant for the *viśeṣa-darśin* who has fully understood the spiritual nature of his own identity, and is thus progressing into the state of *kaivalya* where the separation of *puruṣa* from *citta* is absolute.

4.26 *tadā viveka-nimnaṁ kaivalya-prāg-bhāraṁ cittam*

> Then, when it is immersed in discriminative understanding, the weight of the *citta* moves towards *kaivalya*.

The subject of this *sūtra* is its final word, *citta*, whilst the first word, *tadā*, meaning 'then', indicates that what is said here relates to the state of *citta* when the *yogin* directly perceives the true nature of the self, beyond theoretical teachings received from a text or *guru*. This is expressed in two compounds, the first of which is *viveka-nimna*. We have encountered the term *viveka*, meaning 'distinction', several times before, and the word *nimna*, with which it is connected here, means 'being sunk' or 'immersed', indicating that now the *citta* of the advanced *yogin* is utterly absorbed in the realised sense of distinction between *puruṣa* and *citta*. His whole consciousness is saturated with that direct realisation. Then we have *kaivalya-prāg-bhāra*. *Kaivalya*, as we know, means 'separation' or 'liberation', *prāg* has the meaning of 'towards', and the literal meaning of *bhāra* is 'weight' or 'burden'. Hence the indication here is of the balance of the mind tilting away from absorption in worldly affairs and gravitating strongly towards the ultimate state of *kaivalya*. This is not yet achieved, but the balance is now moving decidedly towards the state of pure spiritual existence.

Vyāsa comments only briefly on this *sūtra*, noting that it indicates a movement of the mind away from ignorance and objects of pleasure by becoming heavily weighted towards *viveka-jñāna*. Śaṅkara describes this as a counter-current to the previous flow, whilst Vācaspati Miśra merely states that there is no need for any further comment, as the meaning is self-evident. Vijñāna Bhikṣu is equally brief, but adds that the movement of the mind towards discriminating knowledge, *viveka-jñāna*, indicates that the practitioner aspires for liberation from rebirth.

4.27 *tac-chidreṣu pratyayāntarāṇi saṁskārebhyaḥ*

When this state is disrupted, other conceptualisations emerge as a result of existing *saṁskāras*.

What is being discussed here is a level of yogic progression in which the normative state of the *citta* is becoming weighted towards *viveka-jñāna*, but *kaivalya* is not yet fully attained. Hence, at times, interruptions to this elevated condition will occur, and then there will be *pratyaya-antarāṇi*, different thoughts and ideas that arise not from *samādhi* but from the still existing *saṁskāras*, the latent impressions of past experiences, actions, and thought processes, which remain present in the *citta*. It is only when these *saṁskāras* are fully removed that the mind can remain in a constant, unwavering of state of *viveka-jñāna*; this is *kaivalya*, the final goal.

Here again Vyāsa is succinct with his comments, but suggests that thoughts such as 'I am this', 'I know this', and 'I do not know this' can be taken as examples of the thought processes that intrude when there is an interruption of the consciousness of *viveka-jñāna*. On this *sūtra*, Śaṅkara merely summarises Vyāsa's comments, but Vācaspati Miśra explains that thoughts such as 'I know' or 'I do not know', are indicative of the liberated and non-liberated mind respectively. Vijñāna Bhikṣu adds that the expression *asmi*, 'I am', cited by Vyāsa as an example of an intruding thought, means 'I am a man', or 'I am a god'. Because all such ideas pertain solely to the present form of embodiment, they are to be recognised as a product of *avidyā*, ignorance of one's true spiritual identity. When it is applied to the knowledge 'I am *puruṣa*', however, *asmi* is an example of true discriminative awareness, the perfection of *viveka-jñāna*.

4.28 *hānam eṣāṁ kleśavad uktam*

> It is said that these can be negated in the same way as the afflictions mentioned earlier.

In the previous *sūtra*, there was an indication of a problem that will arise whenever there is a pause or break of continuity in the consciousness of discriminative knowledge that fully recognises the distinctive identity of *puruṣa* as separate from its embodiment. The problem rests on the continued existence of *saṁskāras* within the *citta,* which give rise to further movements of the mind during these pauses. In this *sūtra,* Patañjali offers a solution for this problem by stating that the remaining *saṁskāras* can be nullified in the same way as was advocated previously with regard to the *kleśas,* the afflictions or obstacles that impede the successful practice of the techniques of Yoga. This must be a reference back to the beginning of Chapter 2, the *Sādhana-pāda,* where *sūtras* 2.3 to 2.14 first define the *kleśas* as *avidyā, asmitā, rāga, dveṣa,* and *abhiniveśa,* ignorance, egotism, hankering, aversion, and attachment to life, and then offer a means of nullifying them. The connection between the *kleśas* and *saṁskāras* is apparent from *sūtras* 2.12 and 2.13 of the *Sādhana-pāda,* which assert that it is the *kleśas* that are the cause of the progression of karma, which, as we have seen, is also attributed to the *saṁskāras.* The *hāna,* or nullification, of the *saṁskāras* being mentioned here is therefore achieved by the three methods mentioned in the *Sādhana-pāda.* First of all, there is the *kriyā-yoga* described in *sūtras* 2.1 and 2.2, then there is *dhyāna,* which overcomes their coarse activities and makes them subtle, and thirdly, there is the turning them back to the source when they have been made subtle. While the first two refer to the weakening of the *kleśas,* their final nullification was described in 2.10, which, in Vyāsa's interpretation, states that when they have been reduced to a subtle state, a state similar to burnt seeds, they will dissolve in their source along with the mind. This is the process of reversed creation where everything that is not *puruṣa* dissolves back into the undifferentiated state of *prakṛti.* Following the logic of Patañjali's presentation here, we must presume that these three methods are to be understood as effective in nullifying all remaining *saṁskāras.*

Presumably to avoid repetition of what he has said in the *Sādhana-pāda*, Vyāsa does not take up this line of consideration, and merely remarks that the nullification of the *saṁskāras* is achieved by reducing them to the burnt-seed stage where they cannot fructify, a point he made in reference to *kleśas* when commenting on *sūtra* 2.2 of the *Sādhana-pāda*. He also makes the point that this does not apply to the *jñāna-saṁskāras*, the *saṁskāras* of knowledge, which will be maintained up to the point of absolute *kaivalya*. Śaṅkara gives a further explanation of this latter point, stating that the *jñāna-saṁskāras* do not generate further movements of the mind because their presence nullifies action. Vācaspati Miśra suggests that what is being mentioned in these *sūtras* relates to degrees of advancement in *viveka-jñāna*. It is when such discriminative knowledge is well established that residual *saṁskāras* are in the form of burnt seeds, but for those who are less advanced, the methods referred to here are required. Vijñāna Bhikṣu refers back to the *Sādhana-pāda* as discussed above, but does not include *kriyā-yoga* as one of three methods, mentioning only turning back and meditation. He also explains that the *jñāna-saṁskāras* disappear naturally without the need for any means to remove them, for at the point of *kaivalya*, the mind is dissolved, and the *jñāna-saṁskāras* along with it.

Sūtras 4.29–4.34: Achieving Kaivalya

Here, at last, we find the full conclusion of the *Yoga Sūtras* as a whole, as Patañjali briefly describes the state of *kaivalya*, which is liberation from rebirth. At this point, the successful *yogin* becomes freed from the afflictions, the *kleśas*, which give rise to the perpetual progression of karma. And when this cycle of action and reaction is terminated, then there is no more rebirth and absolute knowledge is attained, for this is the natural state of *puruṣa* when its true identity is no longer covered by the veils of *avidyā*. The constant movement of the *guṇas* that shape all lives then also comes to an end, for the adept in Yoga has transcended *prakṛti*, and thus transcended the *guṇas* with which *prakṛti* is imbued. In this liberated state, *puruṣa* becomes what it truly is, purely spiritual and so free of the sufferings of life in this world; according to the *Bhagavad-gītā* (5.21, 6.21), this is a state of pure, unadulterated joy. As with most Indian texts, little detail is given about this liberated state of *kaivalya*, *mokṣa*, *mukti*, or *nirvāṇa*, with the emphasis consistently placed on the idea of freedom from the blight of human bondage; one presumes that this is because the state of liberation is located in a domain of existence beyond the power of words to describe or thoughts to conceptualise.

4.29 *prasaṁkhyāne 'py akusīdasya sarvathā viveka-khyāter dharma-meghaḥ samādhiḥ*

For one who seeks nothing at all, even from his practice of meditation, the *samādhi* called 'cloud of *dharma*' then appears through discriminative insight.

This *sūtra* refers to the adept in Yoga who has reached the ultimate stage of achievement through the yogic cultivation of *viveka-khyāti*, perfect knowledge that brings full awareness of the spiritual identity of *puruṣa* as distinct from its material embodiment. The precise meaning is, however, open to some doubt and, in this case, Vyāsa's commentary is not particularly illuminating. The word *prasaṁkhyāna* usually means 'an enumeration', and hence it might be taken in the sense of 'a high count', but it can also mean 'calculation', 'knowledge' or 'contemplation'; a person can be referred to as *akusīda* if he seeks no personal gain from his endeavours, whilst the addition of *sarvathā* adds the sense of 'in any way whatsoever'. While Vyāsa does not explain the word *prasaṁkhyāna* in more detail, he confirms that this state, achievement, or practice is something that one should ultimately become disinterested in (*virakta*). Vyāsa uses the word *prasaṁkhyāna* in his commentary to other *sūtras*, and there it seems to mean 'knowledge' or 'insight'. It is possible that Vyāsa intends to refer back to the *sūtras* 3.49-50, where 3.49 claims that the insight into the difference between *sattva* and *puruṣa* brings about omnipotence and omniscience and 3.50 claims that *kaivalya* occurs when the *yogin* becomes disinterested even in these.

I am not certain of the precise meaning intended here, as Patañjali could be saying 'he seeks nothing even from the elevated state he has achieved', or he could be saying, 'he seeks nothing at all from the insight he has gained', or he could be saying 'he seeks nothing at all, even from his practice of meditation'. What convinced me to go with the latter reading is finding that in his *Upadeśa Sāhasrī* (18.12, 17), Śaṅkarācārya (definitely the real Śaṅkarācārya) uses the word *parisaṁkhyāna* to indicate a form of meditational practice by which the truth of the *ātman* is realised. Then *viveka-khyāteḥ* would mean 'from his discriminating enlightenment', giving us a clear sense of the general meaning that the fully enlightened *yogin* seeks nothing at all from his high achievements in Yoga. Here one is reminded of the wonderful mystical powers outlined in the *Vibhūti-pāda*, and so the indication seems to be that at the point of ultimate yogic perfection, all desires and aspirations, material and spiritual, simply melt away into the acquired state of perfect being.

We are then told that when such desires are wholly transcended, there appears the *dharma-megha samādhi*, the *samādhi* that takes the form of a raincloud filled with *dharma*. Exactly why it is that this highest form of *samādhi* is designated as *dharma-megha* is unclear, as the term *dharma* has a number of different meanings, and on this point Vyāsa offers no guidance at all. The two main possibilities would seem to be that either *dharma* is being used in its philosophical sense as a knowable object, or else in the more widespread usage of virtuous action. Scholars like Gokhale[3] and O'Brien-Kop[4] have pointed out that this is probably related to the Buddhist notion of the *dharma-meghā*, which is the highest level (*bhūmi*) on the bodhisattva's spiritual path, although it is unclear to what extent the supposed Buddhist background of *dharma-megha* illuminates the exact meaning of *dharma* in this *sūtra*. Each of our three other commentators follows Vyāsa's brevity on this point, though we do get some indication of the line of interpretation they are following. Śaṅkara merely states that the *megha*, the cloud, rains down the supreme *dharma* called *kaivalya*, but Vācaspati Miśra shows an inclination towards the first of the two possible definitions by referring to a 'rain cloud of *dharmas*', the plural form of *dharma* indicating that he is taking it to mean objects existing in this world. Vijñāna Bhikṣu appears to take a different line, however, as he writes, 'It is *dharma-megha* because it rains *dharma* which totally uproots *kleśas* and *karma*' (Trans. Rukmani).

Personally, I prefer to understand the *dharma-megha* as a monsoon cloud that rains down *dharma* in the form of pure, unadulterated virtue. If we turn to the *Mahābhārata*, we can find several explanations of precisely what is meant by *dharma*. Here are three of them:

> *adrohaḥ sarva-bhūteṣu karmaṇā manasā girā anugrahaś ca*
> *dānaṁ ca satāṁ dharmaḥ sanātanaḥ*
>
> Never displaying malice towards any living being through actions, thoughts, or words; acts of kindness; giving

---

3 Gokhale, *The Yogasūtra of Patañjali*.

4 O'Brien-Kop, '*Dharmamegha* in Yoga and Yogācāra: The Revision of a Superlative Metaphor', *Journal of Indian Philosophy*, 48 (2020): 605–635.

> in charity; this is the Sanātana Dharma adhered to by righteous persons (3.281.34)
>
> *sarvaṁ priyābhyupagataṁ dharmam āhur manīṣiṇaḥ paśyaitaṁ lakṣaṇād deśaṁ dharmādharme yudhiṣṭhira*
>
> The wise say that dharma is whatever is based on love for all beings. This is the characteristic mark that distinguishes *dharma* from *a-dharma*, Yudhiṣṭhira. (12.251.24)
>
> *anukrośo hi sādhūnāṁ su-mahad-dharma-lakṣaṇam anukrośaś ca sādhūnāṁ sadā prītiṁ prayacchati*
>
> Amongst righteous persons, compassion is the great characteristic mark of *dharma*, and compassion is always a source of delight for the righteous. (13.5.23)

When we consider these definitions of *dharma* from a roughly contemporary period, we can see that what is being spoken of is not a set of rules or even an ideal mode of conduct, but rather a state of consciousness. Hence *dharma* is perhaps best understood as a state of being in which one abandons self-centred action based on greed, desire, and malice towards others. What we have seen in the *Yoga Sūtras* is a prescription for a transformation of the mind away from such self-centred preoccupations towards an elevated state of spiritual consciousness that is wholly devoid of such negative tendencies. Viewing *dharma* from the *Mahābhārata*'s perspective, we can thus understand why the highest state of yogic realisation should be referred to as *dharma-megha*, for in this state, one's outlook on the world is utterly and absolutely benign, and any thought of rivalry or ill-will towards others is inconceivable for the enlightened mind. At the end of the *Bhagavad-gītā*'s teachings on meditational yoga (6.32), we find the following verse:

> *ātmaupamyena sarvatra samaṁ paśyati yo 'rjuna sukhaṁ vā yadi vā duḥkhaṁ sa yogī paramo mataḥ*
>
> One who thus sees everyone's pleasure and suffering as the same as his own, Arjuna, is considered to be the highest *yogin*.

To find equal joy in the happiness of others and to feel equal sorrow in the suffering of others is the very essence of *dharma* as defined by the *Mahābhārata*, and I think it must be for this reason that the perfection of Yoga is here described as being saturated through and through with the innately benign consciousness of *dharma*.

> 4.30 *tataḥ kleśa-karma-nivṛttiḥ*
>
> And as a result, the afflictions and the influence of karma cease to be active.

Here the opening word *tataḥ* means 'thereupon', or 'from that', indicating that the *sūtra* is commenting on the consequences of *dharma-megha samādhi*. And these consequences are the *nivṛtti* of *kleśa* and karma, where *nivṛtti* means 'ceasing to be active', just as *vṛtti* means 'the movements'. So when the *dharma-megha samādhi* appears, the *kleśas* no longer exert their influence, and we will recall that the primary *kleśa* is *avidyā*, ignorance of our true identity as *puruṣa* distinct from *prakṛti*. When *avidyā* is eradicated, then the *saṁskāras* are nullified and the cycle of karma becomes still. This is *kaivalya*, liberation from karma, and liberation from suffering and rebirth.

Vyāsa here asserts that the *yogin* reaches this state of liberation from *avidyā* and karma even whilst physically existing in this world, the state of *jīvan-mukti*. The root cause of rebirth and karma is a false understanding of one's true nature, and when this is corrected by *viveka-jñāna*, the cycle of transmigration is brought to an end; Śaṅkara confirms this point using the phrase *mithyā-jñāna*, false knowledge, to refer to the ignorance eradicated by Yoga practice. Vācaspati Miśra is very brief here, but he does confirm Vyāsa's statement regarding *jīvan-mukti*, stating that liberation is achieved through the eradication of ignorance, and the moment the *dharma-megha samādhi* appears, ignorance is uprooted. Vijñāna Bhikṣu is also primarily concerned with the question of liberation whilst still living in this world, and takes the opportunity to refute the idea of *jīvan-mukti* as taught by the *ācāryas* of Advaita Vedānta.

4.31 *tadā sarvāvaraṇa-malāpetasya jñānasyānantyāj jñeyam alpam*

> Because of the limitless nature of this knowledge, from which the entire covering of impurity has been removed, there then remains little further to be known.

Here the compound *sarva-āvaraṇa-mala* means 'all the coverings of dirt or impurity', and *apeta* means 'removed'. This phrase refers to the *jñāna-ānantya*, the unlimited nature of knowledge that emerges when the *mala* or *kleśas* headed by *avidyā* are cleared away by *samādhi*. This limitless knowledge is not acquired from any external source but emerges from within as an inherent feature of the true identity of *puruṣa* when the coverings are finally worn away to nothing by Yoga practice. The idea here is very similar to the Śaivite teachings that state that each living being is of the same nature as Śiva, but it is only when the *mala* of ignorance is removed that the omniscient Śiva nature emerges from within the enlightened person. This is not knowing in the sense of learning, thinking, and remembering, but just a state of perfect knowingness that emerges naturally as the *kleśas* melt away. Patañjali states that at this point, *jñeyam alpam*, there is only a small amount that remains to be known, which might appear to be somewhat restrained given that it is the state of perfect yogic enlightenment that is being considered here.

Vyāsa offers little by way of explanation on this latter point, merely adding: 'By the endlessness of knowledge what is to be known becomes like a firefly'. Śaṅkara qualifies this somewhat by saying: 'As there is nothing to find out about fireflies in the sky, so there is nothing to be investigated now' (Trans. Leggett). On that point, one feels that an entomologist might beg to differ. Vācaspati Miśra refers back to his particular understanding of *dharma-megha samādhi*, suggesting that the knowledge possessed by the advanced *yogin* is *ananta*, without limit, because the *dharmas* falling from the cloud are in fact all knowable objects. Vijñāna Bhikṣu understands the *sūtra* in a rather different way, interpreting it to mean that because the unlimited knowledge acquired by the *yogin* is in relation to the twenty-four elements of *prakṛti* along with *puruṣa*, there is in fact a very small range of knowables. Almost certainly, this statement reflects his theistic orientation, and he is suggesting that knowledge of *īśvara* is of a higher nature still.

Gokhale points out that the progression implied in this *sūtra* again resembles that found in Mahāyāna Buddhism. He suggests that 'Patañjali is indirectly referring to the Buddha stage which immediately follows the highest stage of the *bodhisattva*'[5]. While the *dharma-megha* is the highest stage (*bhūmi*) in the path of the *bodhisattva*, for whom the *kleśāvaraṇa*, 'the veil of defilement', is removed, there still remains the *jñeyāvaraṇa*, 'the veil of the knowable' which is only removed when full Buddhahood is reached.

---

5 Gokhale, *The Yogasūtra of Patañjali*, 181.

4.32 *tataḥ kṛtārthānāṁ pariṇāma-krama-samāptir guṇānām*

Then the sequential transformation of the *guṇas* from one to the other comes to an end, for they have fulfilled their purpose.

Again we have a *sūtra* beginning with the word *tataḥ*, meaning 'then' or 'from that', indicating a line of progression in yogic attainment as a result of the appearance of *dharma-megha samādhi*. In this case, the result referred to relates to the three *guṇas*, which now cease their constant transformations that bring about the manifest world. We will recall that the *guṇas* of *sattva*, *rajas*, and *tamas* are the three qualities or attributes that are a pervasive feature of *prakṛti* in all its evolved forms. *Sattva* is the quality of light, virtue, purity, and wisdom, *rajas* is the quality of energy, action, desire, and passion, and *tamas* is the quality of darkness, inertia, sloth, and ignorance. Here then we are informed that another consequence of the appearance of the *dharma-megha samādhi* is that this constant transformation of the *guṇas* comes to an end, and they become inactive or dormant in the mind of the perfect *yogin*.

An interesting point here is the reason given for the *samāpti*, the cessation, of the *pariṇāma-krama* of the *guṇas*, their constant transformations. This is said to be *kṛta-artha*, because they have fulfilled their purpose, which Vyāsa reminds us is that of providing either enjoyment and experience, or else enlightenment and liberation. This idea of *prakṛti* and its *guṇas* having the particular purpose of providing a means by which *puruṣa* can gain liberation is also found in the *Sāṁkhya Kārikā* (vs 63, 66), and is used as a basis for the refutation of the Sāṁkhya system by Śaṅkarācārya in his *Upadeśa Sāhasrī* (16.47–16.49). Śaṅkara's argument is that if *prakṛti* is insentient by nature, then how it can it be understood to be acting for a particular purpose? One answer to this question is to be found in the theistic Sāṁkhya of the *Bhagavad-gītā* (9.10), which offers the teaching that all the movements and evolutions of *prakṛti* take place according the direction of the Deity, so that we are to understand that the *artha*, the purpose, is an expression of the divine will rather than that of the non-conscious *prakṛti*.

Here Vyāsa merely asserts that the *guṇas* give up their active nature because the dual purposes they serve on behalf of *puruṣa* of experiencing the world and gaining liberation have now been completely fulfilled. Śaṅkara adds that the *guṇas* are active within the mind of every person, and so when the mind is transcended through the attainment of *samādhi*, the actions of the *guṇas* automatically cease. Vācaspati Miśra comments that it is the movements of the *guṇas* in the mind which create *saṁskāras* and future karma, so that the cessation of such movements is essential if liberation from all karma is to be achieved. Vijñāna Bhikṣu provides a longer commentary, pointing out references from other works which confirm the point being made here.

4.33 *kṣaṇa-pratiyogī pariṇāmāparānta-nirgrāhyaḥ kramaḥ*

> The sequence of transformations takes place moment by moment, but is perceived only at the end of the transformation.

On the surface, this *sūtra* is just an elaboration on the word *krama*, progression or sequence, used in the previous *sūtra*, but there is a rather more significant meaning lurking behind it. Earlier in this chapter (*sūtras* 4.14 to 4.17), both Patañjali and Vyāsa were emphatic in their rejection of the Buddhist notion of momentariness, which insists that there is no reality to any object because it constantly undergoes a process of transformation. This idea was refuted on the grounds that there is a constant identity to all objects that remains permanent despite the constant transformation. Here, however, the idea of constant transformation is fully accepted, though not, of course, the concomitant implication that this renders all objects non-real. Such transformations generally take place to a minute degree moment by moment, but because the rate of transformation is so gradual, it cannot be perceived until the process of transformation reaches its conclusion. To illustrate this point, Vyāsa uses the example of an item of clothing. We cannot observe such an item ageing before our eyes, but eventually we will see that the new dress I bought has now become old.

The real significance of the *sūtra*, however, rests on the question of whether a process of constant transformation can be fully arrested, for this is a question that reflects precisely on the idea of liberation from the *krama* of karma and rebirth. Vyāsa begins his explanation by stating that *puruṣa* is permanently unchanged, and experiences no progression; the *guṇas* are the exact opposite, for it is in their very nature to be constantly fluctuating. He then poses the question of whether or not the cycle of rebirth, a perpetual sequence, will reach an end point, and responds by saying that this question cannot be answered with a simple 'yes' or 'no'. The point is that for one who lacks *viveka-jñāna*, the knowledge that distinguishes *puruṣa* from *prakṛti*, there is no end to rebirth, but for the enlightened *yogin*, the apparently endless sequence now has a clearly defined end point. Śaṅkara notes a possible objection from one who points out that even the enlightened *yogin* must die, so how can it be said that the sequence of deaths has been ended? To this, Śaṅkara responds with the answer we might expect, saying that for *puruṣa* there is no death, and the enlightened one exists wholly within the identity of *puruṣa*.

Vācaspati Miśra makes the point that despite constant transformations, the *guṇas* are also to be regarded as permanent simply because their nature of being in a state of constant flux is permanent. We might observe that it was said in the previous *sūtra* that for the *yogin*, the sequence of *guṇa*-movement does come to an end at the point of liberation, but what Vācaspati Miśra is saying is that the fundamental nature of the *guṇas* has not been transformed; the *guṇas* remain as *guṇas* with their particular identities. He also makes the point that the creation and destruction of the world, which occur repeatedly, do not mark a break in the sequence, for in the new creation, the embodied *puruṣa* simply resumes its cycle of rebirth, guided by the fluctuating *guṇas*. Vijñāna Bhikṣu goes to some length to consider the question of permanence or transience in relation to *prakṛti*, concluding that its essential nature is permanent, but that it simultaneously exists in a state of constant transformation. On the other hand, it may appear that *puruṣa* is also in a state of constant transformation, but this understanding is based on the superimposition of a material identity, which does undergo change, onto the changeless *puruṣa*.

4.34 *puruṣārtha-śūnyānāṁ guṇānāṁ pratiprasavaḥ kaivalyaṁ svarūpa-pratiṣṭhā vā citi-śaktir iti*

> *Kaivalya* means the return of the *guṇas* to their original source, when they no longer have a purpose for *puruṣa*. Or *kaivalya* can be said to be the potency of the true consciousness when it achieves its natural position.

And so we come at last to the final *sūtra* of Patañjali's great work, and, as an apt conclusion, he gives us a twofold definition of *kaivalya*, one positive and the other negative. From a negative perspective, *kaivalya* means the termination of the present form of life that is predominated by the fluctuations of the *guṇas*. *Kaivalya* means that these constant movements come to an end as they are absorbed in their original source, undifferentiated *prakṛti*, and this will in turn bring about the termination of the progression of karma from action to reaction to action once more. And from a positive perspective, the *citi-śakti*, the power of the consciousness of *puruṣa* finds its true identity, which is wholly spiritual. There it is said to be *svarūpa-pratiṣṭhā*, fixed in its own true identity. What this means is that when *puruṣa* is afflicted by *avidyā*, it exists in association with *prakṛti* as an embodied entity, and in this condition, the inherent spiritual potency of *puruṣa* is covered over. As we have heard, *kaivalya* means the removal of such coverings so that the full spiritual glory of *puruṣa* shines forth. This also is to be understood as the state of *kaivalya*.

Vyāsa comments only briefly, merely summarising the *sūtra*, but Śaṅkara detects a relationship of cause and effect between the two interpretations of *kaivalya* given here; it is the inhibition of the flow of the *guṇas* that allows the *citi-śakti* of *puruṣa* to become fully manifest. Vācaspati Miśra explains the meaning of the word *pratiprasava*, stating that this does not merely mean an inhibition of the flow of the *guṇas*, but a turning back of the *guṇas* so that they return to their original state of equilibrium within primal *prakṛti*. Likewise, each component of the *yogin*'s mental faculties, the intellect or *buddhi*, the mind or *manas*, and the sense of ego, *ahaṁkāra*, is withdrawn one back into the other, and then finally back into *prakṛti*. In this way, the liberation of the *yogin* is enacted as a microcosmic inversion of the manifestation of the world in which each of these elements evolves one from the other out of primal *prakṛti*. Vijñāna Bhikṣu explains that the emergence of the full potency of consciousness, the *citi-śakti*, is due to 'an absence of the limitation of *buddhi*'. The association of *puruṣa* with *buddhi*, and *puruṣa*'s misidentification of itself as *buddhi*, imposes limitations on its natural potency, but when these are removed at the point of *kaivalya*, then the full *citi-śakti* emerges. In this state of *kaivalya*, there is no possibility that *puruṣa* will again fall prey to *avidyā* and resume its association with *prakṛti*.

Conclusion

In the opening *sūtras* of the *Kaivalya-pāda,* Patañjali emphasised the connection between the *saṁskāras* left on the mind by thoughts and actions and the constant progression of karma, which in turn perpetuates the cycle of death and rebirth. We can then observe the contribution made by the *Yoga Sūtras* to the debate over the established reality of the objects of this world, the *dharmas,* with Patañjali rejecting the Buddhist view of momentariness and seeking to establish the idea of permanent reality. This understanding is important to the Yoga tradition because of the centrality to that tradition of the understanding of *puruṣa,* or *ātman,* as a permanent reality that exists in association with its material embodiment, whilst remaining unchanging and untouched by that state of embodiment. *Puruṣa* is established as a permanent reality in contrast to the Buddhist doctrine of *an-ātman.* Following his assertion of the reality of the changeless *puruṣa,* Patañjali then teaches that the liberation of *puruṣa* from its state of bondage in this world is achieved through the cultivation of discriminative knowledge by means of the techniques of Yoga practice. It is the total absorption of this *viveka-jñāna* that draws *puruṣa* towards *kaivalya,* the ultimate goal of Yoga. This achievement of *kaivalya* engulfs the *yogin* in the pure consciousness of *dharma,* it puts an end to the influence of the three *guṇas,* it entails the removal of all impurities, and it allows *puruṣa* to exist as it truly is, a pure, spiritual entity entirely free from any association with the miseries of life in this world. And it is on this positive note regarding absolute spiritual enlightenment that Patañjali brings the progression of his discourse on Yoga to a close.

Glossary of Sanskrit Terminology*

abhiniveśa: Longing for life. 2.9

abhyāsa: Regular practice. 1.12

adhyātma: In relation to the *ātman* or to personal identity. 1.47

advaita: The philosophical idea of absolute unity between the world, individual living beings, and Brahman, the absolute reality.

Advaita Vedānta: The particular schools of Indian thought based primarily on the teachings of Śaṅkarācārya who sought to show that the Upaniṣads and *Bhagavad-gītā* reveal the truth of *advaita*.

āgama: Literally 'that which has come down'; inherited wisdom or sacred texts. 1.7

ahaṁkāra: (1) That part of the mind that creates a sense of selfhood in relation to the present embodied identity. 1.2; (2) pride, arrogance, and egotism.

ahiṁsā: Not harming; acting to relieve others from suffering. 2.35

ānanda: Joy, usually the joy of spiritual awakening. 1.17

an-ātman: (1) That which is not *ātman*. 2.5; (2) the Buddhist doctrine that denies the existence of the spiritual *ātman*. 4.19

antarāya: Obstacle, obstruction. 1.29

anumāna: Knowledge based on inference derived from previous perceptions. 1.7

anuśāsana: Teaching or instruction. 1.1

aparigraha: Not grasping; removing hankering for material acquisitions. 2.39

* Numbering after entry indicates the *sūtra*(s) most relevant to the term concerned.

asaṁprajñāta: The state of meditation or *samādhi* in which the mind transcends the object of meditation and has no specific object. 1.18, 3.8

āsana: A seat or sitting posture, one of the eight limbs of Yoga. 2.46

aṣṭāṅga: 'having eight limbs', Yoga system that has eight limbs (*aṣṭa aṅga*) or stages, as taught by Patañjali.

asmitā: Egotism, self-centredness. 1.17

asteya: Not stealing. 2.37

ātman: The true spiritual self. An equivalent term for *puruṣa*. 1.23, 1.47, 2.41. The nature of something. 2.18, 2.21, 4.13

avasthā: The particular status or condition of an object at a given time. 3.13

avidyā: Ignorance, lack of knowledge, usually in relation to the true spiritual identity. 2.4, 2.5

avyakta: Literally invisible or non-manifest. A term used for *prakṛti* in its primal unitary state before it evolves into the variegated world. 1.45

Bhagavad-gītā: A passage of the *Mahābhārata* in which Kṛṣṇa gives instruction on a range of spiritual ideas and practices, including Yoga techniques.

bhakti: The spiritual path centred on devotion to the Deity. 1.23, 2.45

bhāṣya: A commentary providing an explanation of the meaning of an authoritative text.

bhūta: The physical elements of space, air, fire, water, and earth. 2.18, 3.44

brahmacarya: Celibacy, restraint of sexual desires. 2.38

Brahma Sūtras: An alternative title for the *Vedānta Sūtras*.

buddhi: That feature of the mind that engages in reflection and decision making and can be used in Yoga practice when brought under volitional control. 1.2

cakras: Energy centres within the body as taught in later Yoga teachings.

citta: The mental faculties or thinking process. 1.2

dhāraṇā: Concentration of the mind on a single point; one of the eight limbs. 1.40, 2.53, 3.2

dharma: (1) Right action or proper conduct. 2.31; (2) an attribute. 3.13, 3.14, 3.45, 4.12, 4.13

dharmin: That which possesses a *dharma*, an unchanging substance that can manifest different *dharmas*, thereby manifesting as different objects. 3.14

dhyāna: Meditation. 1.39, 3.2

doṣa: Fault, obstacle, contamination. 3.50

draṣṭṛ: The one that sees or perceives; a term used for *puruṣa*. 1.3, 2.17, 2.20

dṛśya: That which is seen or perceived; the external world. 2.17, 2.18

duḥkha: Misery, suffering. 1.31, 1.33

dveṣa: Loathing, distaste, hatred. 2.8

ekāgra: Fixed on a single point, also *ekāgratā*. 1.28

guṇas: The three pervasive qualities of all things material, designated as *sattva*, *rajas*, and *tamas*. 1.2, 2.19, 4.32, 4.34

hāna: Literally, 'giving up', 'abandoning'. Here translated as 'escape' or 'nullification'. 2.25, 2.26, 2.27, 4.28

hetu: The cause or causal factor. 2.17, 2.23

heya: Literally, 'to be given up', thus to be destroyed, to be prevented, to be escaped from. Defined as suffering in 2.16. See also 2.17, 2.27

hṛdaya: The heart. 1.36, 3.34

indriyas: The five senses of external perception (sight, touch, smell, hearing, and taste). 2.18, 2.54, 3.37

īśvara: The Lord; the Supreme Deity in a monotheistic sense. 1.23, 1.24, 1.26

īśvara-praṇidhāna: Devotion to the Deity or meditation on the Deity. 2.1, 2.45

japa: Internal or audible recitation of a mantra or prayer. 1.28

jīva: The living being. Equivalent to *puruṣa* and *ātman*, though usually when the living being is existing in a state of bondage in this world.

jñāna: Knowledge, specifically the spiritual realisation that brings liberation from rebirth. 1.38

jyotis: Light, radiance, or effulgence. 1.36

kaivalya: Literally 'separation' in the sense of sepatation of *puruṣa* from *buddhi*. This is liberation from rebirth; an equivalent term for *mokṣa* and *mukti*. 2.25, 3.50, 3.55, 4.34

kāma: Desire for the pleasures of sensual delights. 2.3

karma: Literally 'action'. The law of karma postulates that good or righteous acts will produce a positive effect in the form of an elevated rebirth and good fortune in the life to come, whilst iniquitous deeds will produce the opposite result. 2.12, 2.13, 4.7, 4.30

karma-yoga: Performance of actions for the welfare of the world without any self-centred desire or attachment, as taught in the *Bhagavad-gītā*. 2.1, 2.32, 4.7

kleśa: Obstruction, fault, or affliction. 2.2, 2.4

kriyā-yoga: Yoga based on prescribed activities. 2.1

krodha: Anger. 2.34

kṣaya: Diminution, dwindling, wasting away. 2.43

kṣetra: Field, ground (of). 2.4

kumbhaka: The inward retention of the breath during *prāṇāyāma*. 1.34, 2.50

lakṣaṇa: The qualities or characteristics of an object. Here: its position in relation to time. 3.13

liṅga: The characteristic mark of an object that defines its identity or fundamental nature. 1.45

lobha: Greed. 2.7, 2.34

Mahābhārata: An extensive ancient text that tells of the conflict between two factions of the same royal family and includes a number of important passages of instruction on Yoga.

mahā-bhūtas: The great elements: earth, space, fire, water, and air.

mahat: The great element. The first element to emerge from primal *prakṛti* as the world comes into being. Equated with the mental faculty known as *buddhi*. 2.19

mahā-vrata: Great vow. 2.31

mala: Dirt, contamination, material, ethical, or spiritual. 1.48

manas: That part of the mind that receives all sensory perceptions, identifies them, and then passes them on to *buddhi* for further reflection. 1.35

Mīmāṁsā: A system of philosophy that emphasises the primacy of Vedic ritual practices.

moha: Delusion, confusion. 2.34

mokṣa: Release, liberation from rebirth. Equivalent term for *kaivalya*.

nāḍīs: Veins or channels along which subtle energy can be transmitted. 1.36

nidrā: Sleep or, more specifically, deep dreamless sleep. 1.10, 1.38

nirbīja: Literally 'without any seed'; a type of meditation, *samādhi*, that transcends any focus on a specific object. 1.51

nirodha: Restraint or suppression. 1.2

niyama: Positive observances that are spiritually beneficial. 2.32

om: The sacred syllable which is said to be the verbal expression of *īśvara*.1.27

pāpa: Wickedness, action that is harmful to others. 1.47

pariṇāma: Change or transformation. 3.9-3.16 As *pariṇāma-duḥkha*: Misery that comes from inescapable change and transformation inherent in all phenomena. 2.15

pariṇāma-vāda: The philosophical doctrine that states that the world comes into being through a process of transformation from one element to another. 3.13

phala: Fruits, results, consequences. Usually as *karma-phala,* the results of morally good or bad action (karma). 2.14

pradhāna: Prakṛti in its primal undifferentiated state. 1.45

prajñā: Knowledge, realisation, understanding, wisdom. 1.20, 1.48, 2.27

prakṛti: The total material substance out of which this world is formed, including the physical bodies of living beings and their mental faculties. 1.19, 1.45

pramāṇa: A valid source of proof or knowledge in philosophical debate. 1.7

praṇava: The mantra or sound vibration *oṁ*. 1.27

prāṇāyāma: Restraint or regulation of the breathing process. 1.34, 2.49

prasāda: Grace or serenity. 1.33

prātibha: Intuitive knowledge that comes from within rather than from any external source. 3.33

pratyāhāra: Withdrawal of the senses from external perception, one of the eight limbs. 2.54

pratyakṣa: Direct sensory perception; a source of valid knowledge. 1.7

puṇya: Virtue, righteous action for the welfare of others, or religious rituals. 2.14

pūraka: The inhalation of the breath during *prāṇāyāma*. 1.34, 2.50

Purāṇas: A genre of Hindu literature which is one of the main sources of Hindu mythology. For the most part, the Purāṇas are believed to be later than the *Yoga Sūtras*.

puruṣa: The true identity of every living being that is a purely spiritual entity, wholly distinct from its physical and mental embodiments. An equivalent term for *ātman*.

rāga: Desire, passion, hankering. 2.7

rajas (rajo-guṇa): The *guṇa* of *rajas*, which relates to action, passion, desire, and endeavour.

recaka: The exhalation of the breath during *prāṇāyāma*. 1.34, 2.50

ṛta: Truth, virtue, an established rule. 1.48

śabda: (1) Sound. (2) A source of knowledge coming from scriptural revelation or an enlightened teacher.

sabīja: Literally along with a seed; usually meditation, *samādhi*, employing a specific object. 3.9

sādhana: Regular practice to achieve a set goal. Chapter 2

samādhi: The ultimate stage of the Yoga system in which the mind becomes totally absorbed in the object of meditation. For different types of *samādhi* see *asaṁprajñāta*, *saṁprajñāta*, *sabīja*, *nirbīja*. See also *samāpatti*. 1.20, 3.3

samāpatti: The state of mind achieved when the movements of the mind and senses are stilled; the preliminary stage of *samādhi* equated with *sa-bīja samādhi*. 1.41, 2.47, 3.42

śakti: Power, energy, potency.

Sāṁkhya: A major school of Indian religious philosophy that examines the composition of the world and emphasises the distinction between the spiritual entity, *puruṣa*, and the material embodiment formed out of *prakṛti*.

Sāṁkhya Kārikā: The foundational text of the Sāṁkhya system composed by Īśvara Kṛṣṇa, probably later than the *Yoga Sūtras*.

saṁprajñāta: The state of meditation or *samādhi* in which the mind is focused on a particular object. 1.17

saṁskāra: The subtle impressions left on the mind by all thoughts, ideas, and motivations, which later emerge from a latent state and become manifest in the form of future karma. 1.18, 1.50

saṁyama: Collective term for the practice of *dhāraṇā, dhyāna,* and *samādhi.* 3.4

saṁyoga: Unity, proximity, contact. 2.17, 2.23

Śānti-parvan: The twelfth book of the *Mahābhārata,* which contains most of its teachings on Yoga.

satkārya-vāda: The philosophical doctrine that states that all effects are pre-existent in a latent form within their cause. 3.13

sattva (sattva-guṇa): The highest of the three *guṇas* that opens up the path to enlightenment when properly cultivated. It is represented by goodness, purity, light, joy, and wisdom.

satya: Truthfulness, honesty. 2.36

śauca: Purity or cleanliness of body and mind.

siddhi: Success, perfection, supernatural powers. 2.43

smṛti: Memory or mindfulness. 1.20, 1.43

śraddhā: Faith. 1.20

sthiti: State of steadiness. 1.13

śuddha: Pure, free of any blemish. 2.20

sukha: Happiness, joy. As an adjective: happy, easy, comfortable. 2.8, 2.46

svādhyāya: Recitation or study of sacred texts or mantras. 2.1

svapna: Dreaming. 1.38

svarūpa: True nature. 2.23, 3.44

tamas (tamo-guṇa): The *guṇa* of *tamas,* which relates to ignorance, darkness, sloth, cruelty, and inertia.

tan-mātras: In Sāṁkhya teachings, the subtle or primal sense objects or data, namely sound, aroma, flavour, touch sensations, and form/colour out of which each specific object of sensory perception is formed. 1.44

tapas: Acts or vows of austerity aimed at removing attachment to worldly pleasures. 2.1, 2.43, 4.1

tattva: Truth, reality, a particular subject to be learned.

Upaniṣads: Those sections of the Vedas that deal with knowledge, liberation, and spiritual enlightenment rather than ritual practices.

vaināśika: An adjectival derivative of the term *vināśa* meaning 'destruction' or 'ending'. The term *vaināśika* is applied to Buddhists because of their teaching that there is no *ātman* that survives the death of the body. 4.19

vairāgya: Being free of the worldliness that takes the form of passionate desire. 1.15

vāsanā: Equivalent term for *saṁskāra*, perhaps indicating a group or flow of *saṁskāras* of the same nature. 2.24, 4.8, 4.24

vaśīkāra: Gaining control. 1.15, 1.40

Vedānta Sūtras: A philosophical work that attempts to establish the exact nature of the teachings of the Upaniṣads and is regarded as authoritative by all schools of Vedānta. Also known as the *Brahma Sūtras*.

Vedas: The oldest scriptures of Hinduism. They are mostly concerned with ritual activity as opposed to a pursuit of liberation from rebirth.

vibhūti: Opulences, glories, wondrous abilities, supernatural powers. Chapter 3

vicāra: A characteristic of *samāpatti* or *saṁprajñāta samādhi*. A meditative state with *vicāra* is focused on a subtle object that transcends verbal thought processes. 1.17, 1.44, 1.47

Vijñāna-vāda: See Yogācāra.

vikalpa: Movement of the mind to create a mental construct or formulation when it hears or reads words on a particular subject. 1.9, 1.42

viparyaya: False assessment or misapprehension. An opposite of *pramāṇa*. 1.8

viṣaya: An object such as sound, form, or aroma that is perceived by one of the senses. 1.35, 2.54

viśeṣa: Superior, special, or particular. As a noun: difference. 1.49, 4.25

Viṣṇu Purāṇa: An early text dedicated to the glorification of the Deity Viṣṇu, which gives accounts of the activities of *avatāras* of Viṣṇu.

viśoka: Free from sorrow. 1.36

vitarka: (1) A characteristic of *samāpatti* or *saṁprajñāta samādhi*. A meditative state with *vitarka* is focused on a gross object that can be contemplated by verbal thought processes. 1.42; (2) Perverse tendencies contrary to the *yamas* or *niyamas*. 2.33.

vitṛṣṇa: Being free of hankering. 1.15

vivarta-vāda: The philosophical teaching that indicates that the variegated world and the individuality of each being is not an ultimate reality but a false perception based on ignorance of the one true reality, Brahman.

viveka: Distinction, specifically the distinction between spirit and matter, between the true self and its embodiment, between *puruṣa* and *prakṛti* or, more specifically, between *puruṣa* and *sattva* or *buddhi*.

viveka-khyāti: Realisation of *viveka*, which is the distinction between the true self and *prakṛti* or, more specifically, between *puruṣa* and *sattva* or *buddhi*; also *viveka-jñāna*. 2.28

vṛtti: (1) Movements or fluctuations. 1.2 (2) An equivalent term for *bhāṣya*, meaning a commentary.

yama: Restraint from the exercise of negative actions, thoughts, or words. 2.30

Yogācāra: A school of Buddhist thought which shares many terms with the *Yoga Sūtras*. Its postulates that external objects are unreal and only the mind is real. Also known as Vijñāna-vāda.

yogāṅgas: Limbs of Yoga. 2.28

Bibliography

Burley, Mikel. *Classical Sāṃkhya and Yoga: An Indian Metaphysics of Experience*. London: Routledge, 2007.

Dasgupta, Surendranath. *A History of Indian Philosophy*, vols. 1–5. Cambridge: Cambridge University Press, 1922–1955.

Deshpande, Purushottam Yashwant. *The Authentic Yoga: A Fresh Look at Patanjali's Yoga Sutras with a New Translation, Notes and Comments*. London: Rider, 1978.

Gokhale, Pradeep. *The Yogasūtra of Patañjali: A New Introduction to the Buddhist Roots of the Yoga System*. London: Routledge, 2020.

Larson, Gerald James, and Ram Shankar Bhattacharya, eds. *Encyclopedia of Indian Philosophies*. Vol. 12, *Yoga: India's Philosophy of Meditation*. Delhi: Motilal Banarsidass, 2008.

Maas, Philipp. 'A Concise Historiography of Classical Yoga Philosophy'. In *Historiography and Periodization of Indian Philosophy*, edited by Eli Franco. Vienna: De Nobili Series, 2013.

Maas, Philipp. 'Sarvāstivāda Buddhist Theories of Temporality and the Pātañjala Yoga Theory of Transformation (pariṇāma)'. *Journal of Indian Philosophy*, 48 (2020): 963–1003.

O'Brien-Kop, Karen. '*Dharmamegha* in Yoga and Yogācāra: The Revision of a Superlative Metaphor'. In *Journal of Indian Philosophy*, 48 (2020): 605–635.

O'Brien-Kop, Karen. *Rethinking 'Classical Yoga' and Buddhism: Meditation, Metaphors and Materiality*. London: Bloomsbury, 2021.

O'Brien Kop, Karen. *The Philosophy of the Yoga Sutra: An Introduction*. London: Bloomsbury, 2023.

Wujastyk, Dominik. 'Some Problematic Yoga Sūtra-s and their Buddhist Background'. In *Yoga in Transformation: Historical and Contemporary Perspectives*, edited by. Karl Baier, Karin Preisendanz, and Philipp Andre Maas. Göttingen: V&R unipress, 2018.

INDEX

U

V

W

Y

MANDALA

An Imprint of MandalaEarth
PO Box 3088
San Rafael, CA 94912
www.MandalaEarth.com

Find us on Facebook:
www.facebook.com/MandalaEarth

Publisher Raoul Goff
Associate Publisher Phillip Jones
Publishing Director Katie Killebrew
Project Editor Amanda Nelson
VP Creative Director Chrissy Kwasnik
Art Director Ashley Quackenbush
VP Manufacturing Alix Nicholaeff
Sr Production Manager Joshua Smith

Text © 2024 The Oxford Centre for Hindu Studies

Photographs © 2024 Mandala Publishing, except for pages viii (Courtesy Shutterstock); pages 8, 11, 276 (Courtesy Wellcome Collection); and pages 12, 18, 24, 36, and 44 (Courtesy Wikimedia Commons).

All rights reserved. No part of this book may be reproduced in any form without written permission from the publisher.

ISBN: 979-8-88762-079-4
ISBN: 979-8-88762-135-7 (Export Edition)

Manufactured in India by Insight Editions
10 9 8 7 6 5 4 3 2 1

Library of Congress Cataloging-in-Publication Data
Names: Sutton, Nicholas, author.
Title: Exploring the yoga sutras / Nicholas Sutton.
Description: San Rafael, CA : Mandala, an Imprint of MandalaEarth, [2024] | Series: The Oxford Centre for Hindu Studies Mandala Publishing series | Includes bibliographical references and index. | Summary: "In this sutra-by-sutra translation and study of the Yoga Sutras, Hindu Studies scholar Nicholas Sutton offers an accessible guide to the complex philosophical ideas on which the ancient practice of Yoga is based, illuminating the meaning of Patañjali's seminal Yoga treatise and the manner in which it seeks to integrate Yoga into life as a whole"-- Provided by publisher.
Identifiers: LCCN 2024020023 (print) | LCCN 2024020024 (ebook) | ISBN 9798887620794 | ISBN 9798887621357 (export edition) | ISBN 9798887620800 (ebook)
Subjects: LCSH: Patañjali. Yogasūtra. | Yoga. | BISAC: RELIGION / Hinduism / Sacred Writings | HEALTH & FITNESS / Yoga
Classification: LCC B132.Y6 S84 2024 (print) | LCC B132.Y6 (ebook) | DDC 181/.452--dc23/eng/20240531
LC record available at https://lccn.loc.gov/2024020023
LC ebook record available at https://lccn.loc.gov/2024020024

ROOTS of PEACE

REPLANTED PAPER

Mandala Publishing, in association with Roots of Peace, will plant two trees for each tree used in the manufacturing of this book. Roots of Peace is an internationally renowned humanitarian organization dedicated to eradicating land mines worldwide and converting war-torn lands into productive farms and wildlife habitats. Roots of Peace will plant two million fruit and nut trees in Afghanistan and provide farmers there with the skills and support necessary for sustainable land use.

FSC
www.fsc.org
MIX
Paper | Supporting responsible forestry
FSC® C016779